郭连魁

Guo Liankui

人体解剖学图谱

ATLAS OF HUMAN ANATOMY

主编并绘制　Editor in chief and painting

郭连魁　Guo Liankui

执行主编　Executive chief editors

雒树东　Luo Shudong

陆　利　Lu Li

James R. Augustine

副主编　Assistant editors in chief

魏建宏　Wei Jianhong　　郭　庚　Guo Geng

宋慧芳　Song Huifang　　张卫国　Zhang Weiguo

编　委　Editorial staff

张萌萌　Zhang Mengmeng　　任婷婷　Ren Tingting

毕雪斐　Bi Xuefei　　吴勇强　Wu Yongqiang

王一川　Wang Yichuan　　王树乐　Wang Shule

刘雪芹　Liu Xueqin　　石丽洪　Shi Lihong

周　楠　Zhou Nan　　夏仲年　Xia Zhongnian

崔文丽　Cui Wenli

科学出版社

北　京

内 容 简 介

郭连魁乃国内人体解剖学资深教授中的著名画家，画风细腻而富有生机，画坛独树一帜。

以其擅长的工笔彩绘技法，别具特色的艺术风格，系统解剖学与局部解剖学相结合的创新体系，系列、精确地诠释人体形态结构。

以娴熟流畅的线条，丰富、柔和、得体的彩色绘画，展现美妙真实的人体解剖学画卷，大手笔淋漓尽致地呈现繁复人体独特的视觉世界。

将知识性、艺术性、趣味性、实用性科学地融为一体。本书是学习人体解剖学不可或缺的“利器”，收藏佳作，在标准美式英语名词注释的语境中，正确地提高基础医学外文水平。

图书在版编目（CIP）数据

郭连魁人体解剖学图谱 = Guo Liankui ATLAS OF HUMAN ANATOMY / 郭连魁主编 . — 北京：科学出版社，2019.11

ISBN 978-7-03-062790-2

Ⅰ . ①郭… Ⅱ . ①郭… Ⅲ . ①人体解剖学 – 图谱 Ⅳ . ① R322-64

中国版本图书馆 CIP 数据核字（2019）第 242990 号

责任编辑：朱　华 / 责任校对：郭瑞芝

责任印制：李　彤 / 封面设计：陈　敬

科 学 出 版 社 出版

北京东黄城根北街 16 号

邮政编码：100717

http://www.sciencep.com

北京中科印刷有限公司 印刷

科学出版社发行　各地新华书店经销

*

2019 年 11 月第　一　版　开本：787×1092　1/16

2022 年 1 月第二次印刷　印张：18

字数：412 000

定价：198.00 元

（如有印装质量问题，我社负责调换）

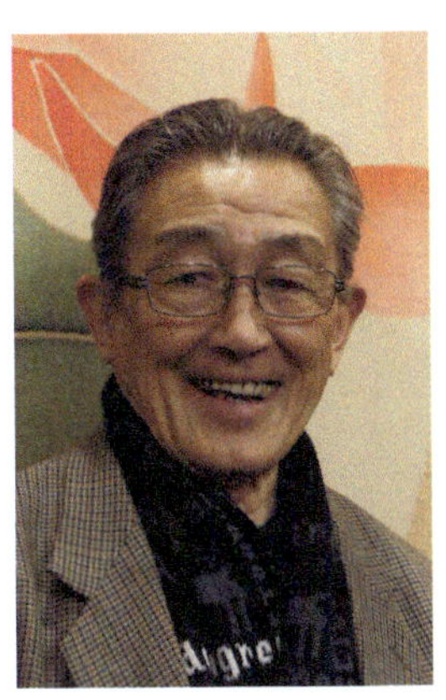

郭连魁　　1929 年 12 月 30 日生于北京顺义。山西医科大学教授，全国先进教育工作者（1960），享受国务院政府特殊津贴（1992）。业余从事美术创作，笔名郭晓，中国工笔画学会会员，山西省当代工笔画艺术研究院名誉院长。

Guo Liankui was born in Shunyi Beijing on Dec. 30th 1929, is a Professor of Shanxi Medical University and a national advanced educator（1960）, Awarded the special government allowance of the State Council（1992）. He Began painting in spare time, pen name is Guo Xiao. He is the Member of Chinese Realistic Painting Society, Honorary President of Shanxi Contemporary Realistic Painting Art Academy.

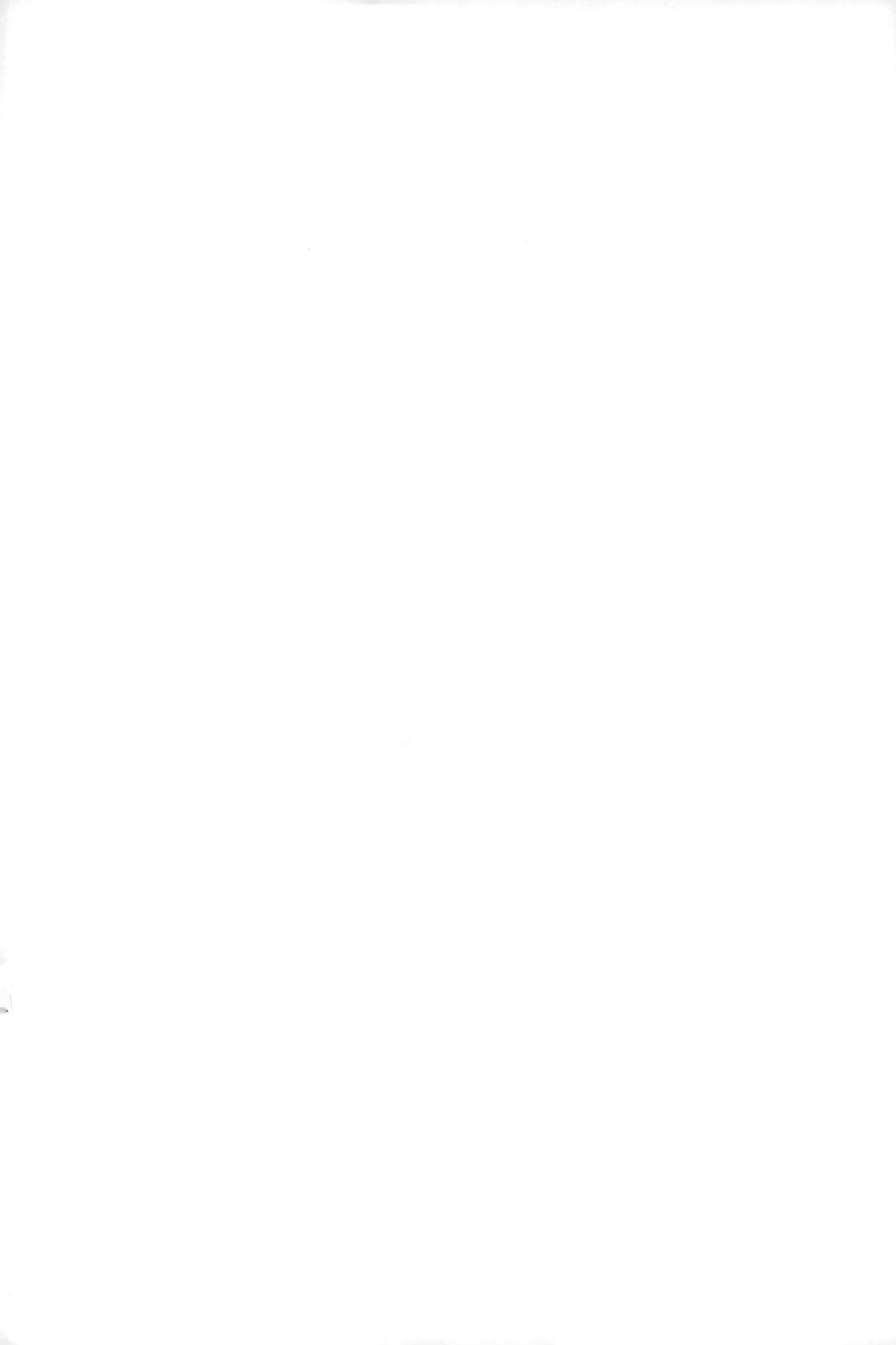

写在前面

我生来嗜画，但我不想成为专业画家。我选择了学医，进入医学院后，我爱上了解剖学，从此，一支画笔和一把解剖刀伴随了我一生。从年轻时候起，就想画一部自己的人体解剖学图谱，并且开始积累资料。此期间，虽然出版过两部人体解剖学图谱，都是依据当时教学需要而绘制的黑白线条图。直到 1995 年退休，我才开始有充分时间对人体结构以彩色进行再创作。时间过得飞快，转瞬间 20 多年过去了，300 多页的人体解剖图稿于 2017 年完成了。然而，将书稿付诸出版，却不是我个人所能完成得了。多亏学校有关领导的大力支持和编委会全体成员两年多来的辛勤劳动，才使得本书得以问世。在这里我表示衷心地感谢！

本书将系统解剖学和局部解剖学组合在一起，而以系统解剖学为主线，即运动系统、内脏学、脉管学、神经系统和感觉器。头颈、躯干、四肢局解置于肌学内，内脏局解分别置于呼吸系统和消化系统内，至于垂体、甲状腺、甲状旁腺等结构则放在各自的解剖位置中叙述；感觉器则放在本书最后。我希望这种安排适合读者的学习需要，我从心底渴望读者的意见和建议。

郭连魁

2019 年 6 月 10 日

Foreword

I have loved painting since I was born. But I didn′t become a specialized painter. I chose to study medicine. After entering medical school, I soon fell in love with Anatomy. One painting brush and one dissection knife accompanied me my whole life since then. I had an aspiration to draw my own anatomic atlas when I was young and began to collect data on anatomy even though there were two anatomy atlases published during my career, but they were both accomplished using line drawings. There was not enough time to do colored pictures until 1995, after I retired. Time flies and now more than 20 years have passed quickly while more than 300 colored anatomic plates were accomplished in 2017. I was not able a published atlas out of those plates by myself. Thanks to the support of the leaders in the university and members of the editorial board, they have worked hard on this atlas for more than two years. I express my wholehearted gratitude to them here.

This book is composed of the systematic anatomy and regional anatomy together while the main emphasis is on the systematic anatomy, that is, the organ systems, splanchnology, angiology and neurology. The regional anatomy of the head, neck, body and appendicular limbs are combined in the myology. The visceral regional anatomy is combined with the respiratory and digestive system, respectively. The pituitary gland, thyroid and parathyroid gland etc. are put in their own regional position. The sensory organs are put at the end of the book. I hope this arrangement is suitable for the reader. I ask for your criticism and suggestions from the bottom of my heart.

Guo Liankui

June 10th 2019

Foreword from South Carolina

It is an honor for me as a fellow human anatomist to write a few words about this excellent Atlas of Human Anatomy produced by my distinguished colleague and friend, Dr. Liankui Guo. With some 270 plates and 516 figures hand-painted by Dr. Guo and carefully labeled for the reader, this atlas demonstrates Dr. Guo′ s extraordinary talents as an artist and as a scientist. I recommend this atlas to all who teach human anatomy as well as to those beginning students who desire to learn human anatomy.

James R. Augustine PhD
Professor Emeritus
University of South Carolina
Columbia, South Carolina

来自南卡罗来纳的几句话

作为一名人体解剖学工作者，能够为我的杰出同事和挚友郭连魁教授所著的《人体解剖学图谱》说上几句，感到非常荣幸。郭教授用自己精心手绘的 516 幅人体解剖学图，组成 270 页并精心注释的人体解剖学图谱，展示了郭教授作为科学家和艺术家的非凡天赋。因此，我向所有从事人体解剖学教学的同行们，和渴望学习人体解剖学的开始学医的学子们推荐本书。

目录 Contents

第 1 章　运动系统 LOCOMOTOR SYSTEM

第 2 章 内脏学 SPLANCHNOLOY

第 3 章　脉管学 ANGIOLOGY

第 4 章　神经系统 NERVOUS SYSTEM

第 5 章　感觉器 SENSORY ORGANS

第1章

运 动 系 统

LOCOMOTOR SYSTEM

Chapter 1

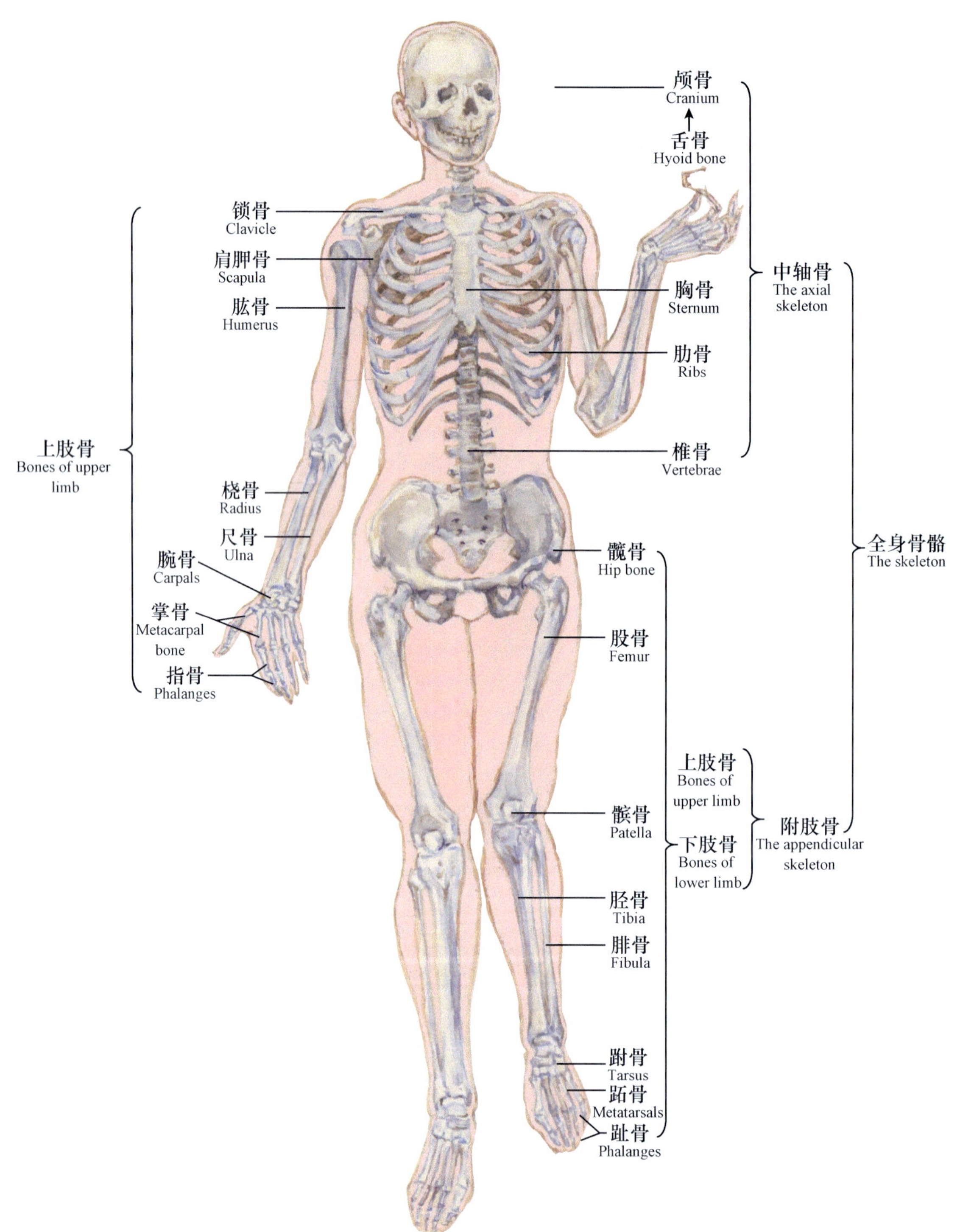

图 1-1　全身骨骼（前面观）
The skeleton (Anterior aspect)

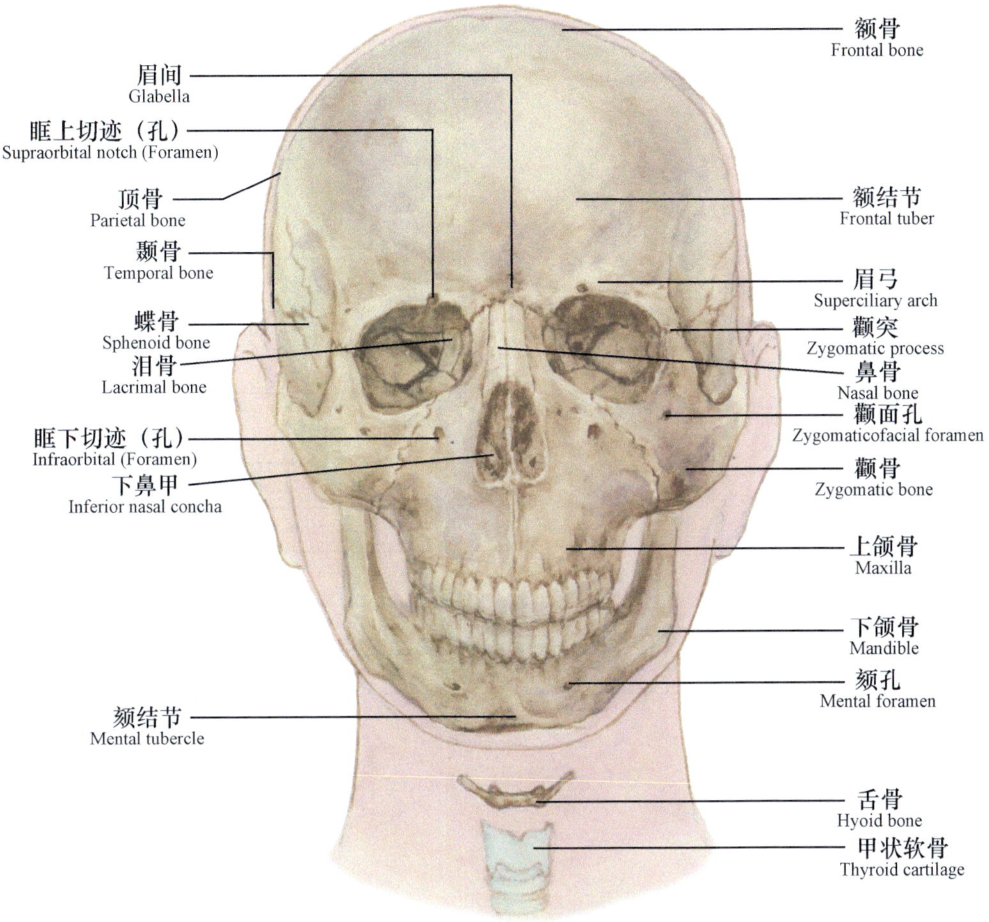

额骨
Frontal bone
眉间
Glabella
眶上切迹（孔）
Supraorbital notch (Foramen)
顶骨
Parietal bone
颞骨
Temporal bone
额结节
Frontal tuber
眉弓
Superciliary arch
蝶骨
Sphenoid bone
颧突
Zygomatic process
泪骨
Lacrimal bone
鼻骨
Nasal bone
颧面孔
Zygomaticofacial foramen
眶下切迹（孔）
Infraorbital (Foramen)
下鼻甲
Inferior nasal concha
颧骨
Zygomatic bone
上颌骨
Maxilla
下颌骨
Mandible
颏孔
Mental foramen
颏结节
Mental tubercle
舌骨
Hyoid bone
甲状软骨
Thyroid cartilage

图 1-2 颅骨（前面观）（1）
The cranium (Anterior aspect) (1)

额骨
Frontal bone
顶骨
Parietal bone
泪骨
Lacrimal bone
蝶骨
Sphenoid bone
筛骨
Ethmoid bone
颞骨
Temporal bone
颧骨
Zygomatic bone
上颌骨
Maxilla
下颌骨
Mandible

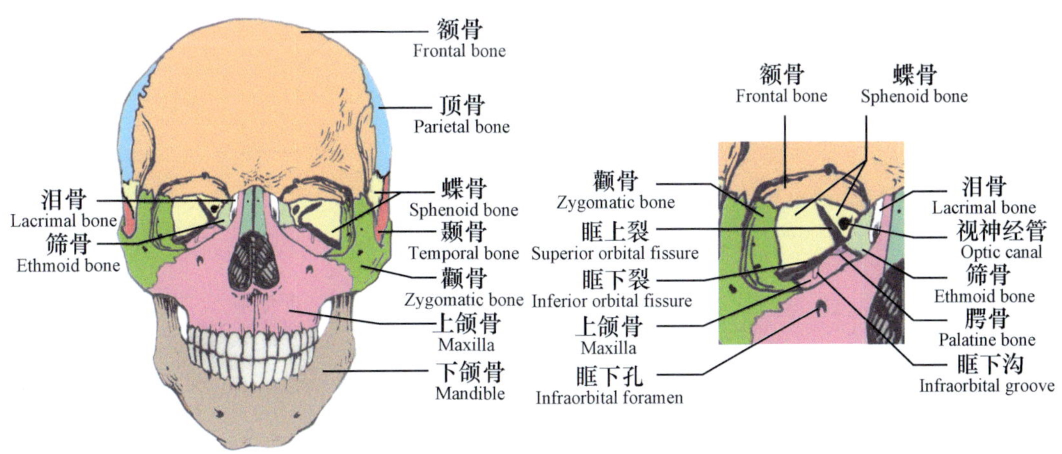

图 1-2 颅骨（前面观）（2）
The cranium (Anterior aspect) (2)

额骨
Frontal bone
蝶骨
Sphenoid bone
颧骨
Zygomatic bone
泪骨
Lacrimal bone
眶上裂
Superior orbital fissure
视神经管
Optic canal
眶下裂
Inferior orbital fissure
筛骨
Ethmoid bone
上颌骨
Maxilla
腭骨
Palatine bone
眶下孔
Infraorbital foramen
眶下沟
Infraorbital groove

图 1-3 眶（前面观）
The orbit (Anterior aspect)

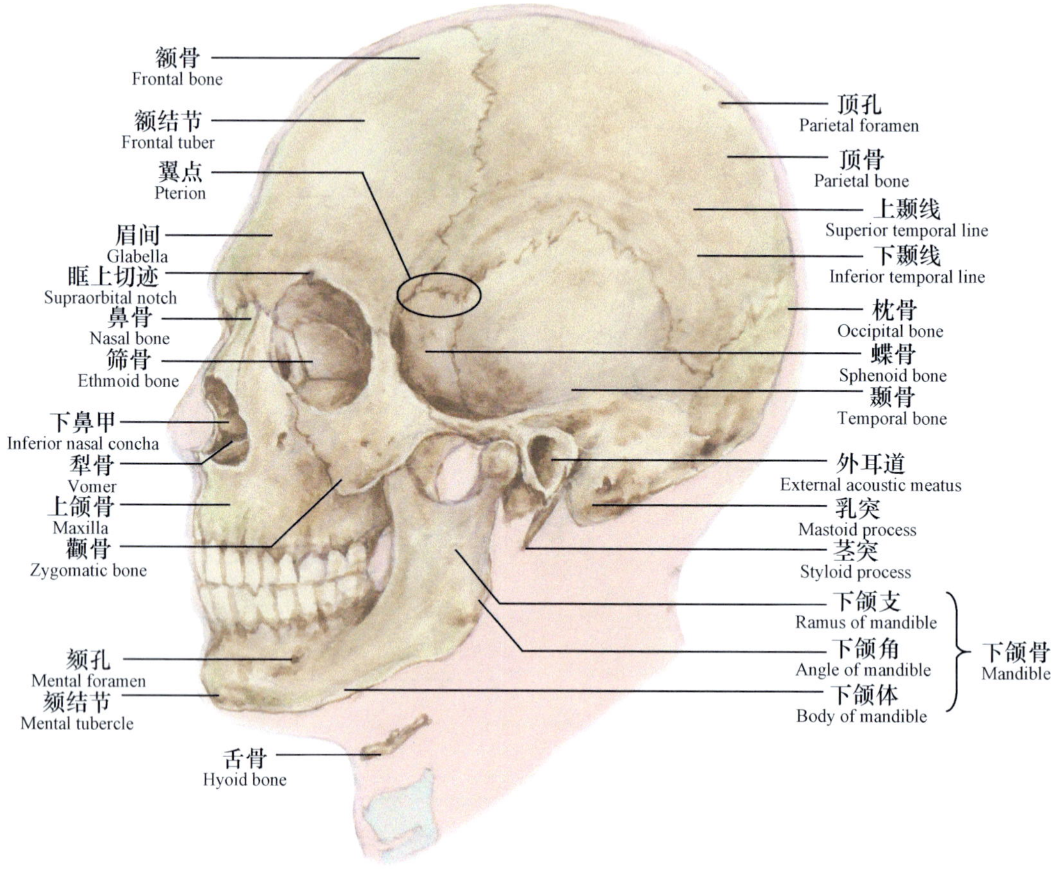

额骨
Frontal bone
额结节
Frontal tuber
翼点
Pterion
眉间
Glabella
眶上切迹
Supraorbital notch
鼻骨
Nasal bone
筛骨
Ethmoid bone
下鼻甲
Inferior nasal concha
犁骨
Vomer
上颌骨
Maxilla
颧骨
Zygomatic bone
颏孔
Mental foramen
颏结节
Mental tubercle
舌骨
Hyoid bone
顶孔
Parietal foramen
顶骨
Parietal bone
上颞线
Superior temporal line
下颞线
Inferior temporal line
枕骨
Occipital bone
蝶骨
Sphenoid bone
颞骨
Temporal bone
外耳道
External acoustic meatus
乳突
Mastoid process
茎突
Styloid process
下颌支
Ramus of mandible
下颌角
Angle of mandible
下颌体
Body of mandible
下颌骨
Mandible

图 1-4 颅骨（侧面观）（1）
The cranium (Lateral aspect) (1)

顶骨
Parietal bone
顶孔
Parietal foramen
上颞线
Superior temporal line
下颞线
Inferior temporal line
颞骨
Temporal bone
枕骨
Occipital bone
外耳道
External acoustic meatus
乳突
Mastoid process
额骨
Frontal bone
翼点
Pterion
筛骨
Ethmoid bone
鼻骨
Nasal bone
泪骨
Lacrimal bone
眶下孔
Infraorbital foramen
上颌骨
Maxilla
颏孔
Mental foramen
茎突
Styloid process
下颌支
Ramus of mandible
下颌角
Angle of mandible
下颌体
Body of mandible
下颌骨
Mandible

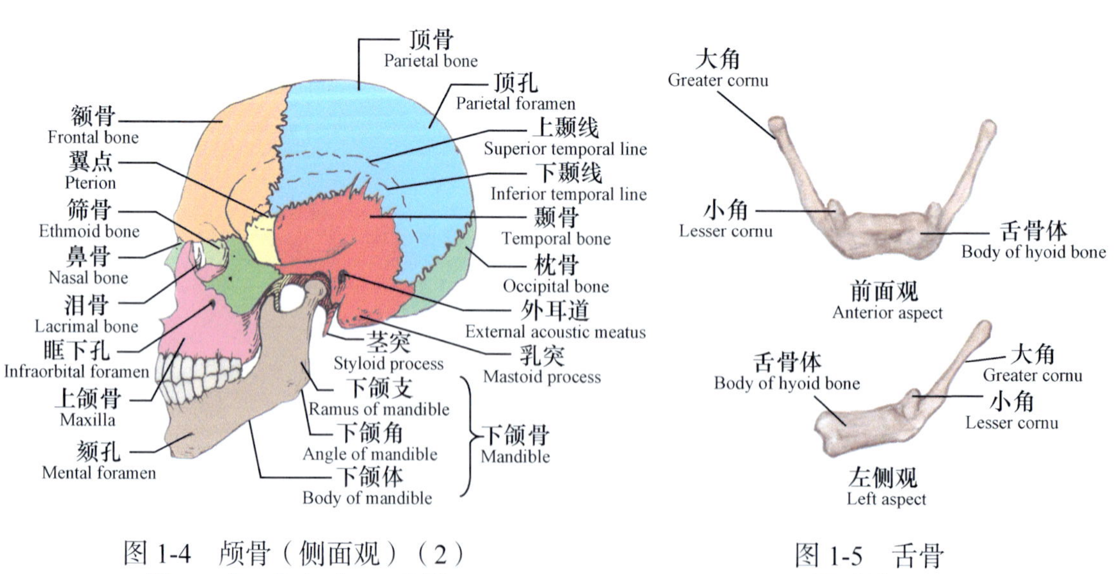

图 1-4 颅骨（侧面观）（2）
The cranium (Lateral aspect) (2)

大角
Greater cornu
小角
Lesser cornu
舌骨体
Body of hyoid bone
前面观
Anterior aspect
舌骨体
Body of hyoid bone
大角
Greater cornu
小角
Lesser cornu
左侧观
Left aspect

图 1-5 舌骨
Hyoid bone

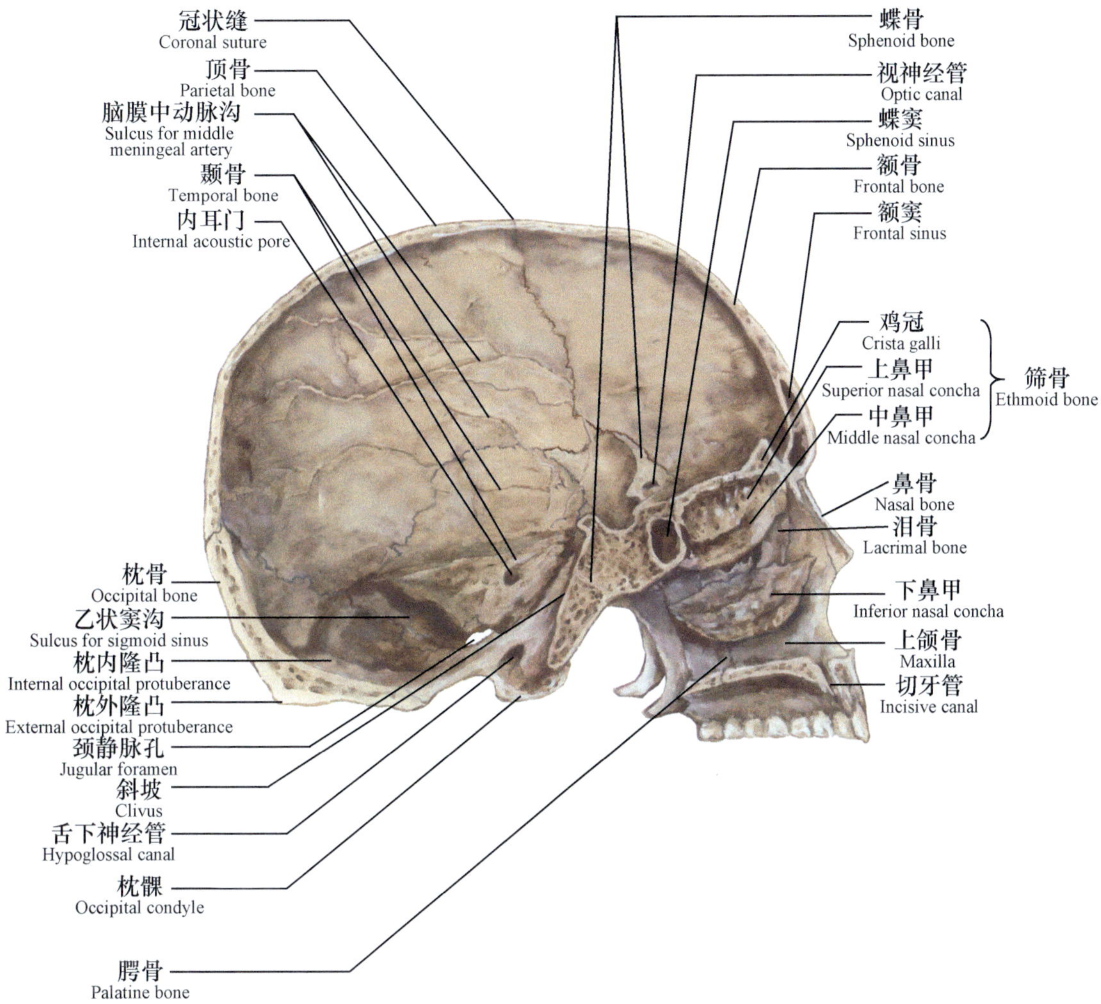

冠状缝
Coronal suture
顶骨
Parietal bone
脑膜中动脉沟
Sulcus for middle meningeal artery
颞骨
Temporal bone
内耳门
Internal acoustic pore
枕骨
Occipital bone
乙状窦沟
Sulcus for sigmoid sinus
枕内隆凸
Internal occipital protuberance
枕外隆凸
External occipital protuberance
颈静脉孔
Jugular foramen
斜坡
Clivus
舌下神经管
Hypoglossal canal
枕髁
Occipital condyle
腭骨
Palatine bone
蝶骨
Sphenoid bone
视神经管
Optic canal
蝶窦
Sphenoid sinus
额骨
Frontal bone
额窦
Frontal sinus
鸡冠
Crista galli
上鼻甲
Superior nasal concha
中鼻甲
Middle nasal concha
筛骨
Ethmoid bone
鼻骨
Nasal bone
泪骨
Lacrimal bone
下鼻甲
Inferior nasal concha
上颌骨
Maxilla
切牙管
Incisive canal

图 1-6 颅骨（正中矢状切面）（1）
The cranium (Midsagittal section) (1)

顶骨
Parietal bone
视神经管
Optic canal
蝶窦
Sphenoid sinus
上颌窦
Maxillary sinus
内耳门
Internal acoustic pore
枕骨
Occipital bone
颈静脉孔
Jugular foramen
舌下神经管
Hypoglossal canal
下颌孔
Mandibular foramen
腭骨
Palatine bone
额骨
Frontal bone
蝶骨
Sphenoid bone
筛骨
Ethmoid bone
鼻骨
Nasal bone
泪骨
Lacrimal bone
下鼻甲
Inferior nasal concha
上颌骨
Maxilla
切牙管
Incisive canal
下颌骨
Mandible

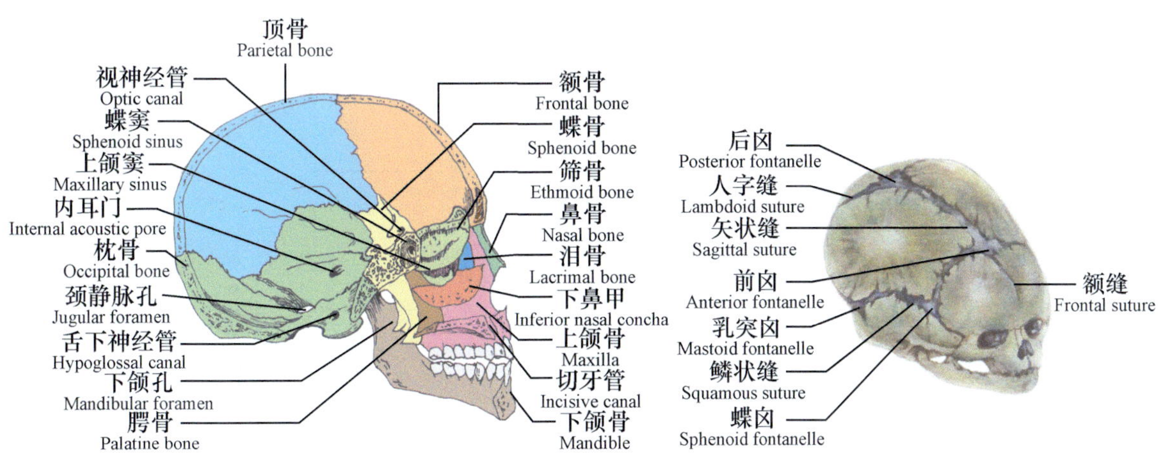

图 1-6 颅骨（正中矢状切面）（2）
The cranium (Midsagittal section) (2)

后囟
Posterior fontanelle
人字缝
Lambdoid suture
矢状缝
Sagittal suture
前囟
Anterior fontanelle
乳突囟
Mastoid fontanelle
鳞状缝
Squamous suture
蝶囟
Sphenoid fontanelle
额缝
Frontal suture

图 1-7 新生儿颅（侧面观）
The cranium of a newborn (Lateral aspect)

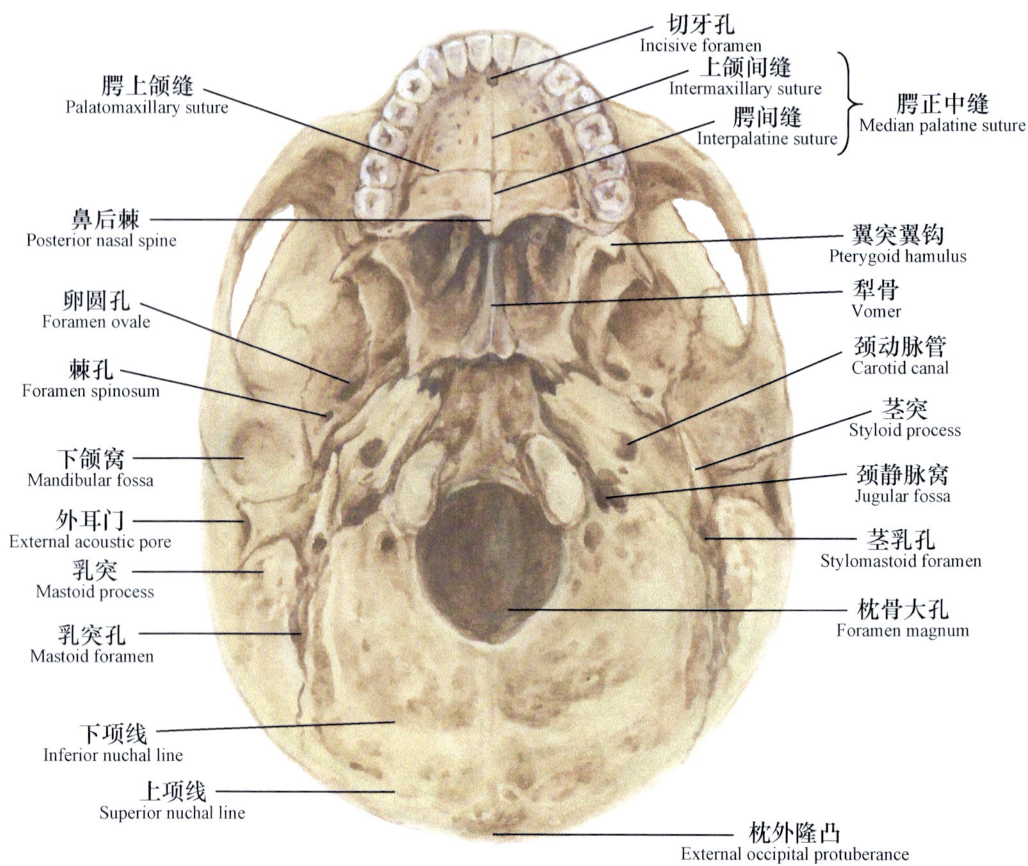

图 1-8 颅底外面观（1）
The external surface of the base of cranium (1)

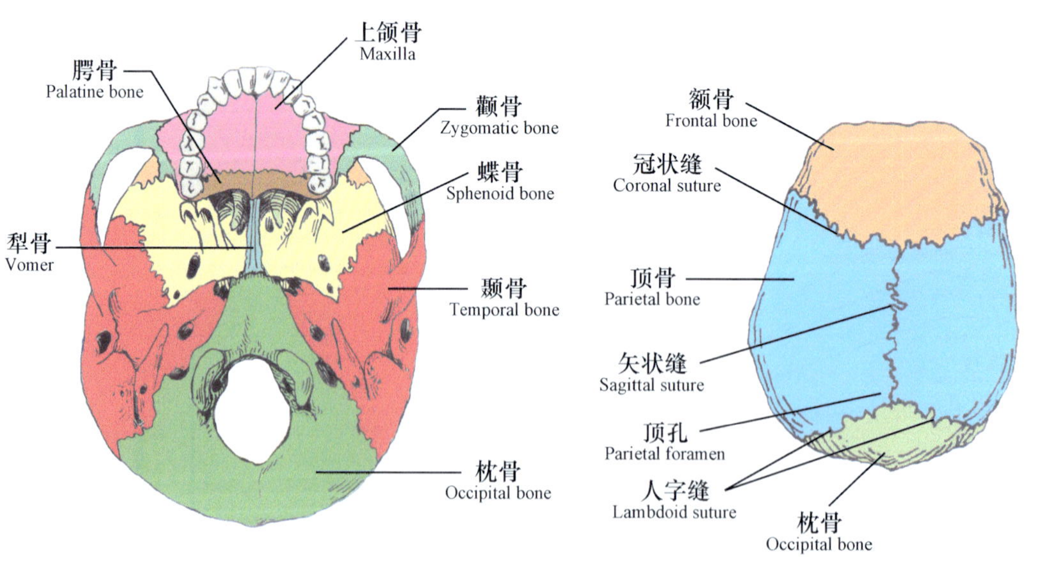

图 1-8 颅底外面观（2）
The external surface of the base of cranium (2)

图 1-9 颅骨（上面观）
The cranium (Superior aspect)

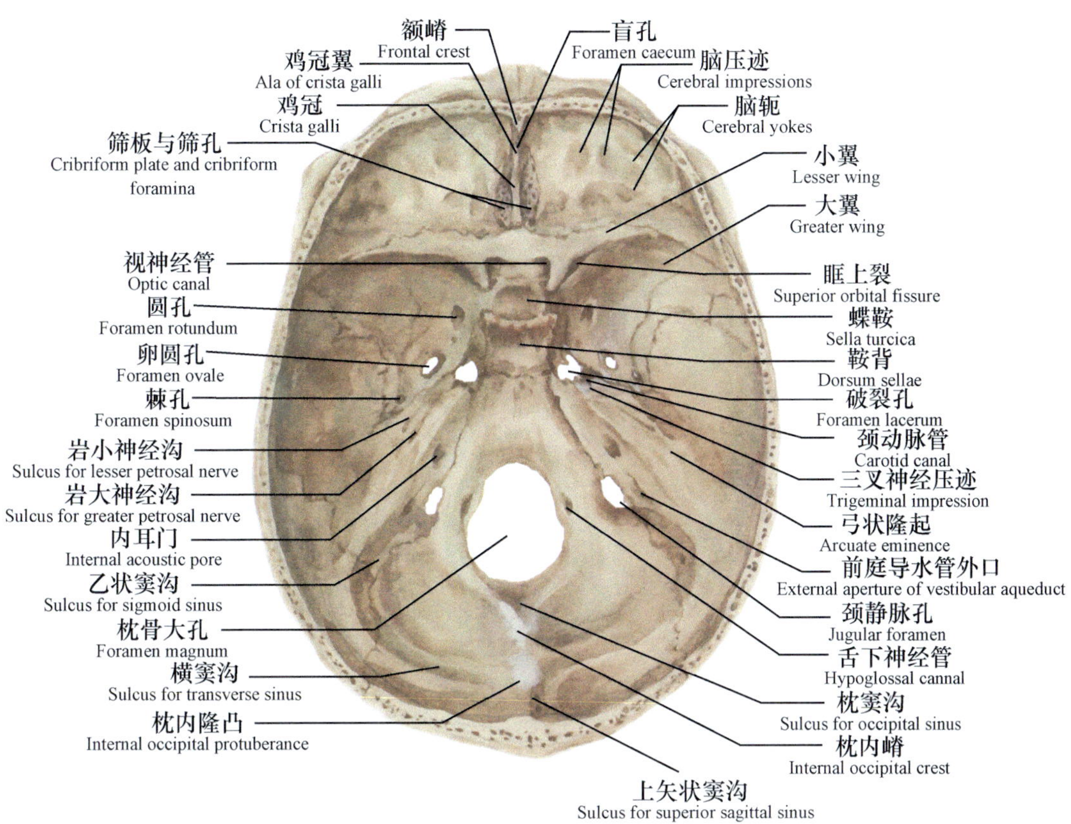

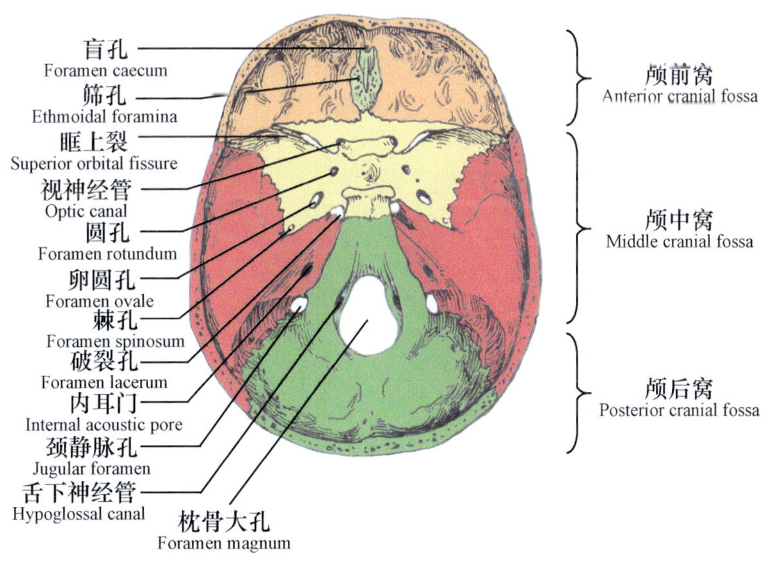

图 1-10　颅底内面观
The internal surface of the base of the cranium

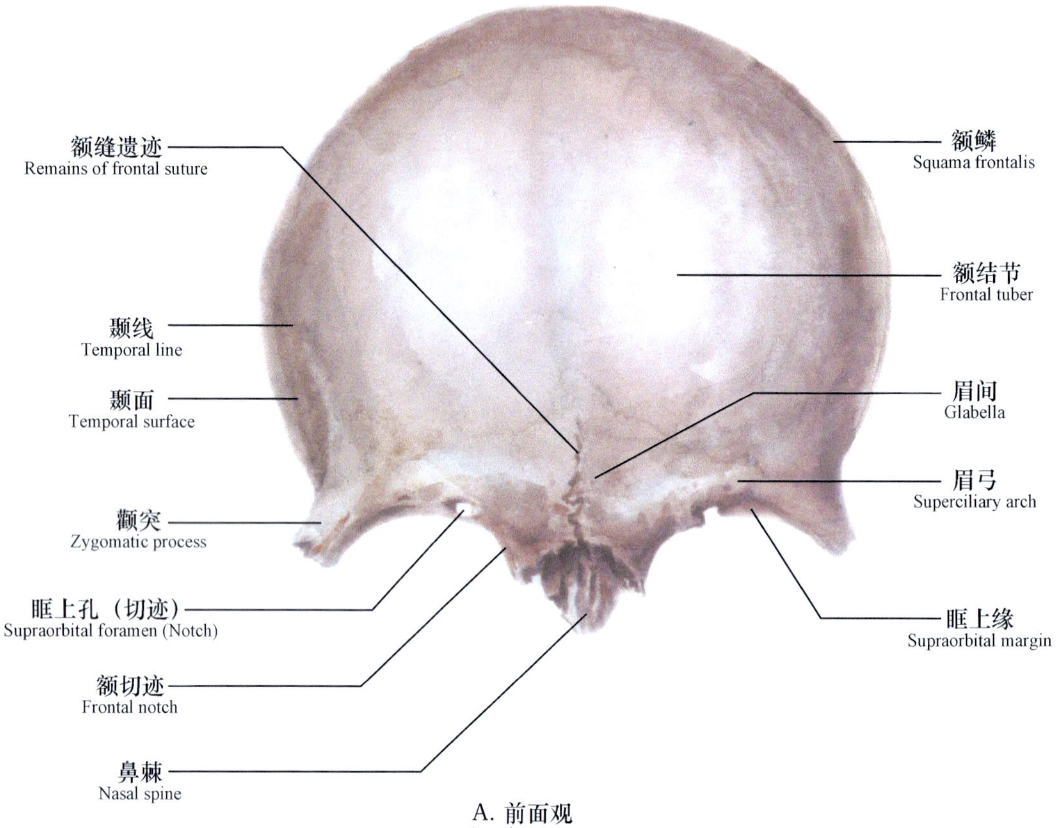

额缝遗迹
Remains of frontal suture
颞线
Temporal line
颞面
Temporal surface
颧突
Zygomatic process
眶上孔（切迹）
Supraorbital foramen (Notch)
额切迹
Frontal notch
鼻棘
Nasal spine
额鳞
Squama frontalis
额结节
Frontal tuber
眉间
Glabella
眉弓
Superciliary arch
眶上缘
Supraorbital margin

A. 前面观
Anterior aspect

鼻缘
Nasal margin
鼻棘
Nasal spine
颧突
Zygomatic process
筛小房
Ethmoidal cellules
泪腺窝
Lacrimal fossa
眶板
Orbital plate
筛切迹
Ethmoidal notch

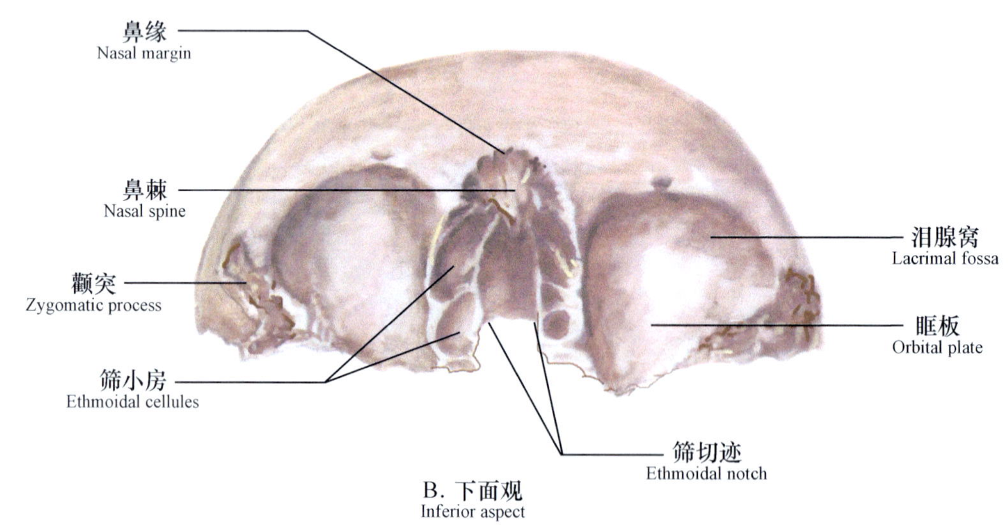

B. 下面观
Inferior aspect

图 1-11 额骨（1）
The frontal bone (1)

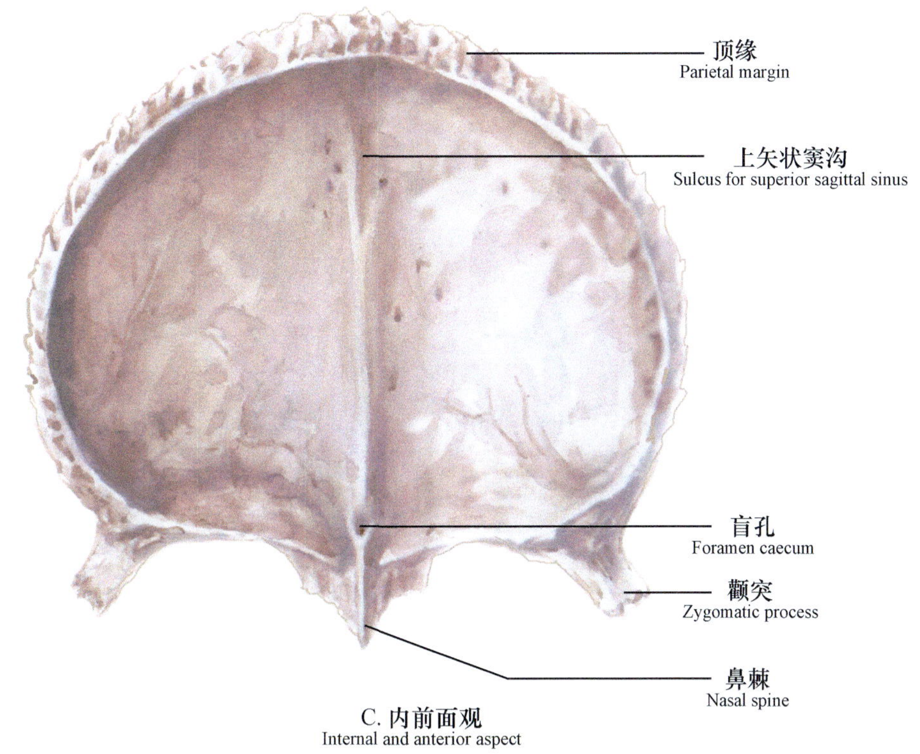

C. 内前面观
Internal and anterior aspect

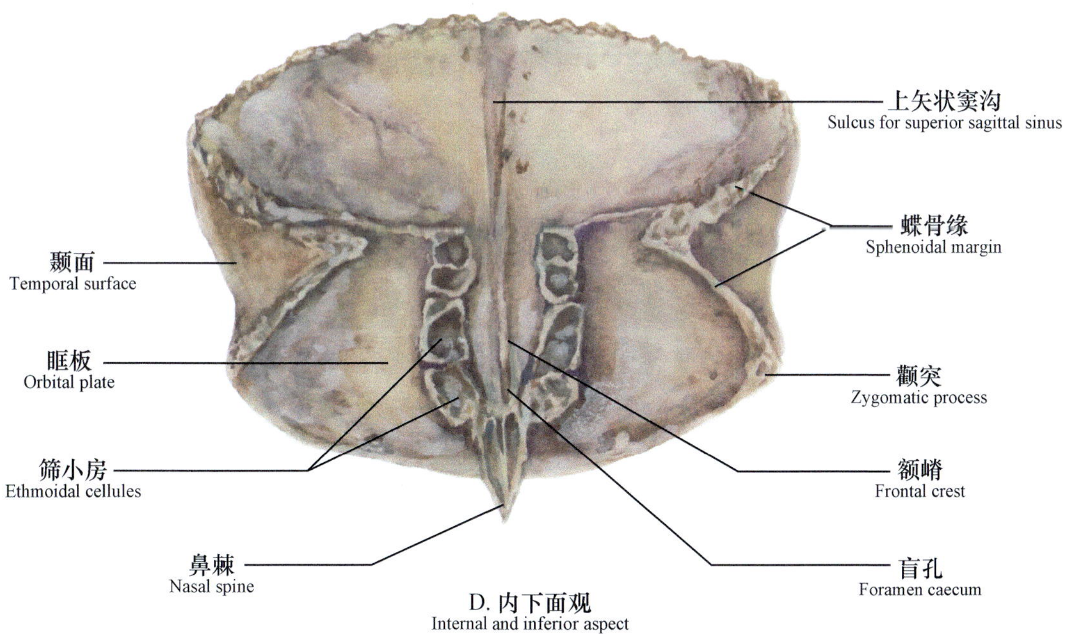

D. 内下面观
Internal and inferior aspect

图 1-11 额骨（2）
The frontal bone (2)

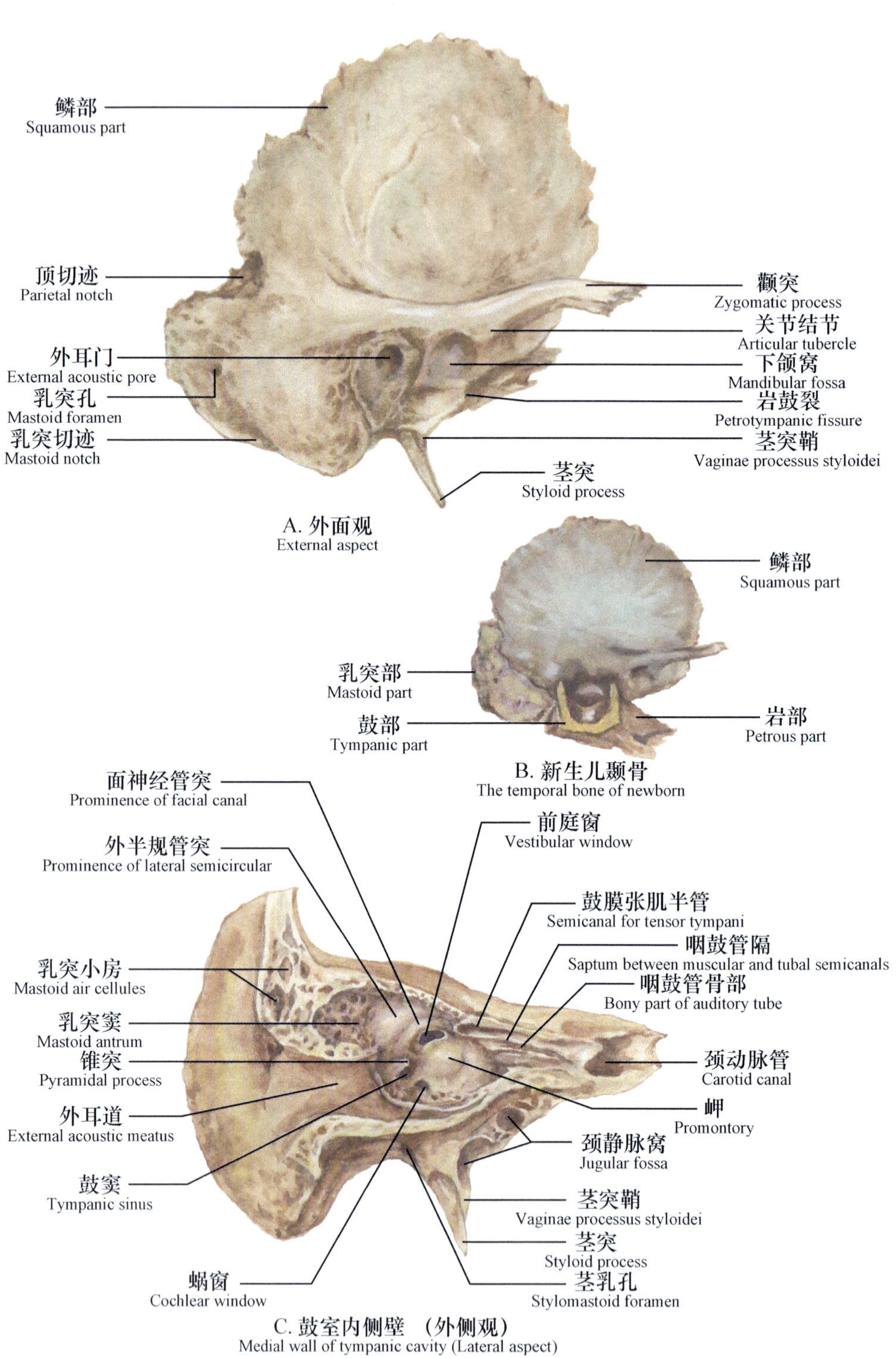

图 1-12 右侧颞骨（1）

The right temporal bone (1)

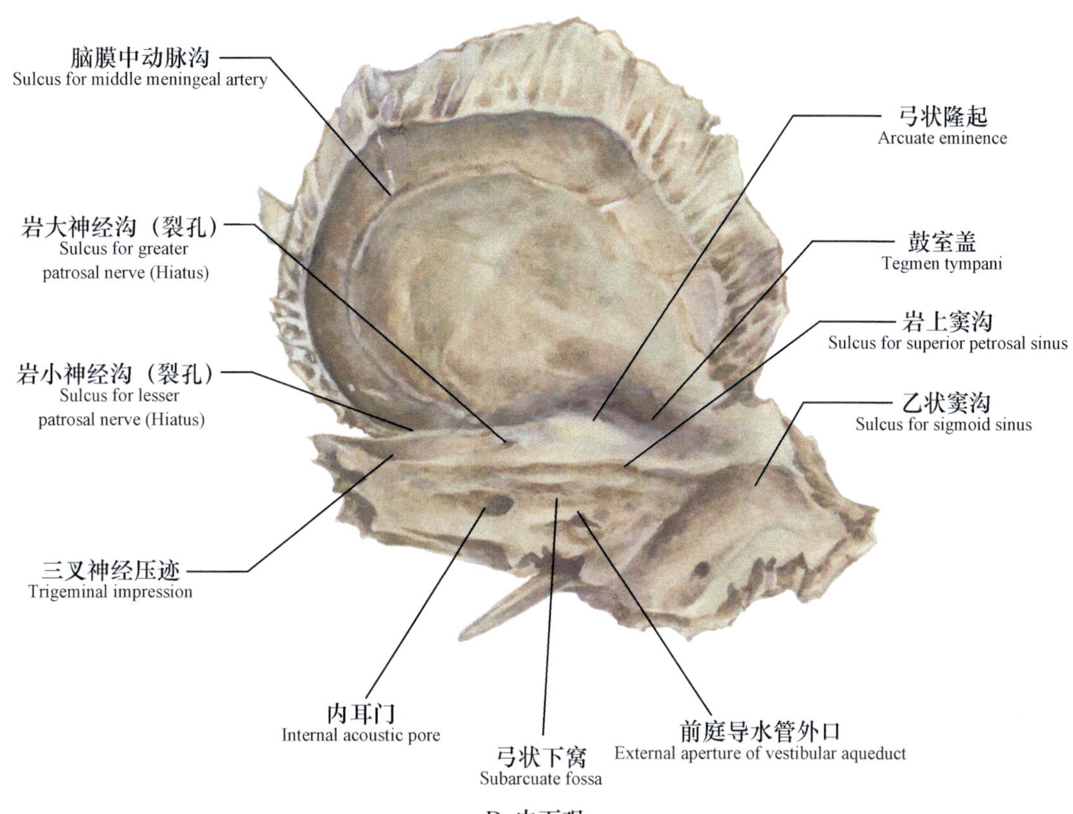

D. 内面观
Internal aspect

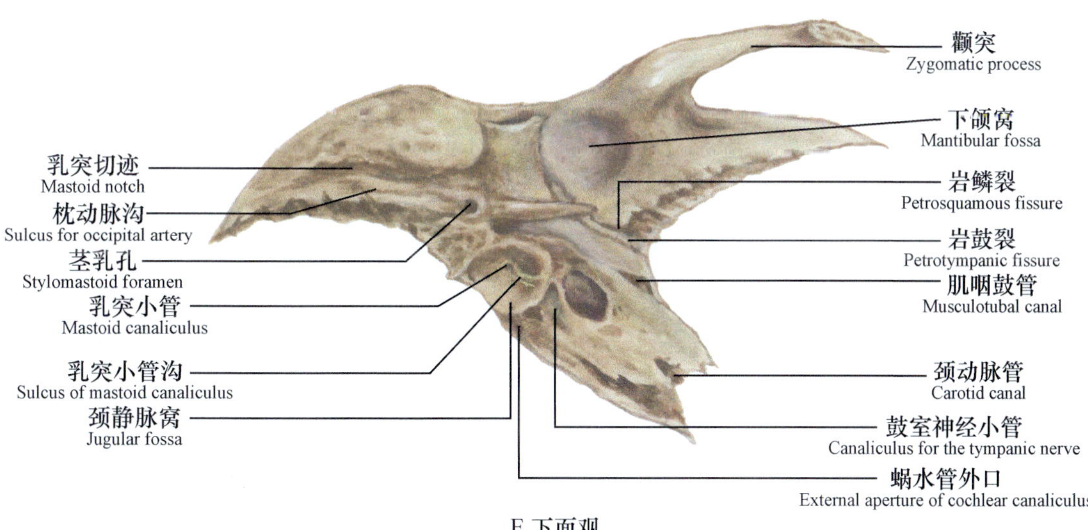

E. 下面观
Inferior aspect

图 1-12 右侧颞骨（2）
The right temporal bone (2)

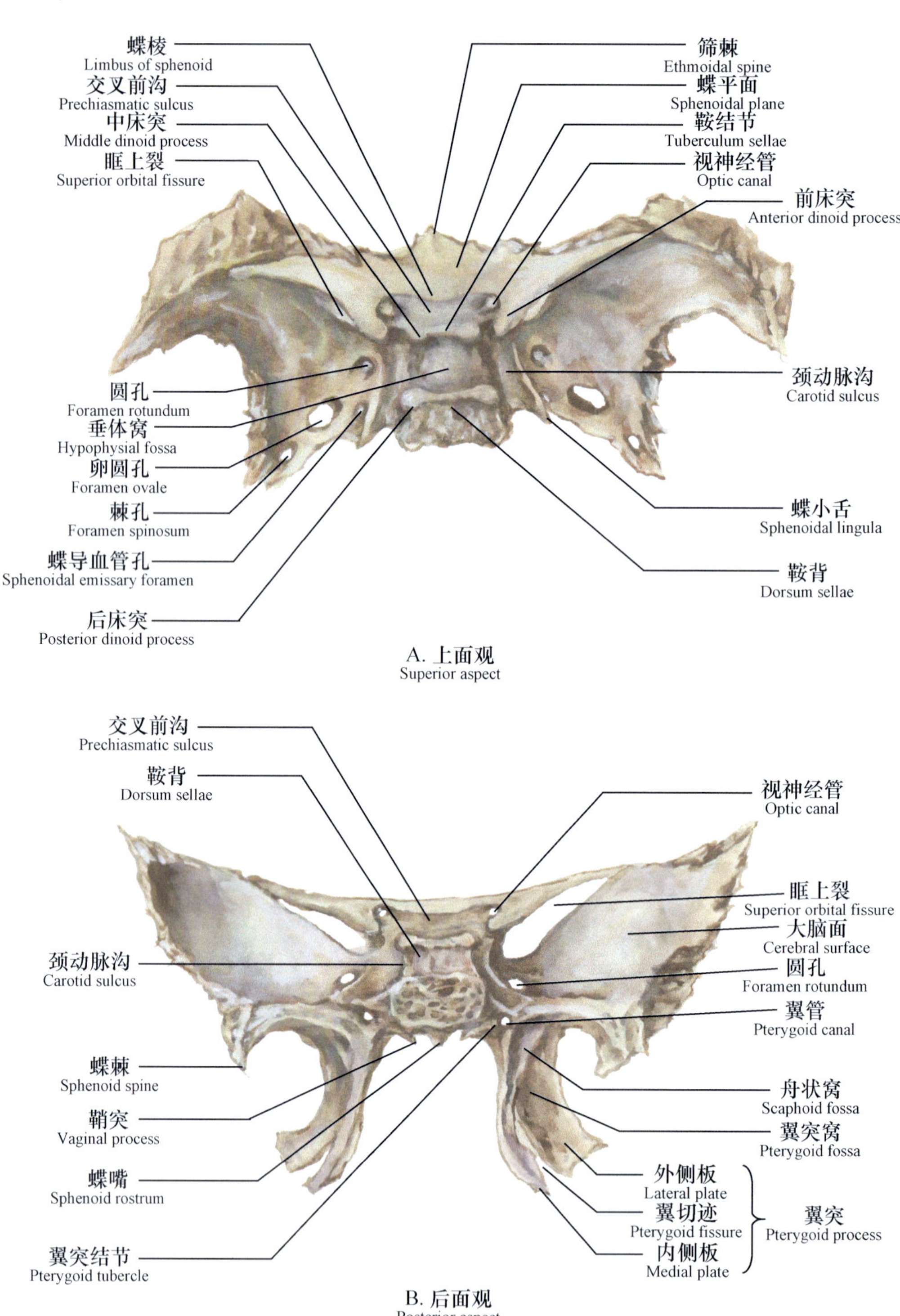

图 1-13 蝶骨（1）
The sphenoid bone (1)

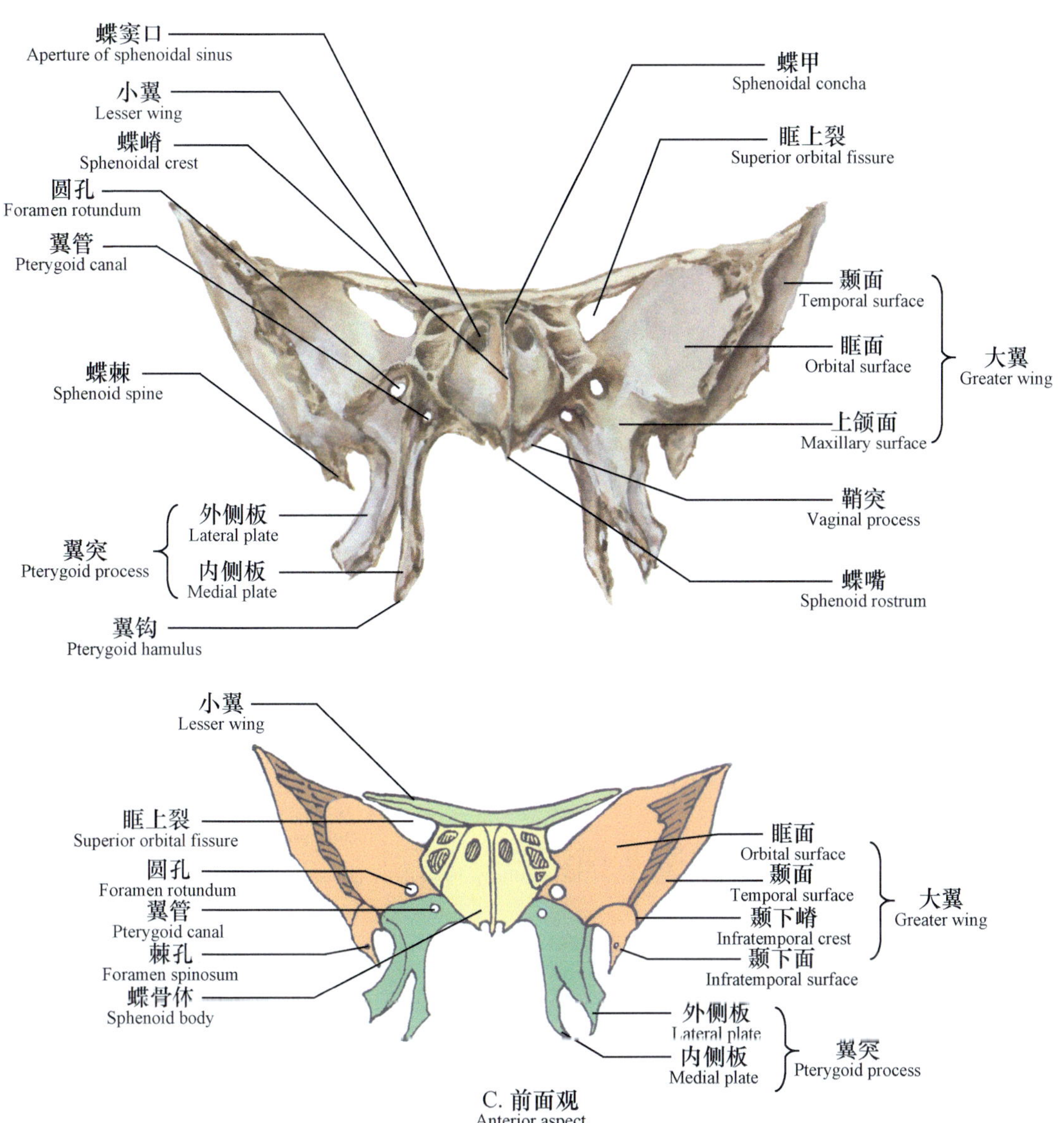

C. 前面观
Anterior aspect

眶上裂（Superior orbital fissure）

- 动眼神经（Oculomotor nerve）
- 滑车神经（Trochlear nerve）
- 眼神经（Ophthalmic nerve）
- 展神经（Obducent nerve）

圆孔（Foramen rotundum）

- 上颌神经（Maxillary nerve）

卵圆孔（Foramen ovale）

- 下颌神经（Mandibular nerve）
- 脑脊膜副血管（Accessory meningeal vessels）

棘孔（Foramen spinosum）

- 下颌神经脑膜支（Mandibular nerve）（V_3）
- 脑脊膜中血管（Middle meningeal vessels）

图 1-13 蝶骨（2）
The sphenoid bone (2)

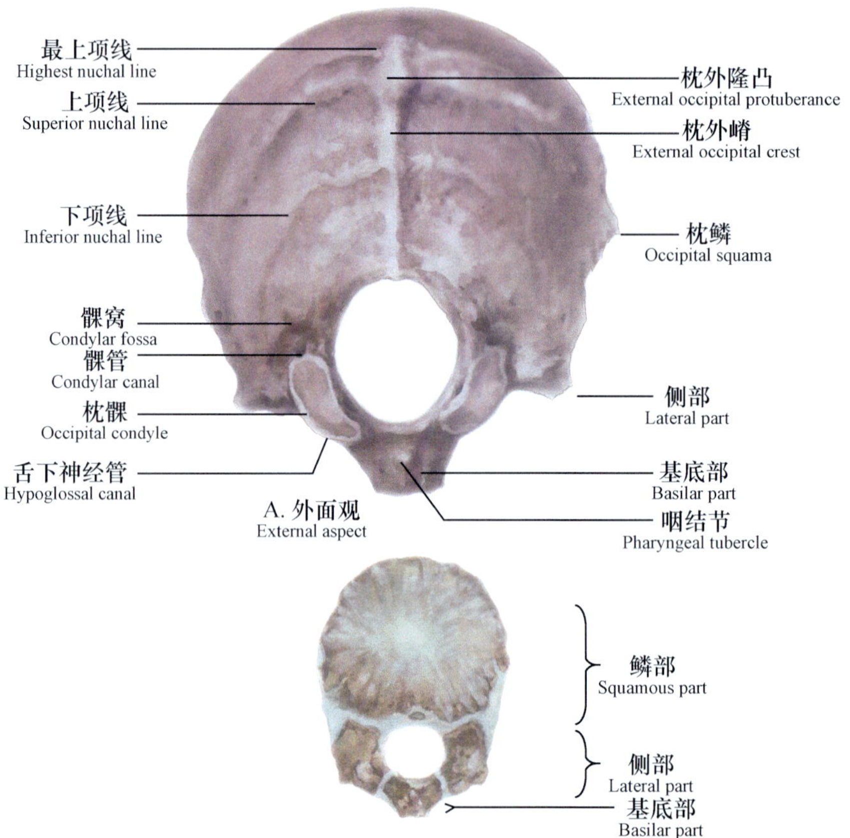

A. 外面观
External aspect

B. 新生儿枕骨（蓝色为尚未骨化部分）
The occipital bone of newborn (The unossified parts are shown in blue)

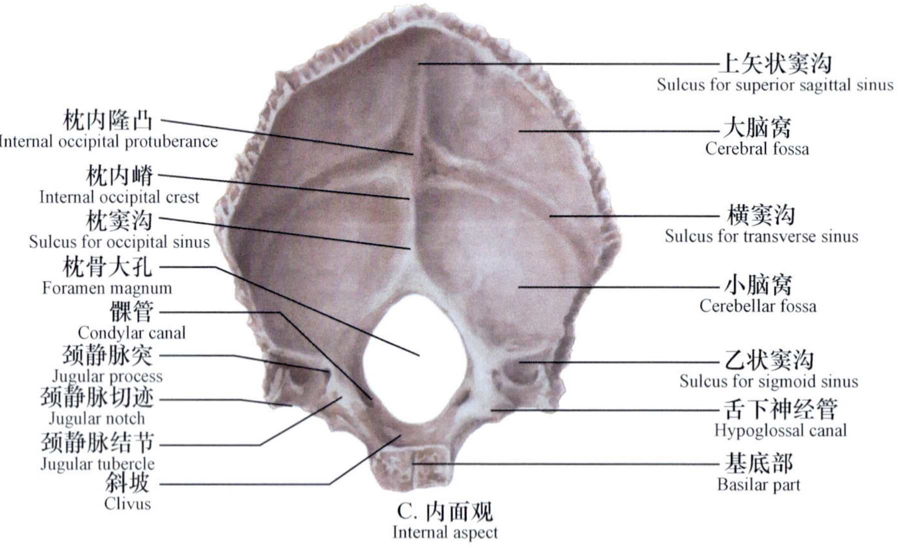

C. 内面观
Internal aspect

图 1-14 枕骨
The occipital bone

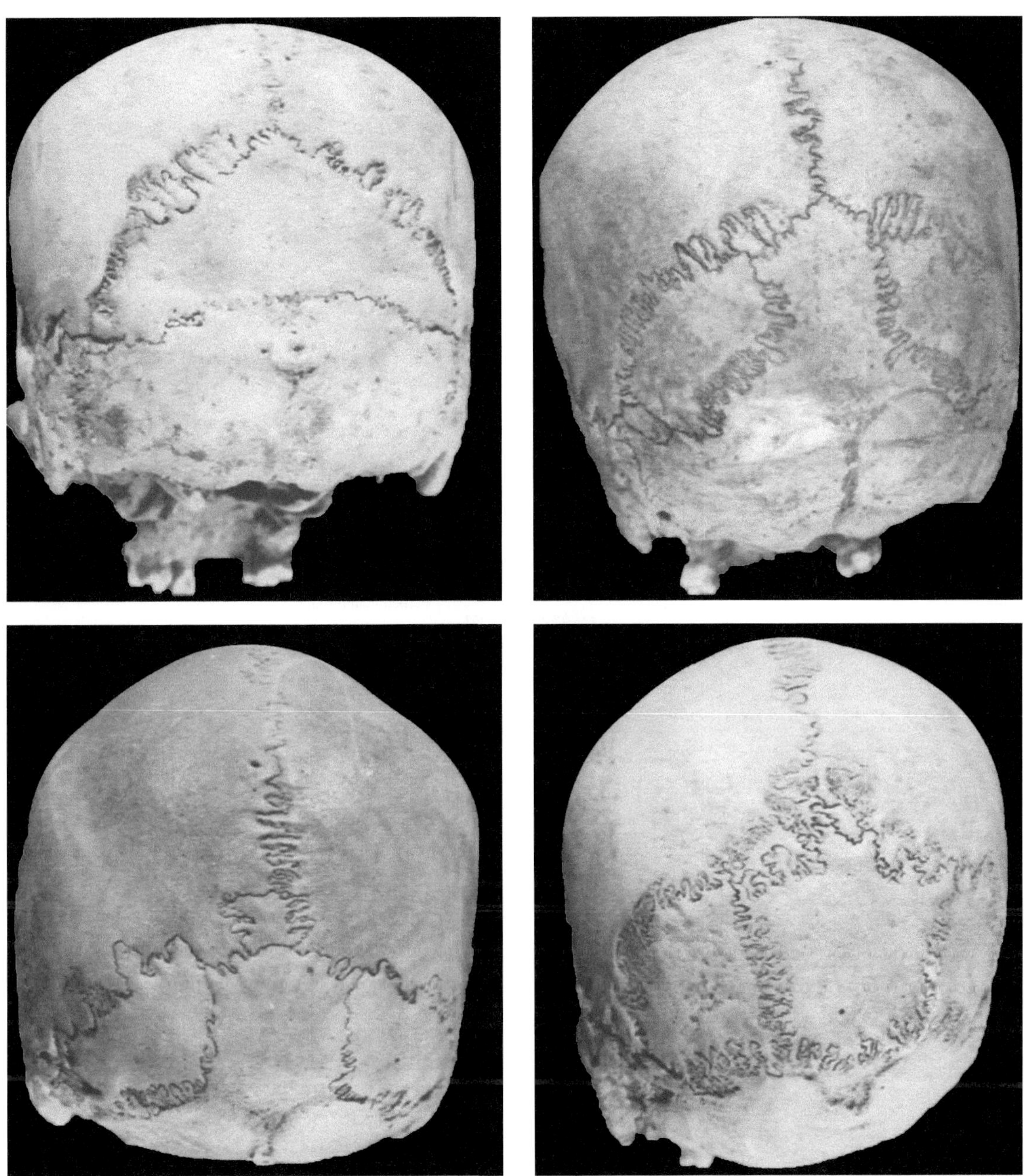

图 1-15　缝骨与顶间骨
Sutural and Interparieta Bone

颅缝内或靠近颅缝处可发生额外附加的骨化中心，形成独立的骨片。出现于两完整顶骨之后的枕鳞上部，纵径及横径均大于 2cm 的游离骨片称为顶间骨，也称印加骨或 Goethe osscle。中国人成年颅骨出现率为 47/1600（2.94%）。人类学家认为，顶间骨可作为民族遗传识别的鉴定标识

Additional extra ossification center may occur within or near the craniosynostosis,forming independent sutural bones.Supraoccipital part appears after two complete parietal bones.The free bone pieces with vertical and horizontal diameters larger than 2cm are called Interparieta Bone,also known as Inca bone or Goethe osscle.The appearance rate of adult skulls in Chinese is 47/1600 (2.94%) .Anthropologists believe that Interparieta Bone can be used as an identification standard for ethnic genetic identification.

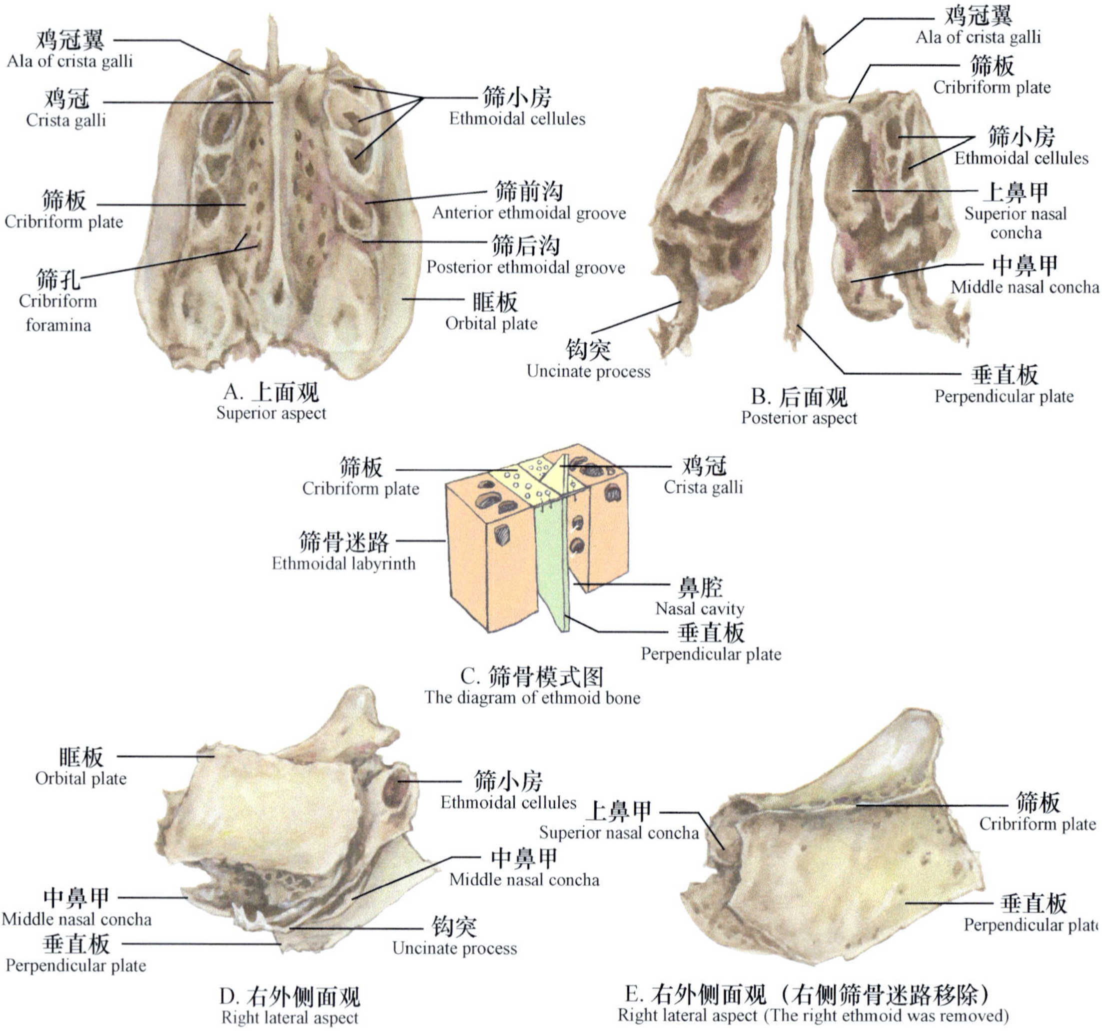

鸡冠翼
Ala of crista galli
鸡冠
Crista galli
筛板
Cribriform plate
筛孔
Cribriform foramina
筛小房
Ethmoidal cellules
筛前沟
Anterior ethmoidal groove
筛后沟
Posterior ethmoidal groove
眶板
Orbital plate

A. 上面观
Superior aspect

鸡冠翼
Ala of crista galli
筛板
Cribriform plate
筛小房
Ethmoidal cellules
上鼻甲
Superior nasal concha
中鼻甲
Middle nasal concha
钩突
Uncinate process
垂直板
Perpendicular plate

B. 后面观
Posterior aspect

筛板
Cribriform plate
鸡冠
Crista galli
筛骨迷路
Ethmoidal labyrinth
鼻腔
Nasal cavity
垂直板
Perpendicular plate

C. 筛骨模式图
The diagram of ethmoid bone

眶板
Orbital plate
筛小房
Ethmoidal cellules
中鼻甲
Middle nasal concha
中鼻甲
Middle nasal concha
钩突
Uncinate process
垂直板
Perpendicular plate

D. 右外侧面观
Right lateral aspect

上鼻甲
Superior nasal concha
筛板
Cribriform plate
垂直板
Perpendicular plate

E. 右外侧面观（右侧筛骨迷路移除）
Right lateral aspect (The right ethmoid was removed)

图 1-16 筛骨
The ethmoid bone

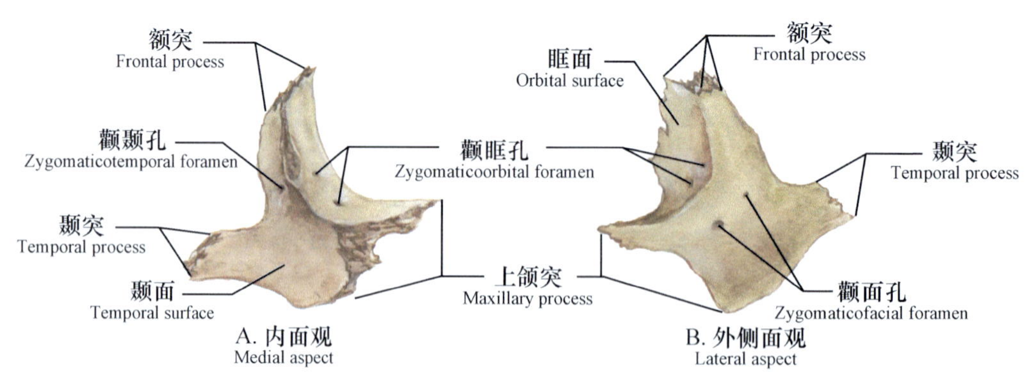

图 1-17 颧骨
The zygomatic bone

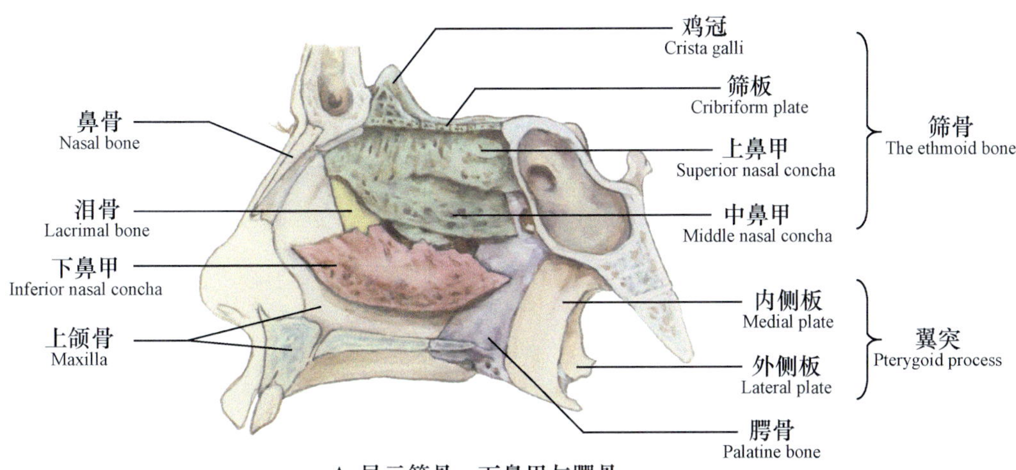

A. 显示筛骨、下鼻甲与腭骨
Showing the ethmoid,inferior turbinate and palatine bone

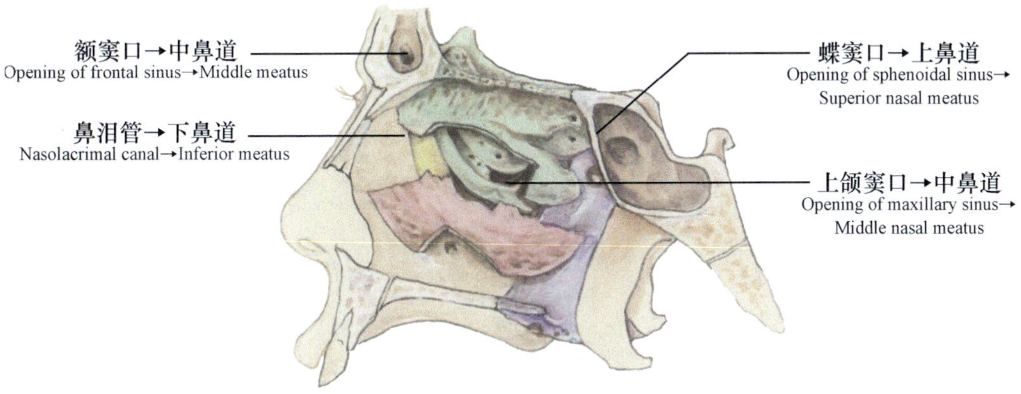

B. 显示气流通道
Showing the passage of the air

图 1-18 鼻腔右侧壁
The right wall of nasal cavity

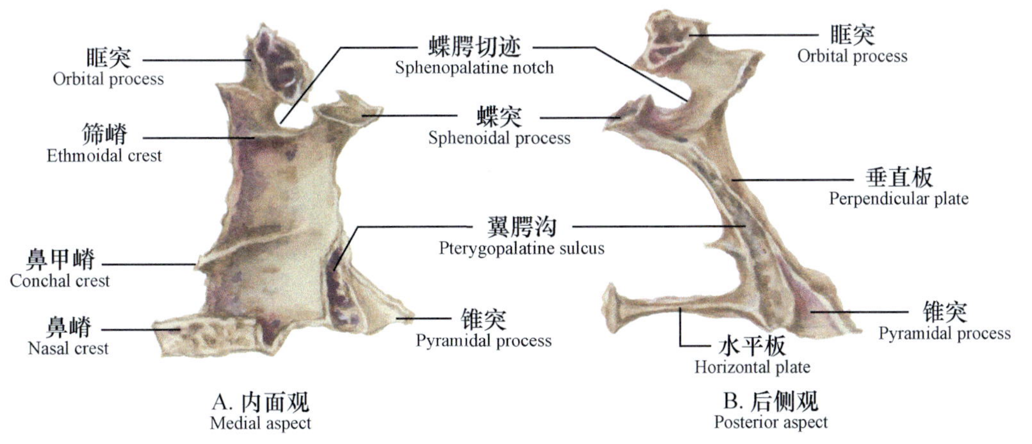

图 1-19 腭骨
The palatine bone

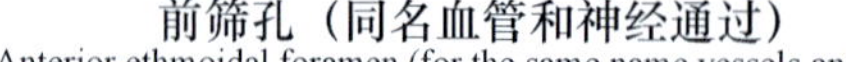

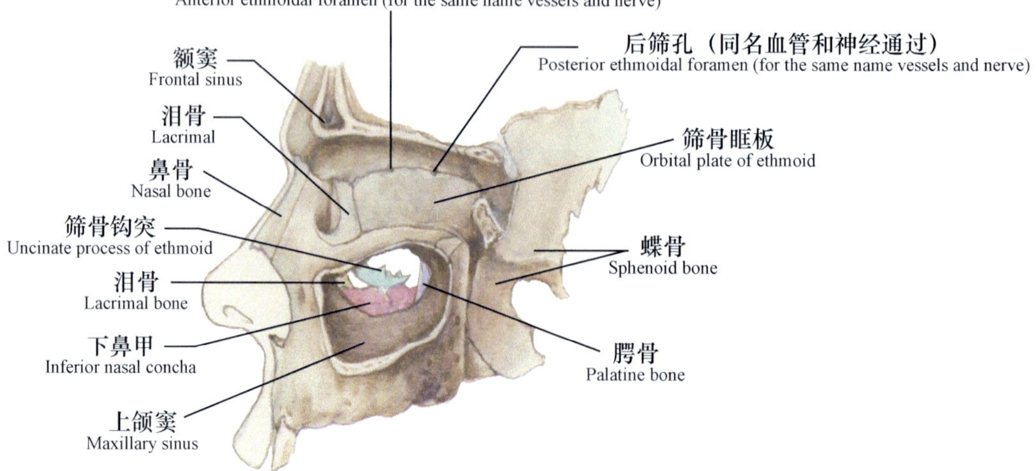

图 1-20　颅骨矢状旁切面（示左上颌窦内面观）
Parasagittal section of the cranium（showing the medial wall of the left maxillary sinus）

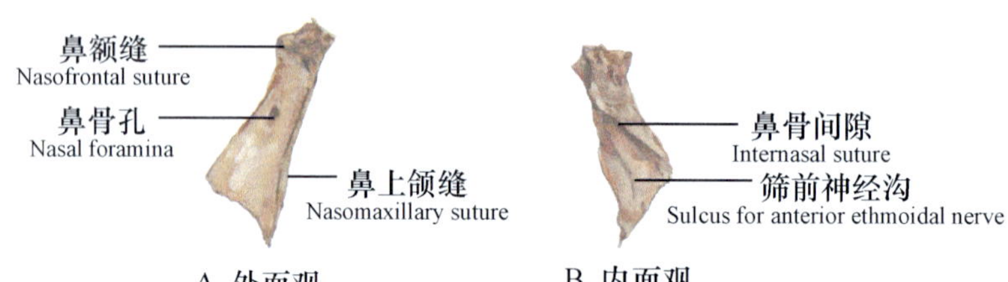

图 1-21　左侧鼻骨
The left nasal bone

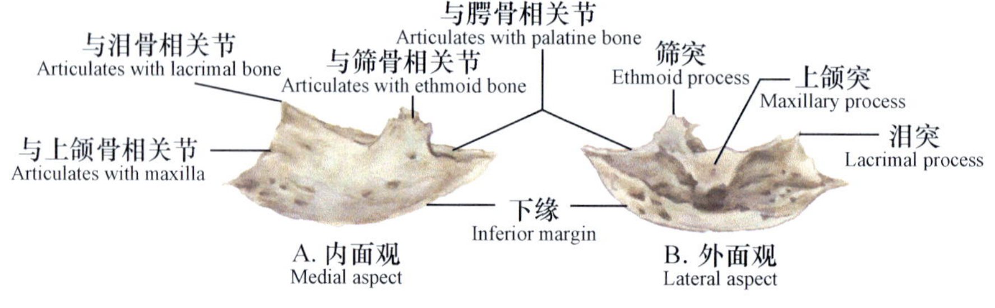

图 1-22　下鼻甲
Inferior nasal concha

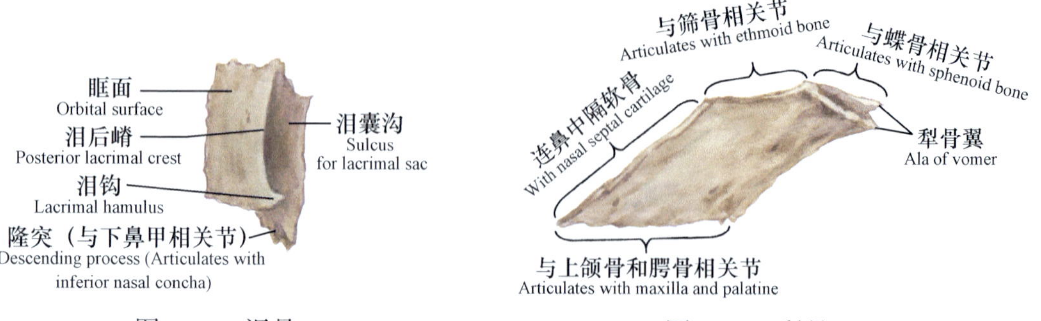

图 1-23　泪骨
Lacrimal bone

图 1-24　犁骨
Vomer

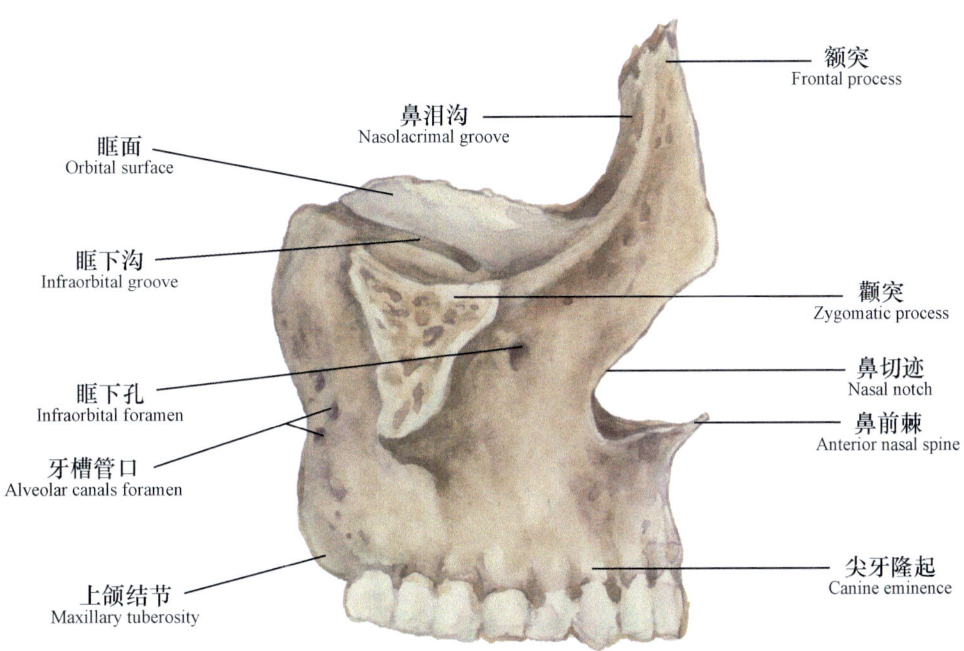

A. 外面观
Lateral aspect

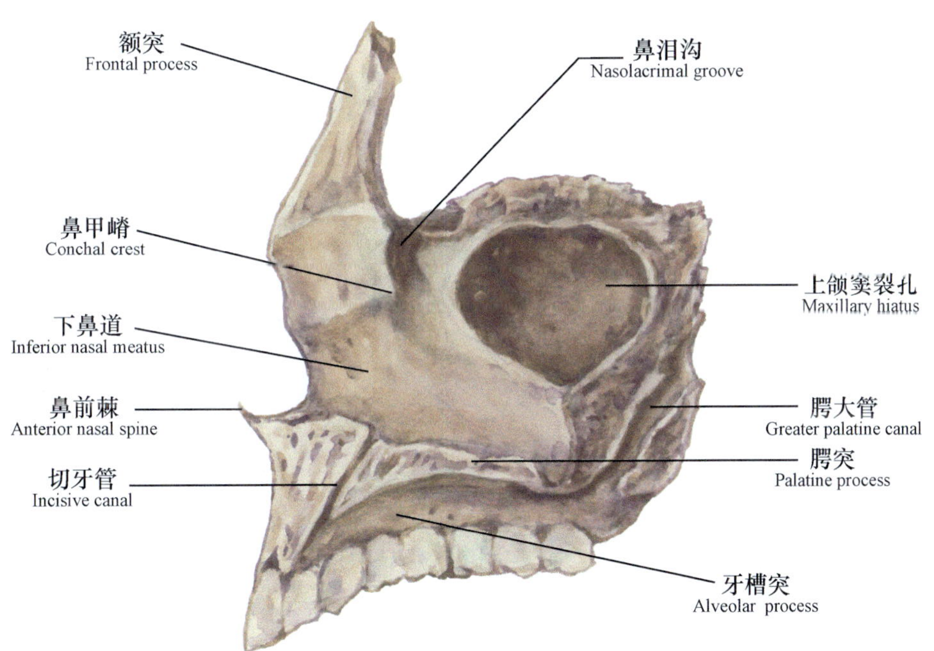

B. 内面观
Medial aspect

图 1-25 右上颌骨
The right maxilla

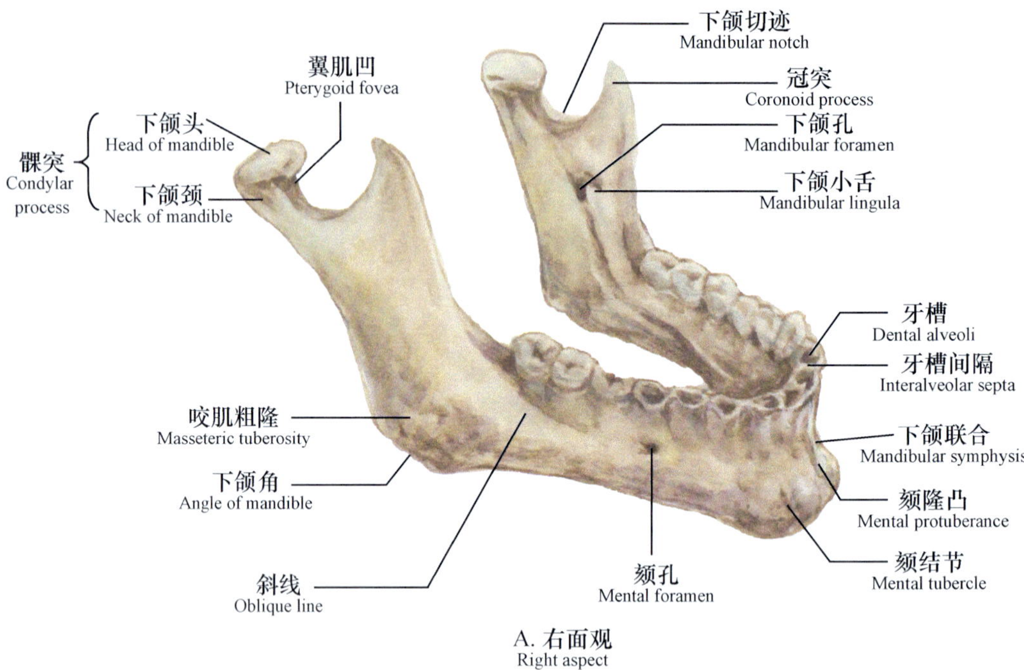

A. 右面观
Right aspect

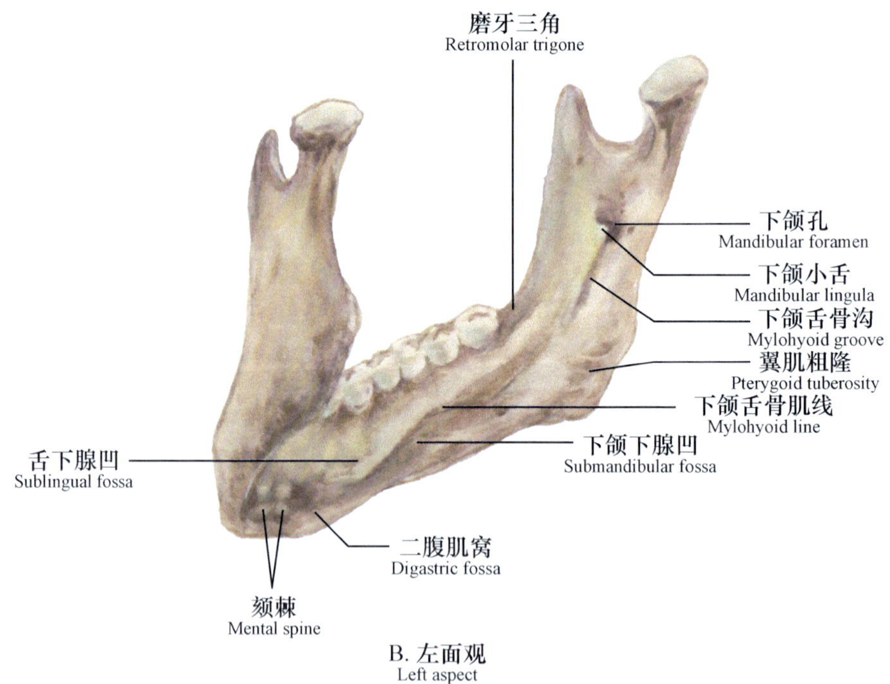

B. 左面观
Left aspect

图 1-26　下颌骨
The mandible

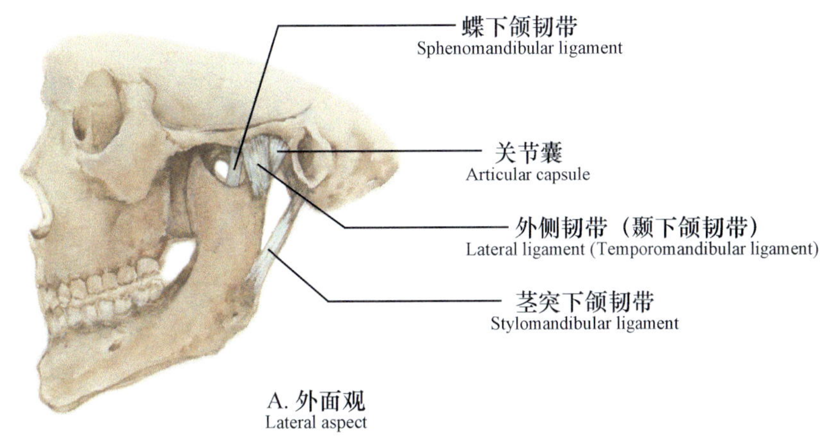

A. 外面观
Lateral aspect

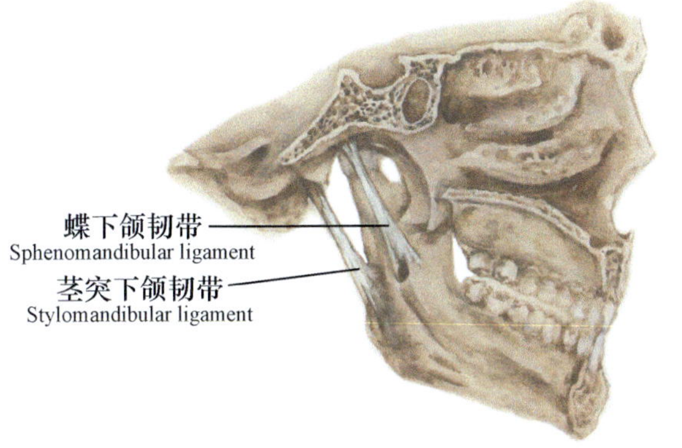

B. 内面观
Medial aspect

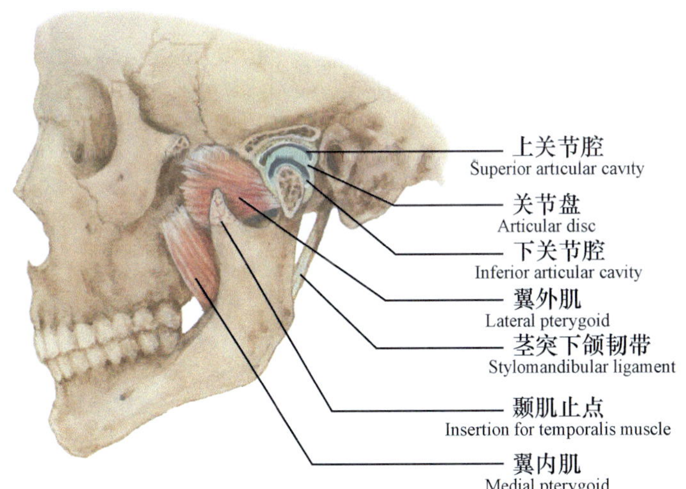

C. 左颞下颌关节矢状切面
A sagittal section through the left temporomandibular joint

图 1-27 左颞下颌关节
Left mandibular joint

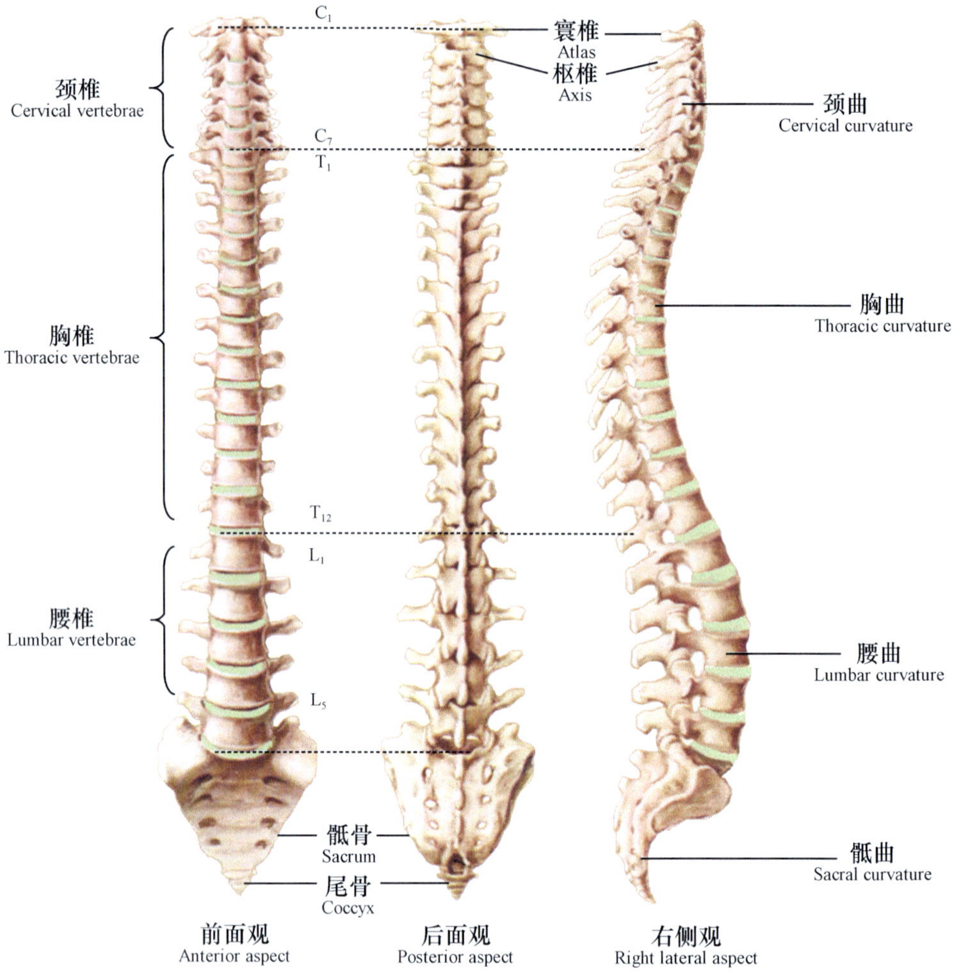

C1
C7
T1
T12
L1
L5

颈椎
Cervical vertebrae

胸椎
Thoracic vertebrae

腰椎
Lumbar vertebrae

寰椎
Atlas

枢椎
Axis

骶骨
Sacrum

尾骨
Coccyx

颈曲
Cervical curvature

胸曲
Thoracic curvature

腰曲
Lumbar curvature

骶曲
Sacral curvature

前面观
Anterior aspect

后面观
Posterior aspect

右侧观
Right lateral aspect

图 1-28 脊柱
Vertebral column

A. 初生（维持胎儿时形成的胸曲和骶曲），当坐位时，脊柱呈弧形；当仰卧位时，脊柱呈水平状
A. At birth (It retains the thoracic and pelvic curves formed during fetal life).When sit position,the vertebral column is present curve.When lie on its back, the vertebral column is horizontal.

B. 出生后4—5个月（婴儿开始抬头看世界），颈曲形成
B. 4-5 months after birth (The child is able to hold up its head and to look at the world).The cervical curvature is formed.

C. 出生后12—18个月（幼儿开始蹒跚学步），腰曲形成
C. 12-18 months after birth (The child begins to walk), and the lumbar curvature is formed.

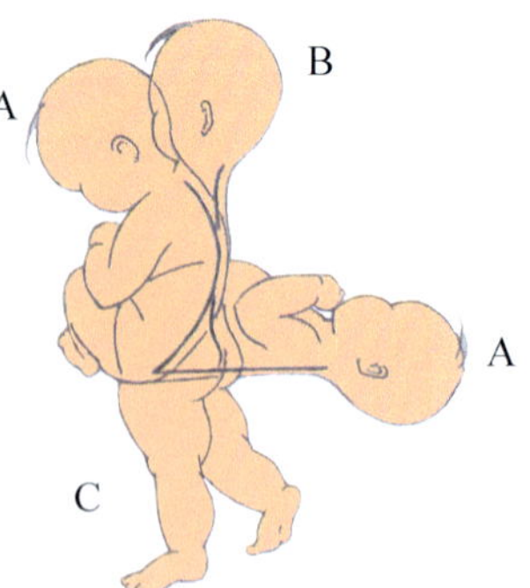

图 1-29 脊柱弯曲的形成
The forming of vertebral curvatures

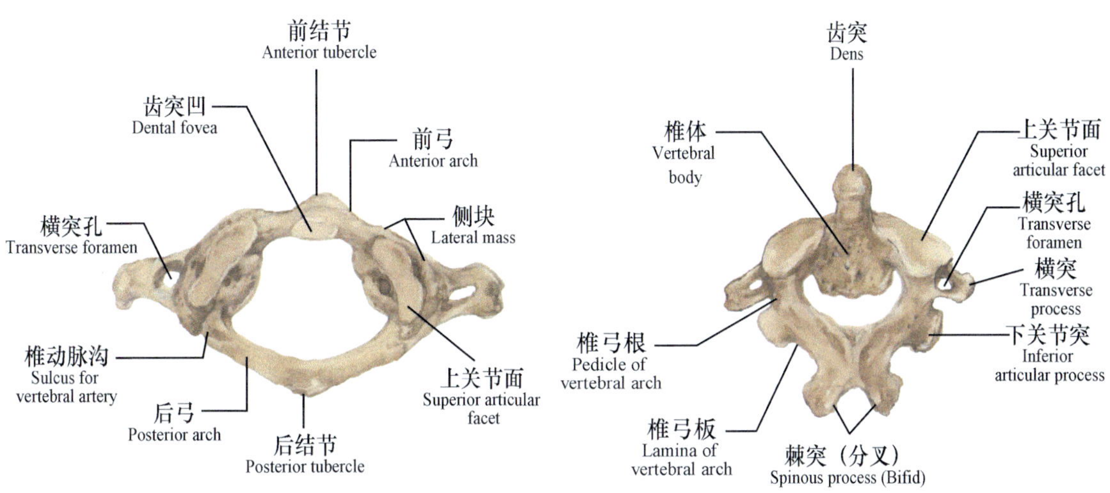

A. 寰椎（第一颈椎）上面观
The atlas (The first cervical vertebra)　superior aspect

B. 枢椎（第二颈椎）上面观
The axis (The second cervical vertebra)　superior aspect

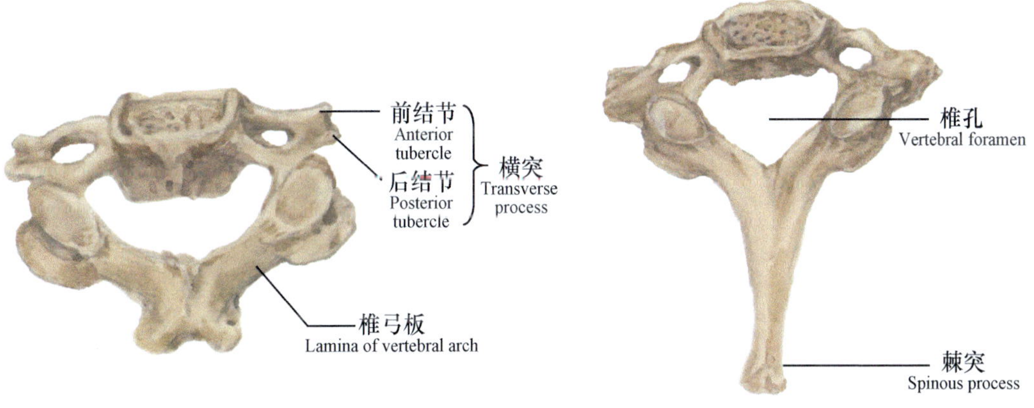

C. 第三颈椎 上面观
（可代表4—6颈椎）
The third cervical vertebra　superior aspect
(which may represent the $C_{4\text{-}6}$)

D. 第七颈椎 上面观
（棘突长，又称“隆椎”）
The seventh cervical vertebra　superior aspect
(which is sometimes called the vertebra prominens for its long spinous process)

图 1-30　颈椎
The cervical vertebra

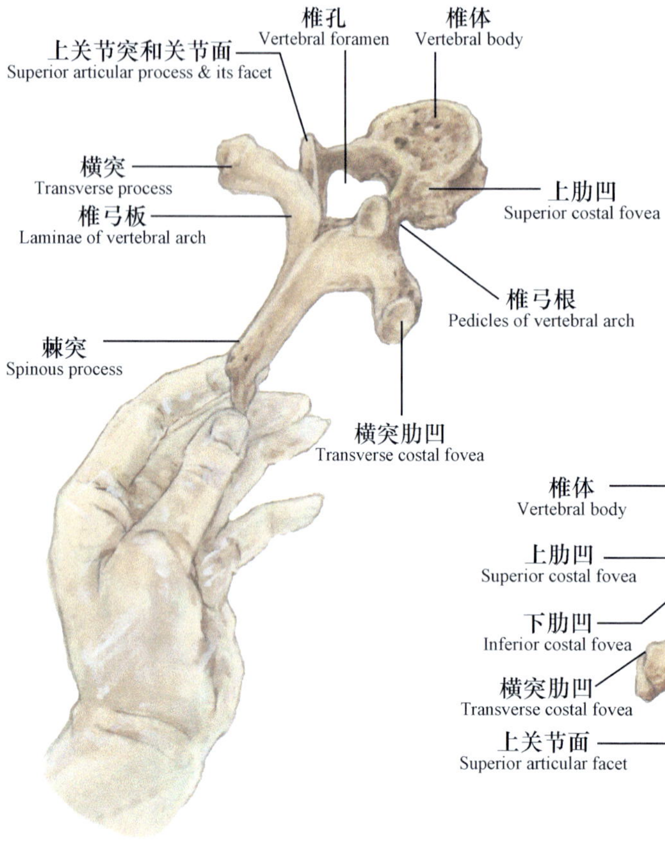

椎孔
Vertebral foramen
椎体
Vertebral body
上关节突和关节面
Superior articular process & its facet
横突
Transverse process
椎弓板
Laminae of vertebral arch
上肋凹
Superior costal fovea
椎弓根
Pedicles of vertebral arch
棘突
Spinous process
横突肋凹
Transverse costal fovea

A. 第六胸椎(具有典型椎体结构)
The sixth thoracic vertebra (which contains a typical vertebral structure)

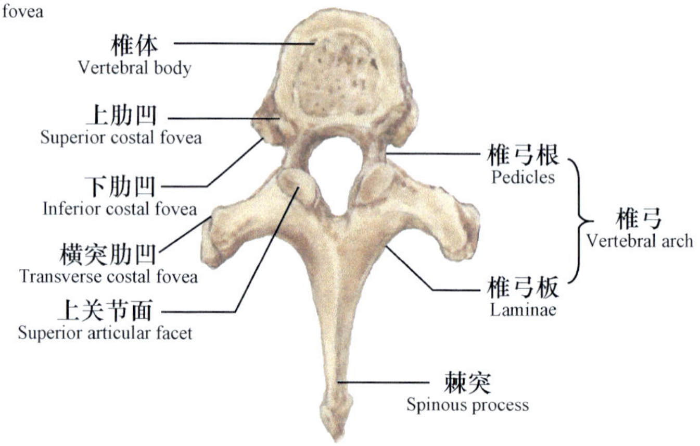

椎体
Vertebral body
上肋凹
Superior costal fovea
下肋凹
Inferior costal fovea
横突肋凹
Transverse costal fovea
上关节面
Superior articular facet
椎弓根
Pedicles
椎弓
Vertebral arch
椎弓板
Laminae
棘突
Spinous process

B. 第六胸椎（上面观）
The sixth thoracic vertebra (Superior aspect)

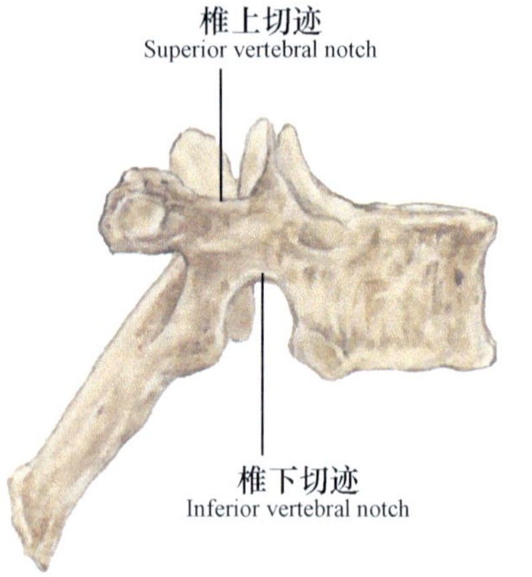

椎上切迹
Superior vertebral notch
椎下切迹
Inferior vertebral notch

C. 第六胸椎（右侧观）
The sixth thoracic vertebra (Right lateral aspect)

下肋凹
Inferior costal fovea
上关节面
Superior articular facet
下关节面
Inferior articular facet

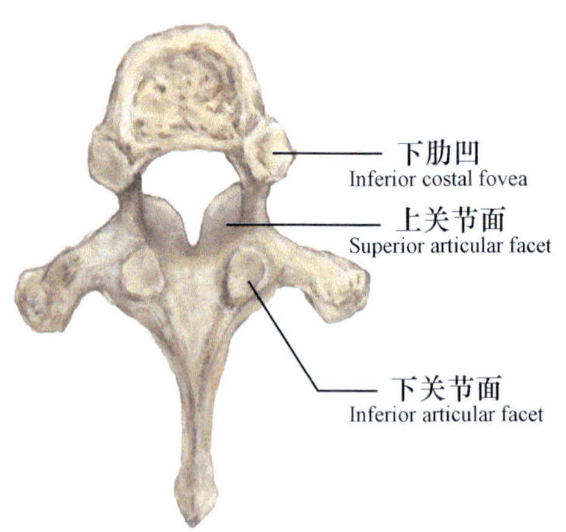

D. 第六胸椎（下面观）
The sixth thoracic vertebra (Inferior aspect)

图 1-31 第六胸椎
The sixth thoracic vertebra

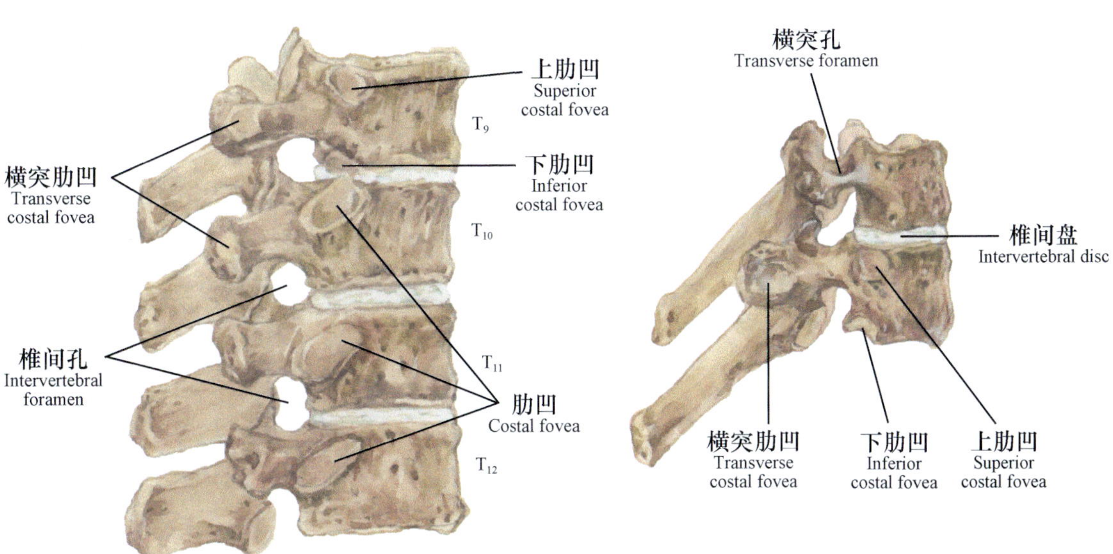

图 1-32　第九至十二胸椎（右侧观）
The ninth to twelfth thoracic vertebra (Right lateral aspect)

图 1-33　第七颈椎与第一胸椎（右侧观）
The seventh cervical vertebra and the first thoracic vertebra (Right lateral aspect)

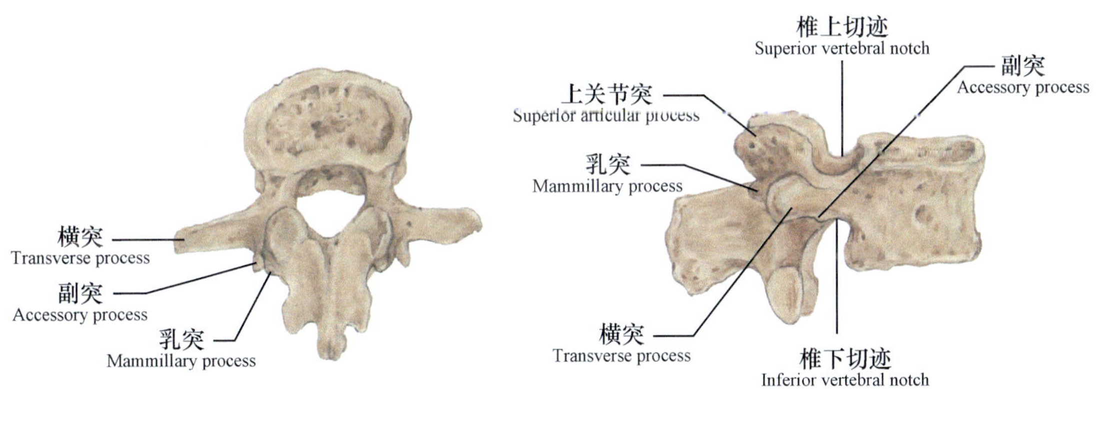

A. 腰椎（上面观）
Lumbar vertebra (Superior aspect)

B. 腰椎（右侧观）
Lumbar vertebra (Right lateral aspect)

图 1-34　腰椎
Lumbar vertebra

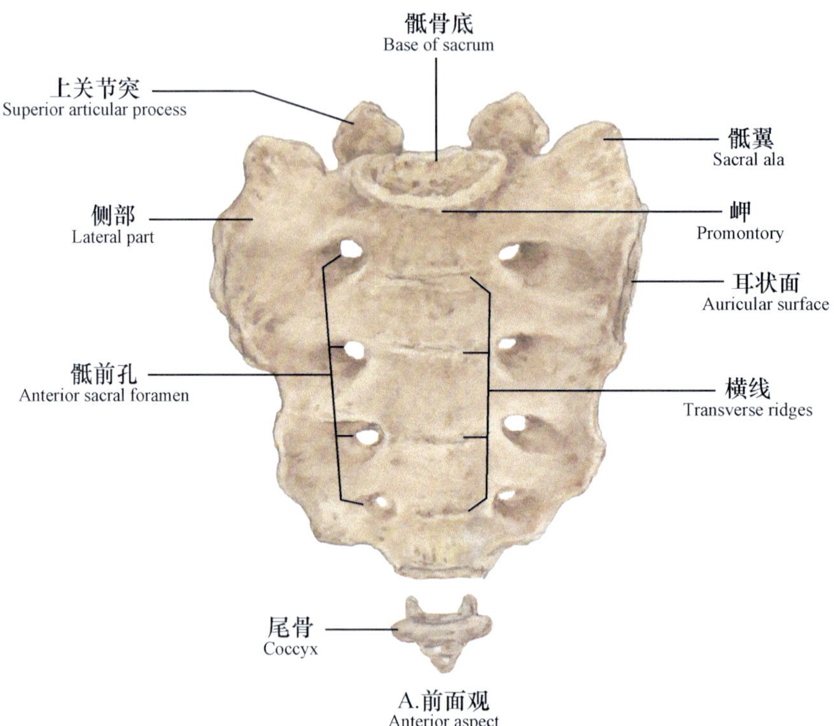

A.前面观
Anterior aspect

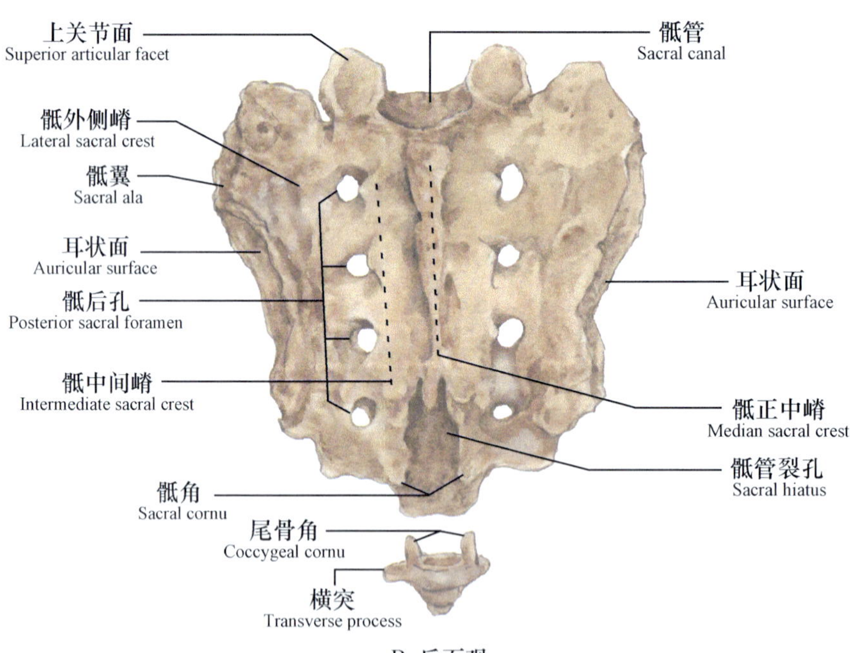

B. 后面观
Posterior aspect

图 1-35 骶骨和尾骨（1）
Sacrum and coccyx（1）

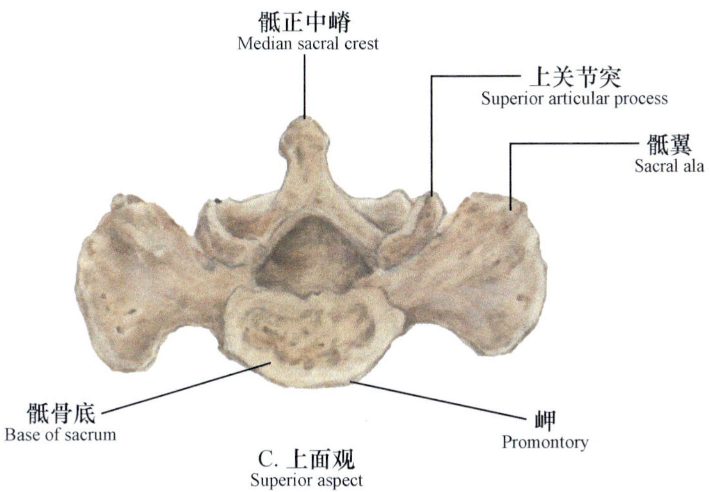

C. 上面观
Superior aspect

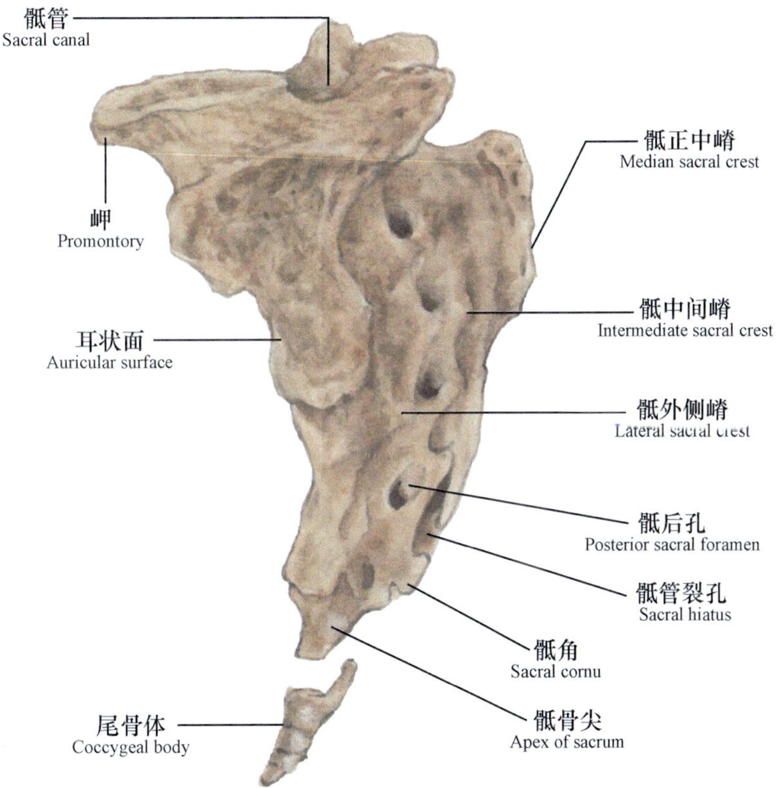

D. 左侧面观
Left lateral aspect

图 1-35　骶骨和尾骨（2）
Sacrum and coccyx（2）

寰椎
The atlas
寰椎横韧带
Transverse ligament of atlas
枢椎
The axis

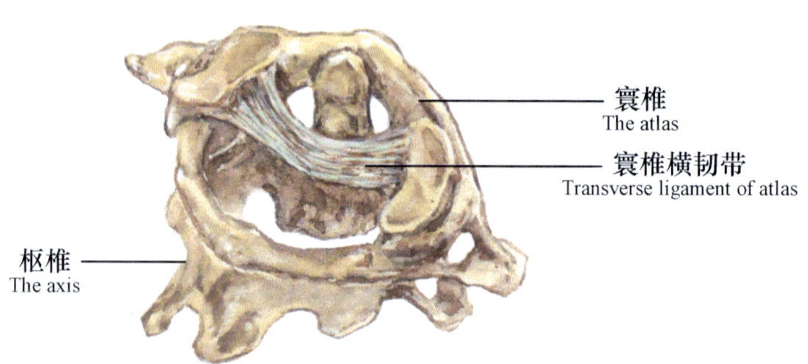

图 1-36 寰椎横韧带与寰椎和枢椎
The atlas and axis with the transverse ligament of atlas

硬膜
Dura mater
覆膜
Tectorial membrane
枕骨基底部
Basilar part of occipital bone
寰枕前膜
Anterior atlantooccipital membrane
齿突尖韧带
Apical ligament of dens
上束
Superior bands
枢椎齿突
Dens of axis
寰椎十字韧带
Cruciform ligament of atlas
寰椎横韧带
Transverse ligament of atlas
寰椎前弓
Anterior arch of atlas
下束
Inferior bands
寰枢前韧带
Anterior atlantoaxial ligament
前纵韧带
Anterior longitudinal ligament
后纵韧带
Posterior longitudinal ligament
舌下神经
Hypoglossal nerve
第一颈神经
1st cervical nerve
椎动脉
Vertebral artery
枕下神经
Suboccipital nerve
寰枕后膜
Posterior atlantooccipital membrane
第二颈神经
2nd cervical nerve
寰枢后韧带
Posterior atlanto-axial ligament
第三颈神经
3rd cervical nerve
黄韧带
Ligamenta flava
第四颈神经
4th cervical nerve

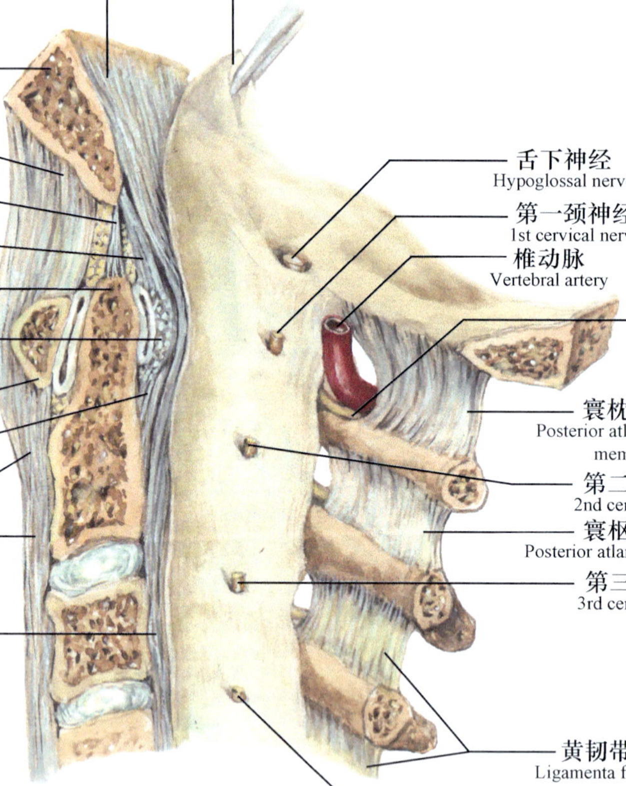

图 1-37 枕骨与上三个颈椎的正中矢状切面（右内侧观）
Median sagittal section through occipital bone and upper three cervical vertebrae (Right medial aspect)

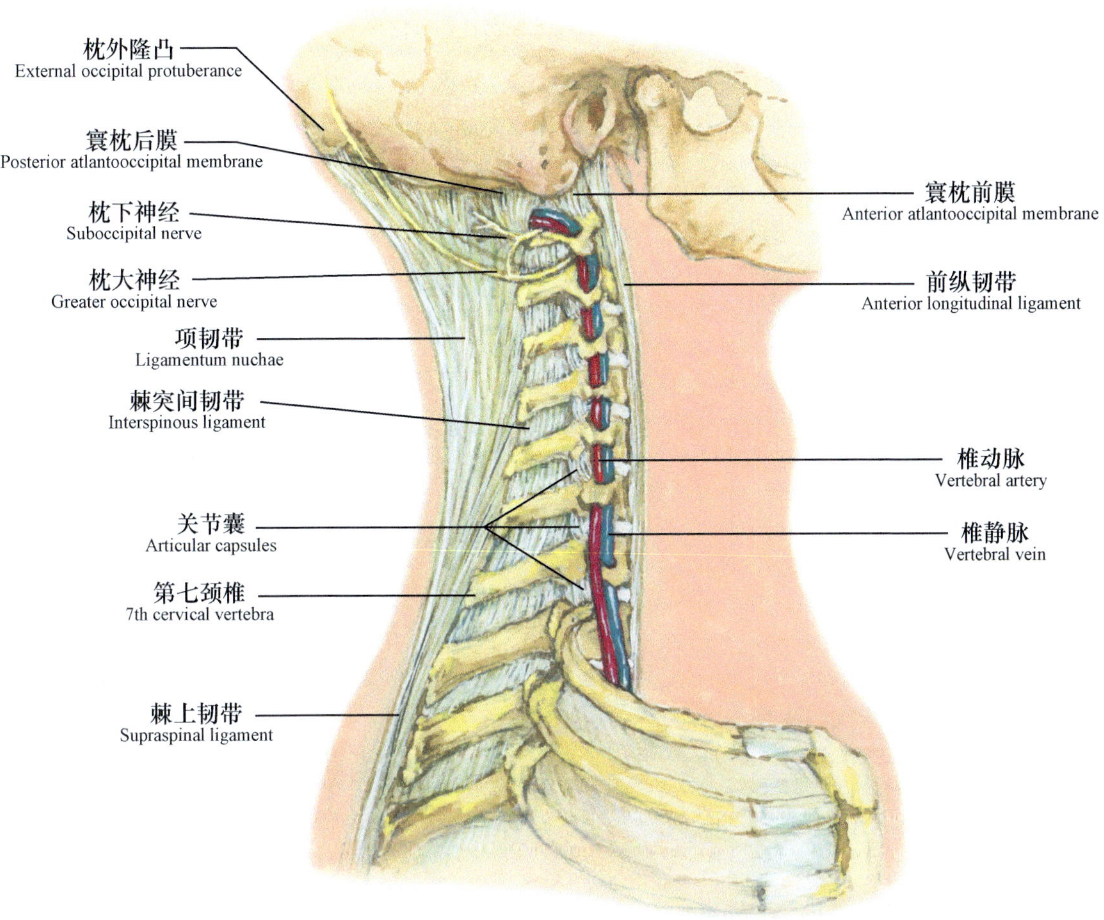

注：枕下神经为第一颈神经背侧支，大于腹侧支，其分支分布于颈后深部枕下三角肌群，并有分支参与第二颈神经后形成枕大神经

The suboccipital nerve is the dorsal division of the first cervical nerve and larger the ventral. It supplies the muscles which bound the suboccipital triangle and has a filament to joining the dorsal division of the second cervical nerve to form the greater occipital nerve.

图 1-38　项韧带（右侧观）

Ligamentum nuchae (Right aspect)

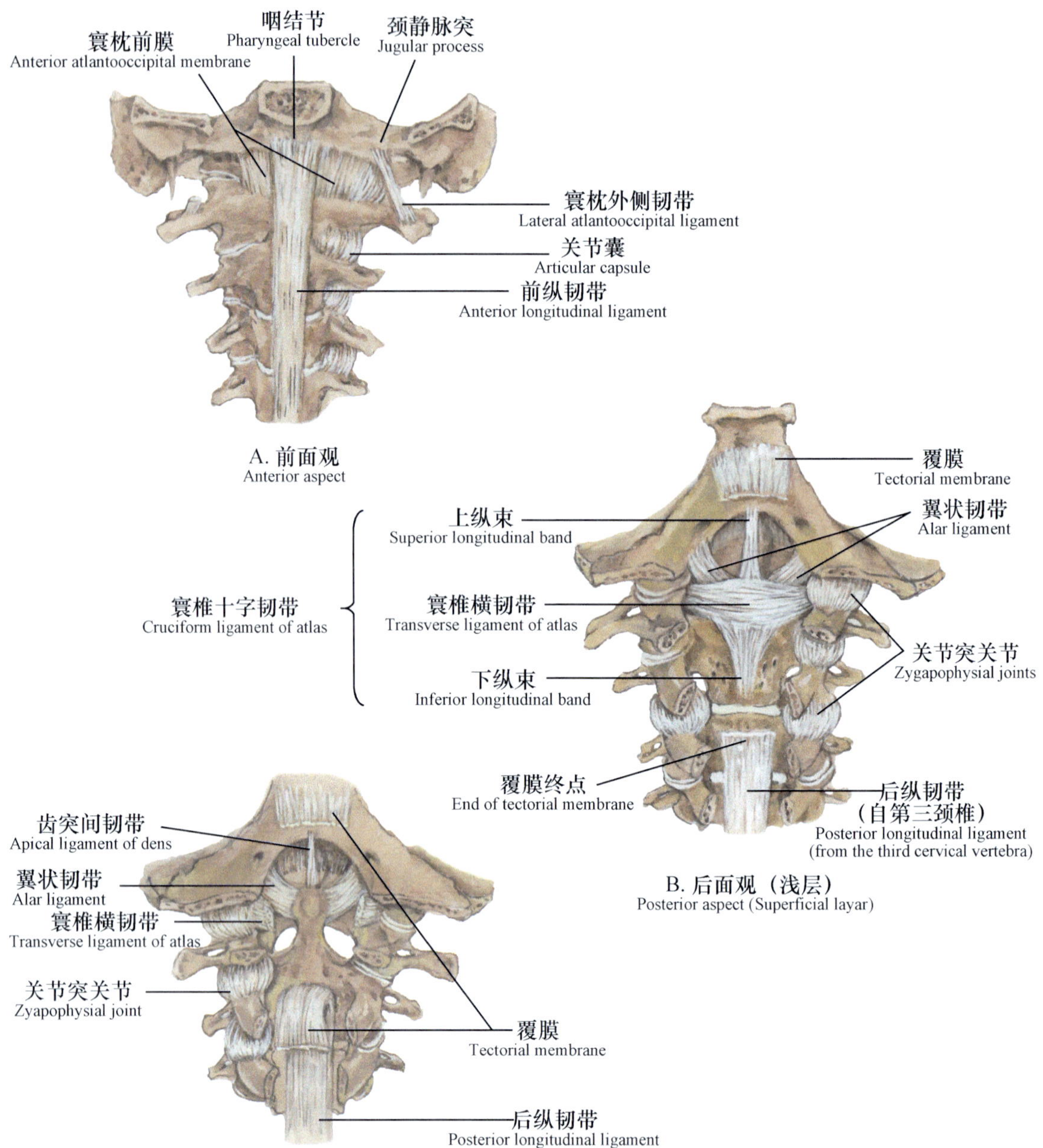

注：①寰枕外侧韧带介于寰椎横突与枕骨颈静脉突之间，有加强关节囊外侧壁的作用
The atlanto-occipital ligaments are attached to the jugular processes of the occipital bone, and to the bases of the transverse processes of the atlas.

②后纵韧带是覆膜位于枢椎椎体后面在椎管内向下的延续
The posterior longitudinal ligament is continous with the tectorial membrane at the dorsal surface of the axial body and extends down within the vertebral canal.

C. 后面观（深层）
Posterior aspect (Deeper layer)

图 1-39 寰枕关节和寰枢关节
The atlantooccipital and atlantoaxial joints

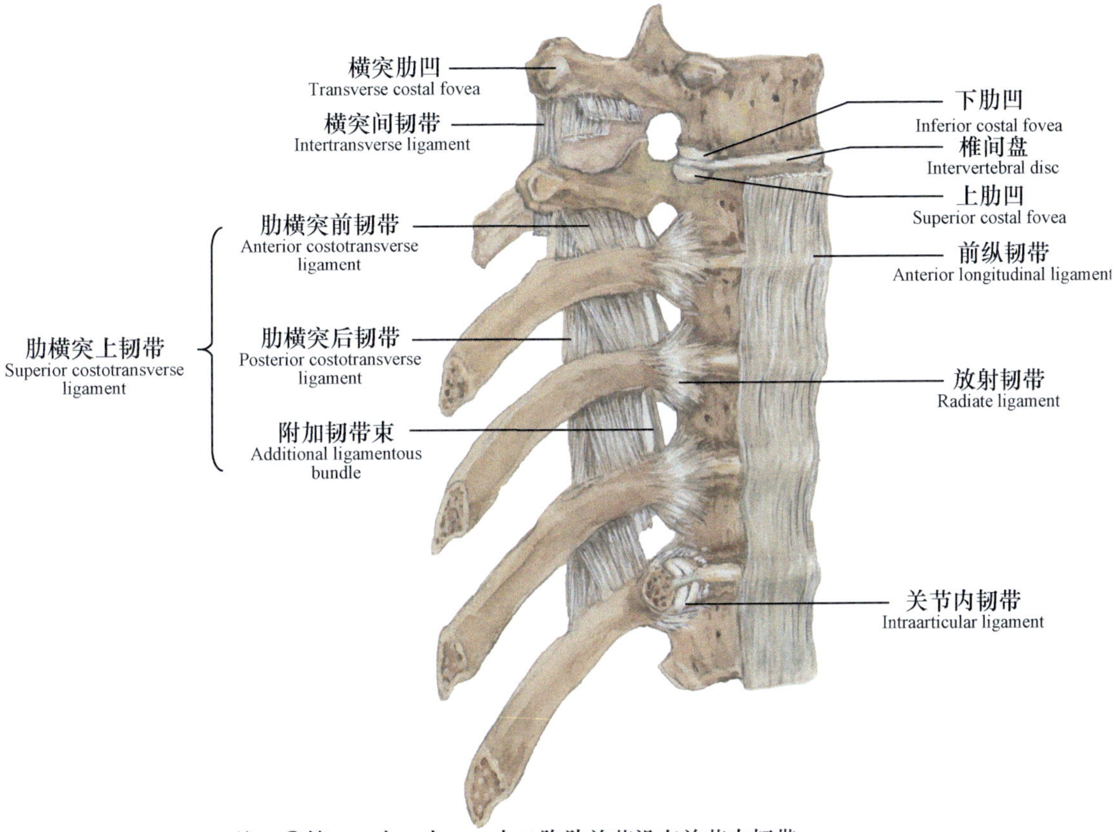

横突肋凹
Transverse costal fovea
横突间韧带
Intertransverse ligament
肋横突前韧带
Anterior costotransverse ligament
肋横突后韧带
Posterior costotransverse ligament
附加韧带束
Additional ligamentous bundle
肋横突上韧带
Superior costotransverse ligament
下肋凹
Inferior costal fovea
椎间盘
Intervertebral disc
上肋凹
Superior costal fovea
前纵韧带
Anterior longitudinal ligament
放射韧带
Radiate ligament
关节内韧带
Intraarticular ligament

注：①第一、十、十一、十二胸肋关节没有关节内韧带
In the joints of the first,tenth,eleventh and twelfth ribs intraarticular ligaments do not exist
②附加韧带束，一般位于肋横突上韧带内侧，被脊神经后支及其伴行血管所分隔
The additional ligamentous band is usually present medial to the superior costotransverse, and separated from it by a dorsal ramus of a thoracic spinal nerve and accompanying vessels

A. 右侧观
Right lateral aspect

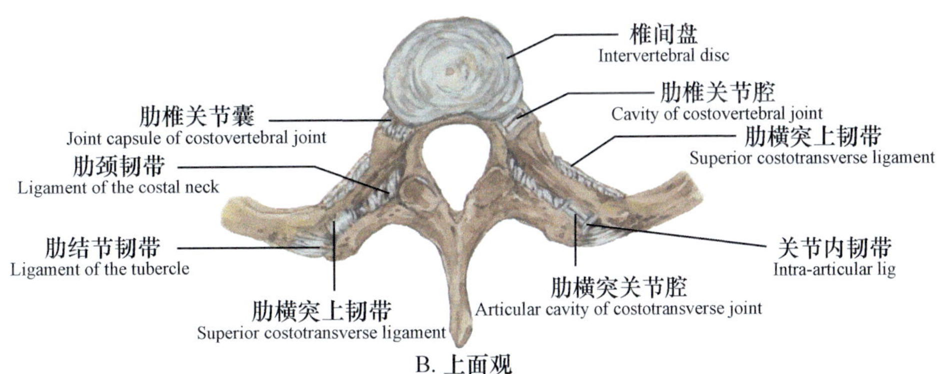

B. 上面观
Superior aspect

图 1-40 肋椎关节
The costovertebral joint

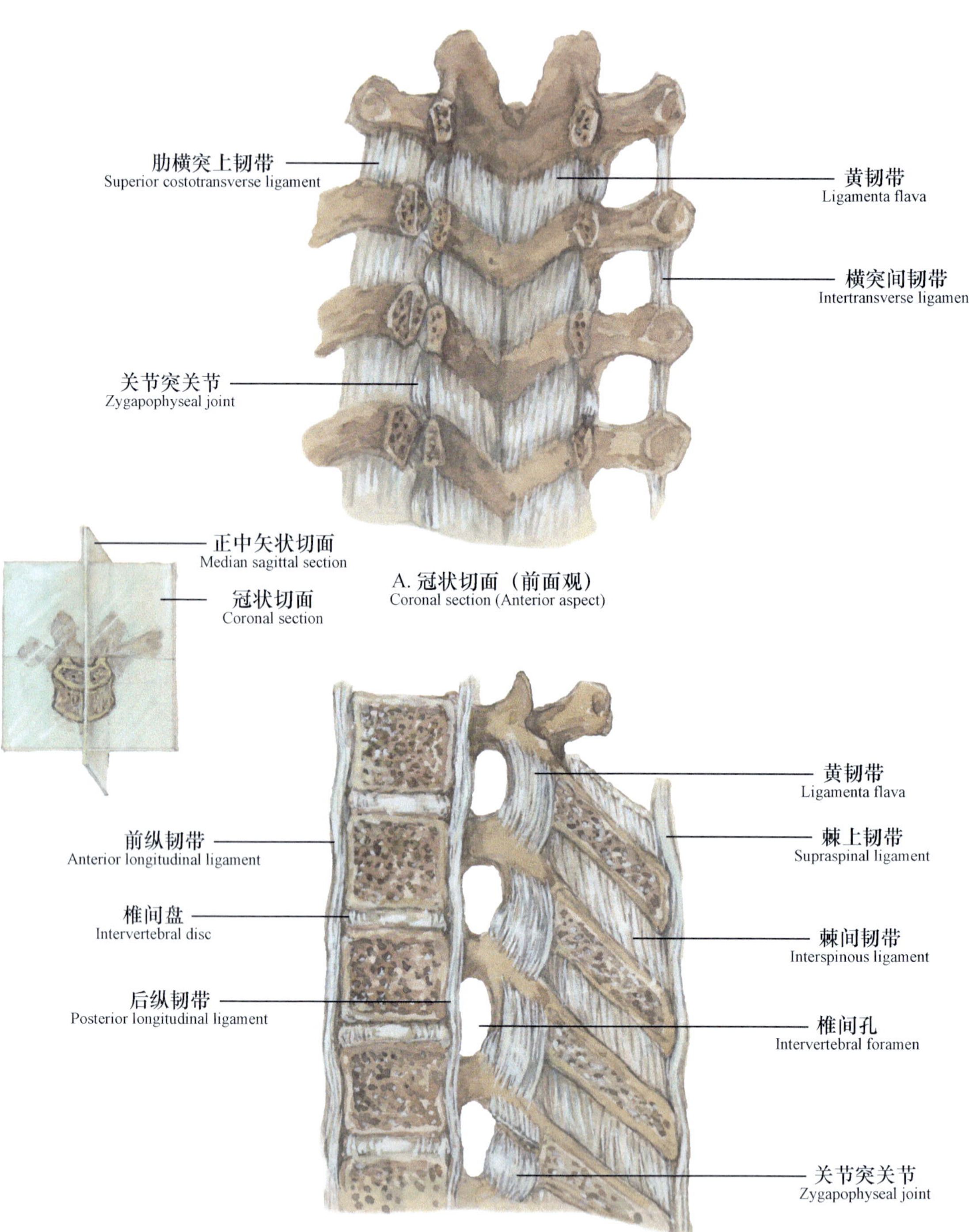

图 1-41　脊柱胸段

The thoracic region of the vertebral column

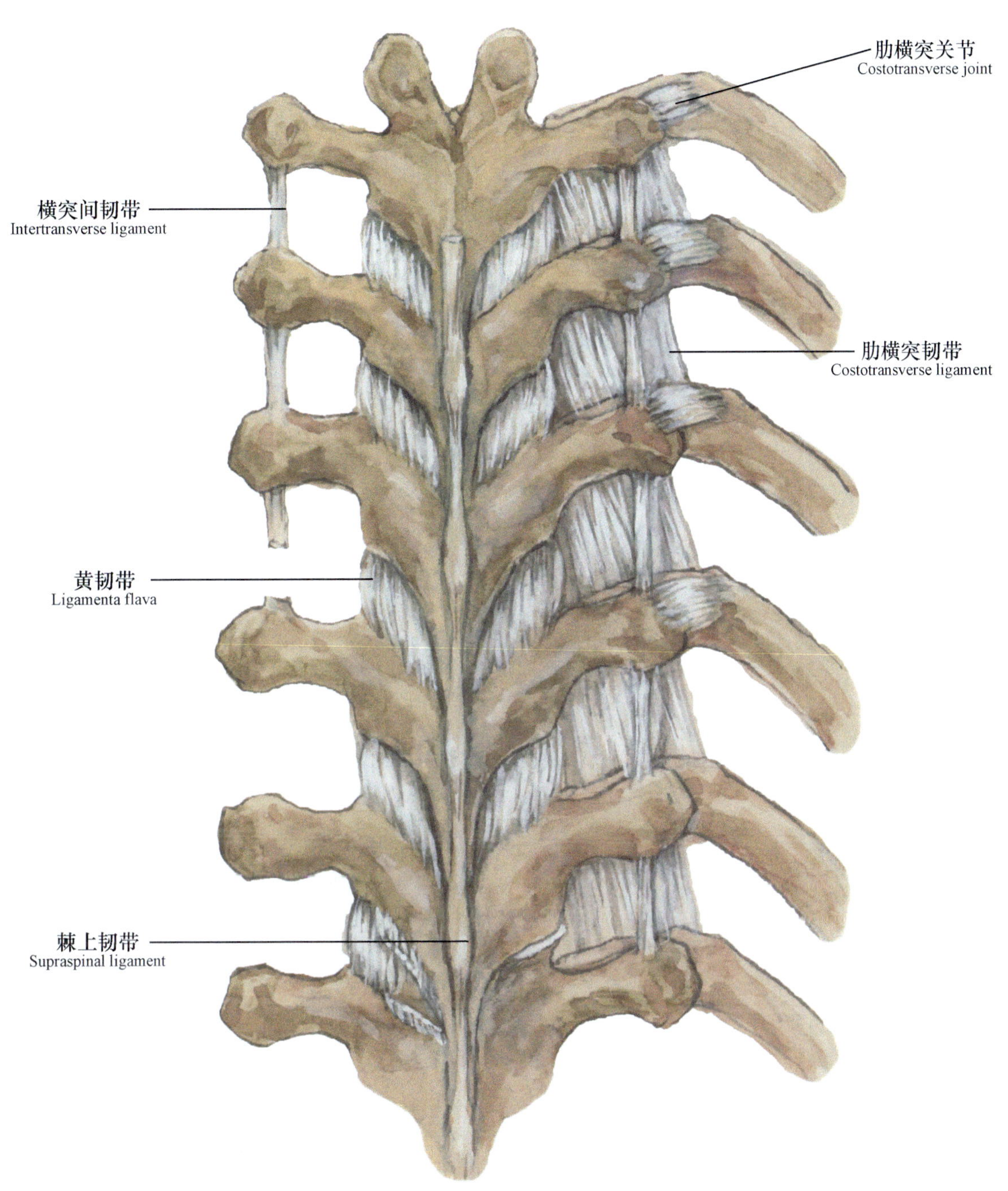

图 1-42 脊柱胸段（后面观）
The thoracic region of the vertebral column (Posterior aspect)

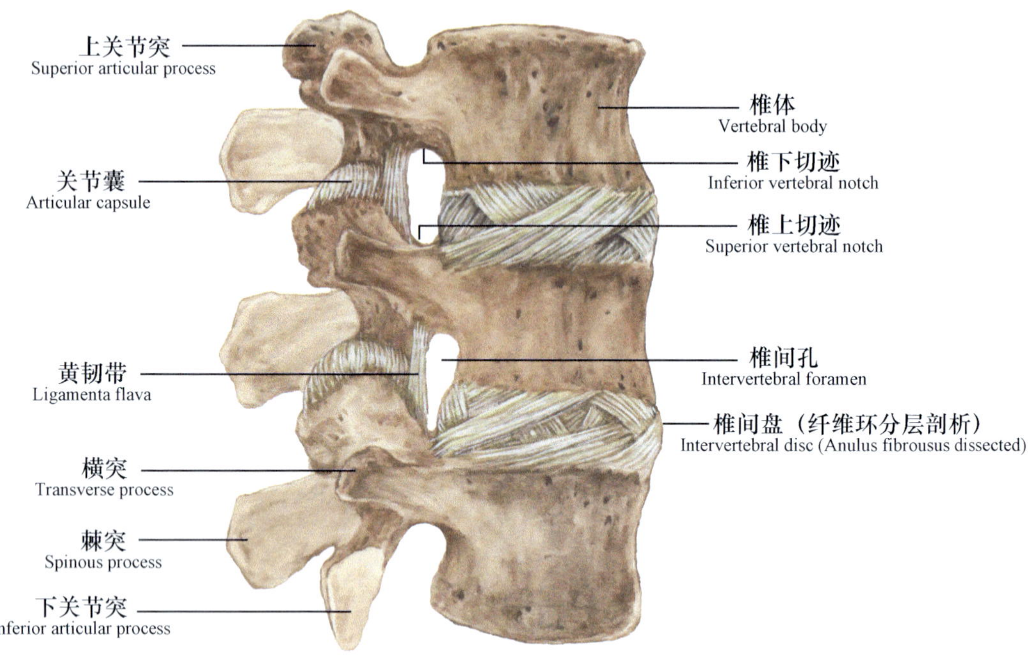

A. 侧面观
Lateral aspect

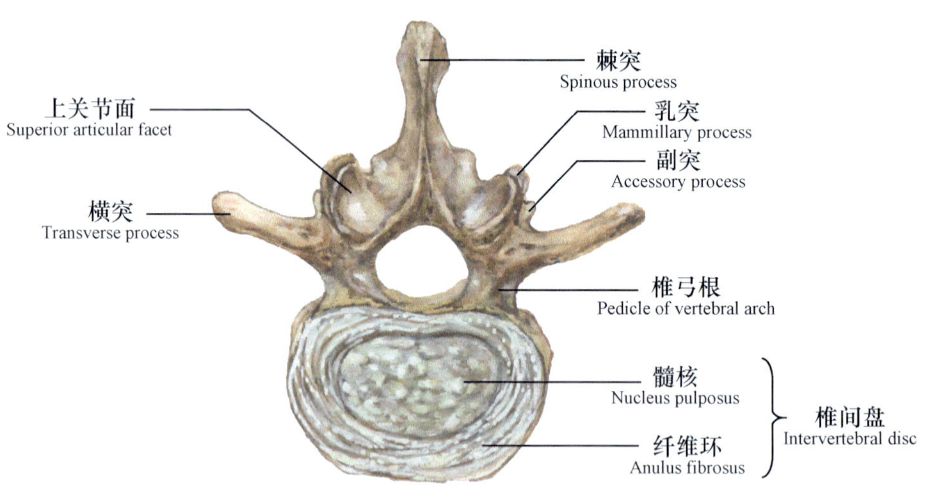

B. 上面观
Superior aspect

图 1-43 腰椎间盘
Lumbar intervertebral disc

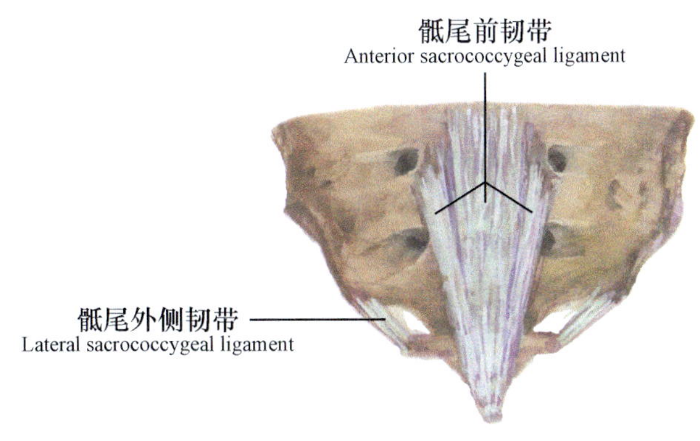

A. 前面观
Anterior aspect

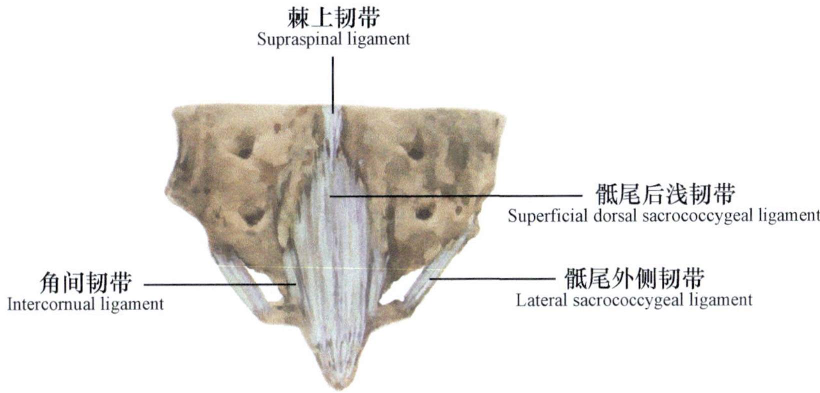

B. 浅层（后面观）
Superficial layer (Posterior aspect)

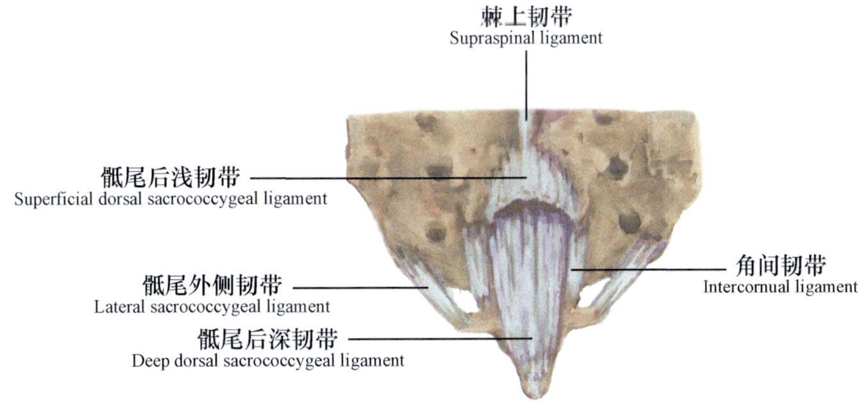

C. 深层（后面观）
The deep layer (Posterior aspect)

图 1-44　骶尾关节
Secrococcygeal joint

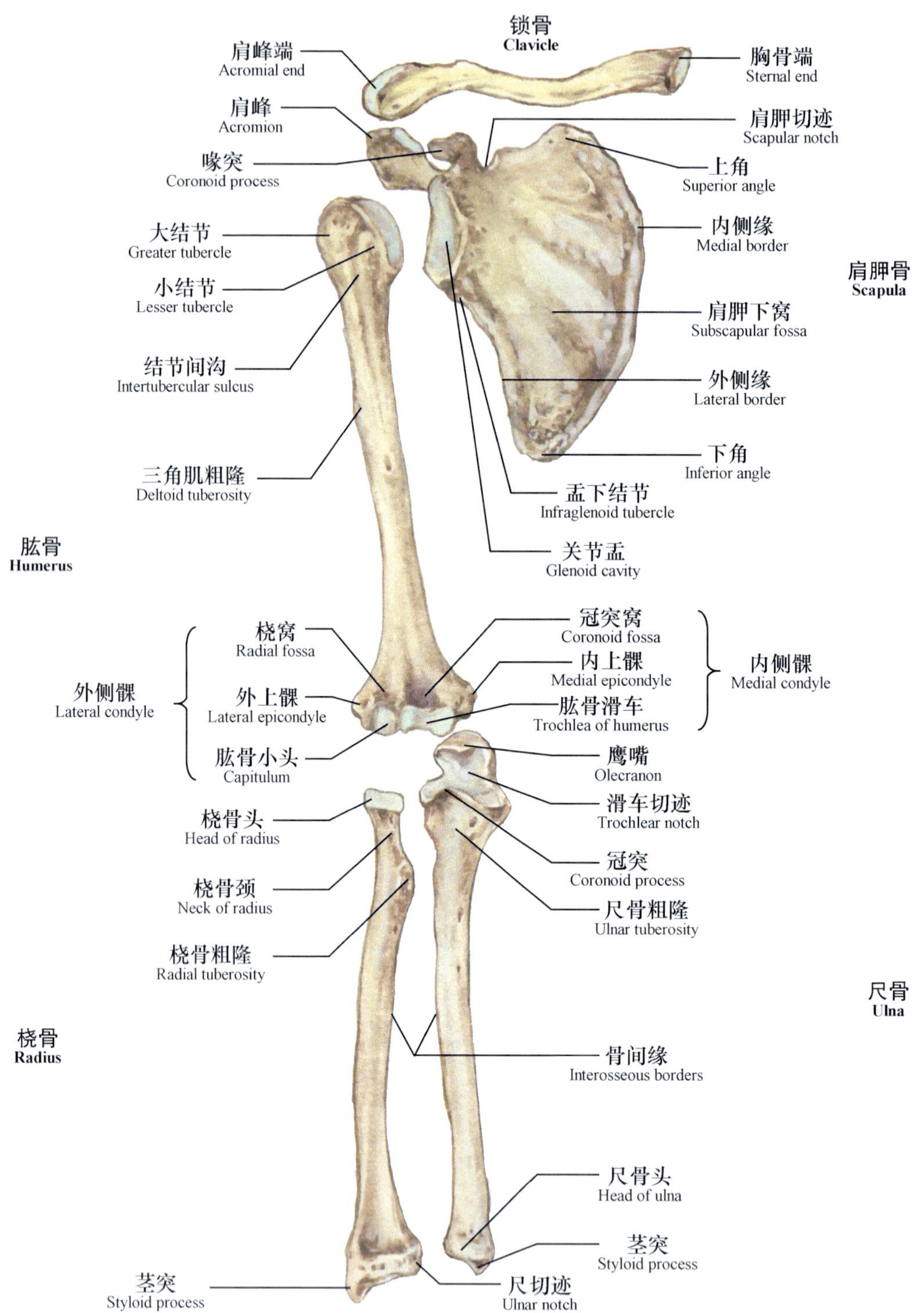

图 1-45 上肢骨（前面观）
Bones of upper limb (Anterior aspect)

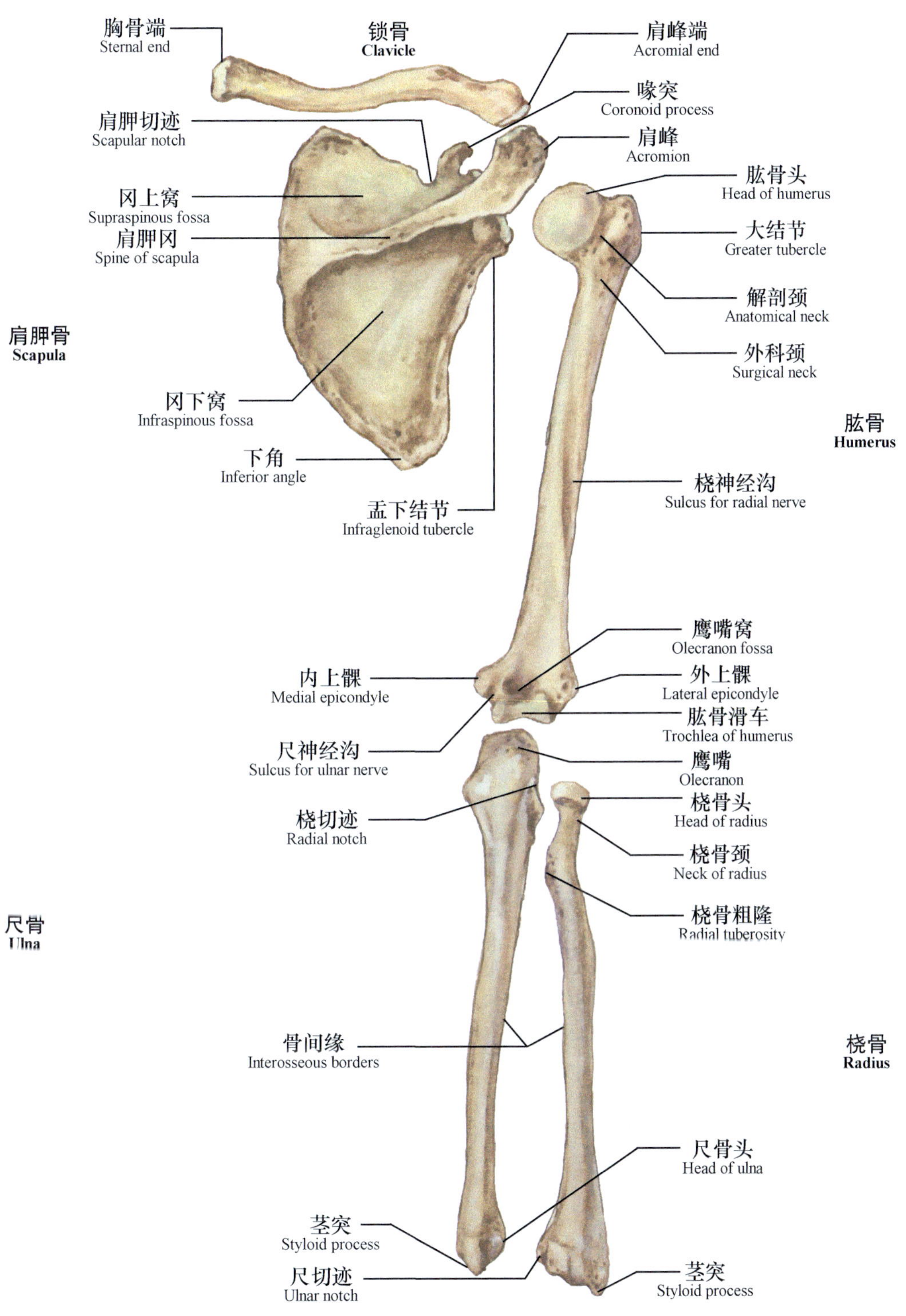

图 1-46 上肢骨（后面观）
Bones of upper limb (Posterior aspect)

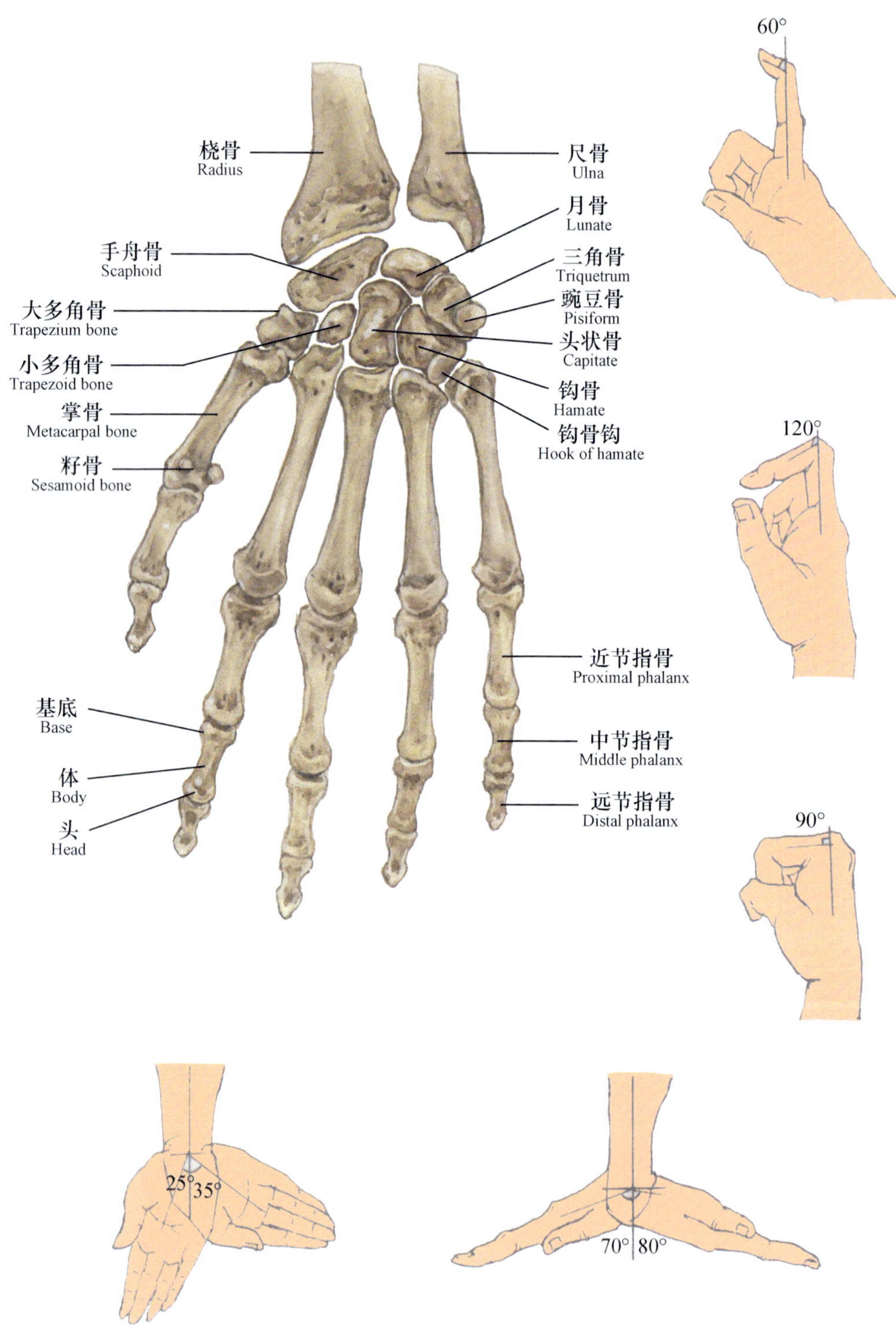

图 1-47　手骨（前面观）
The bones of hand (Anterior aspect)

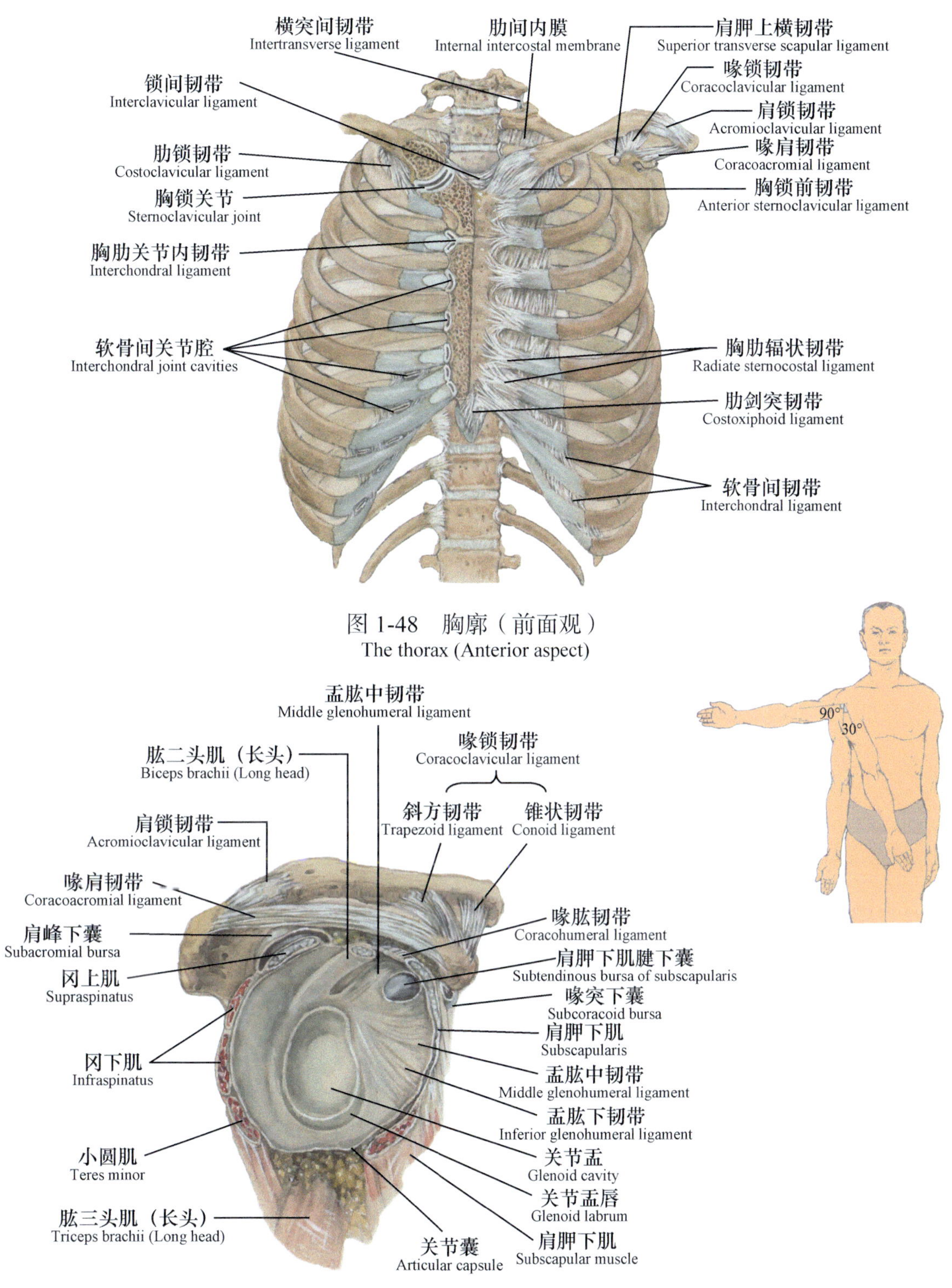

图 1-48　胸廓（前面观）
The thorax (Anterior aspect)

图 1-49　肩关节（内面观）
The shoulder joint (Internal aspect)

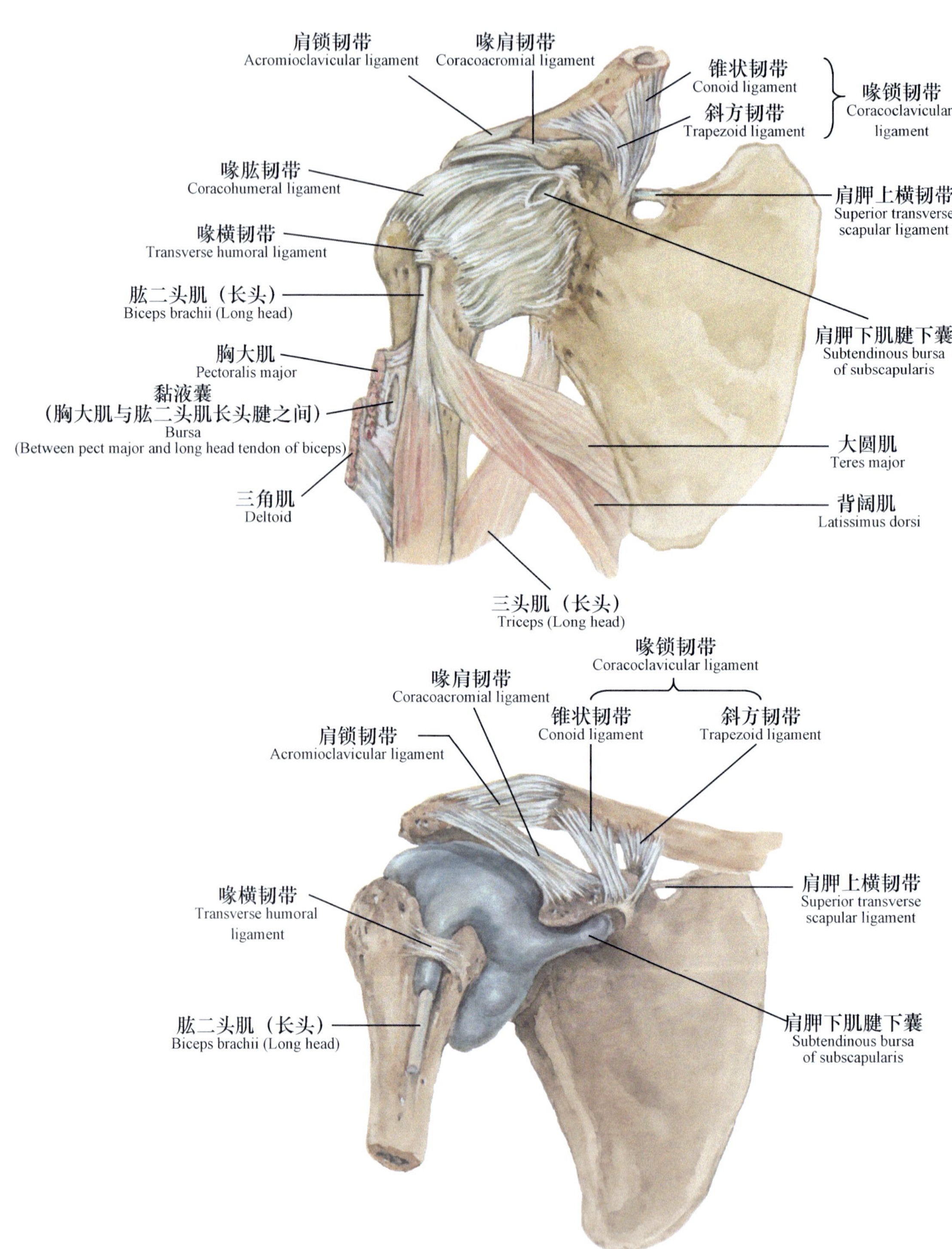

图 1-50　肩关节（前面观）
The shoulder joint (Anterior aspect)

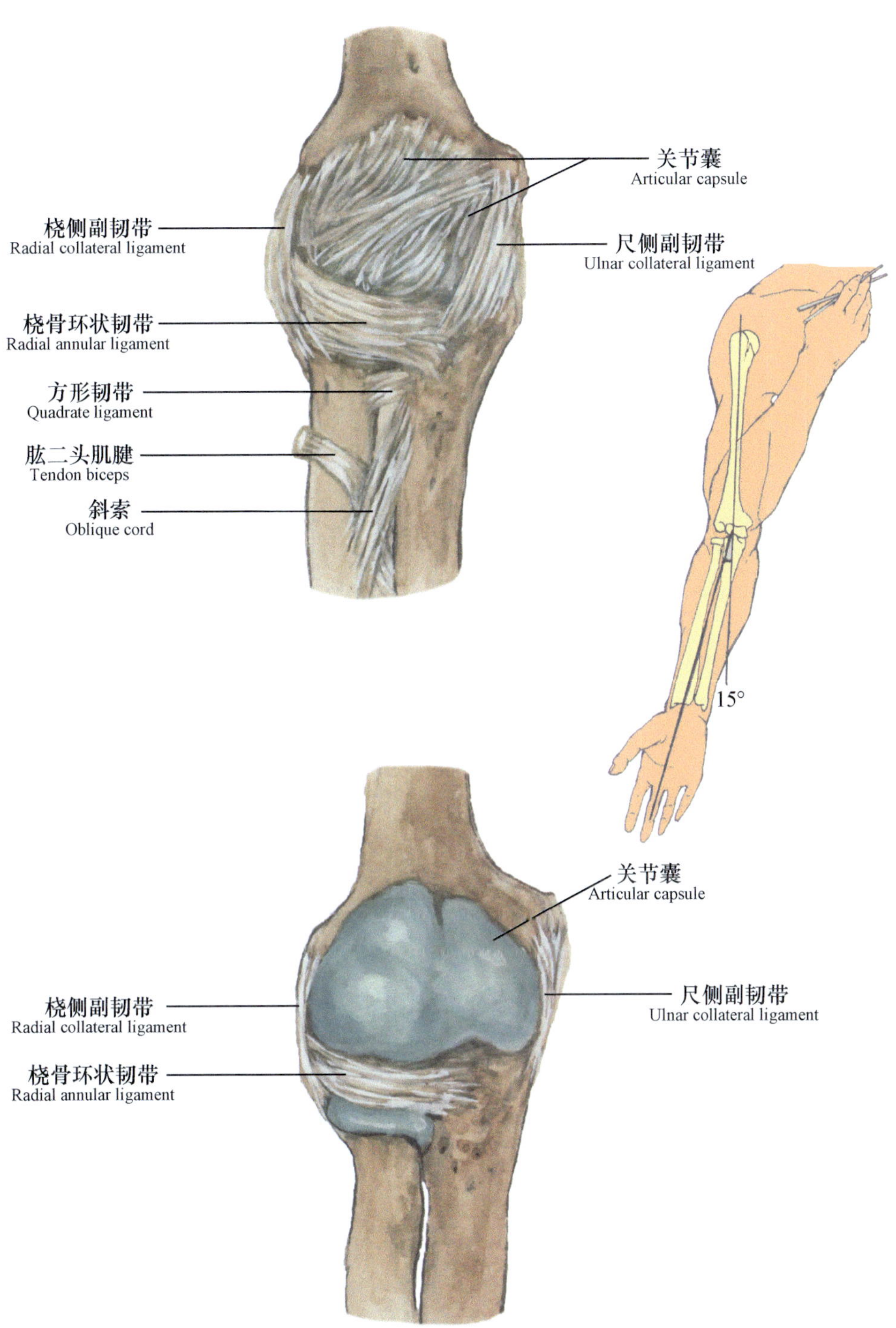

图 1-51 肘关节（1）
The elbow joint (1)

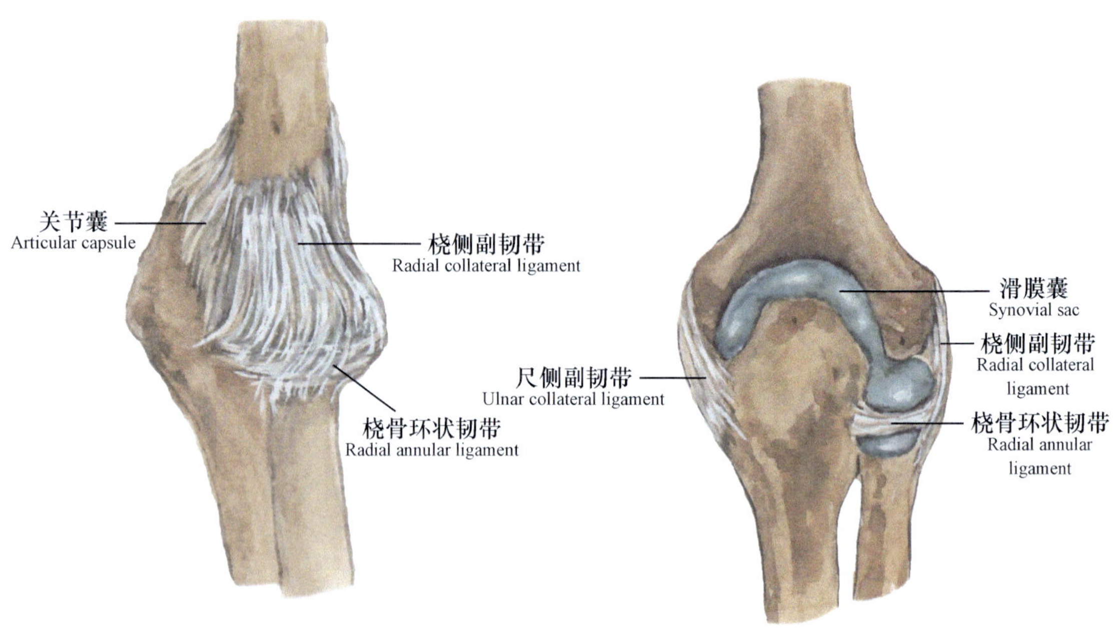

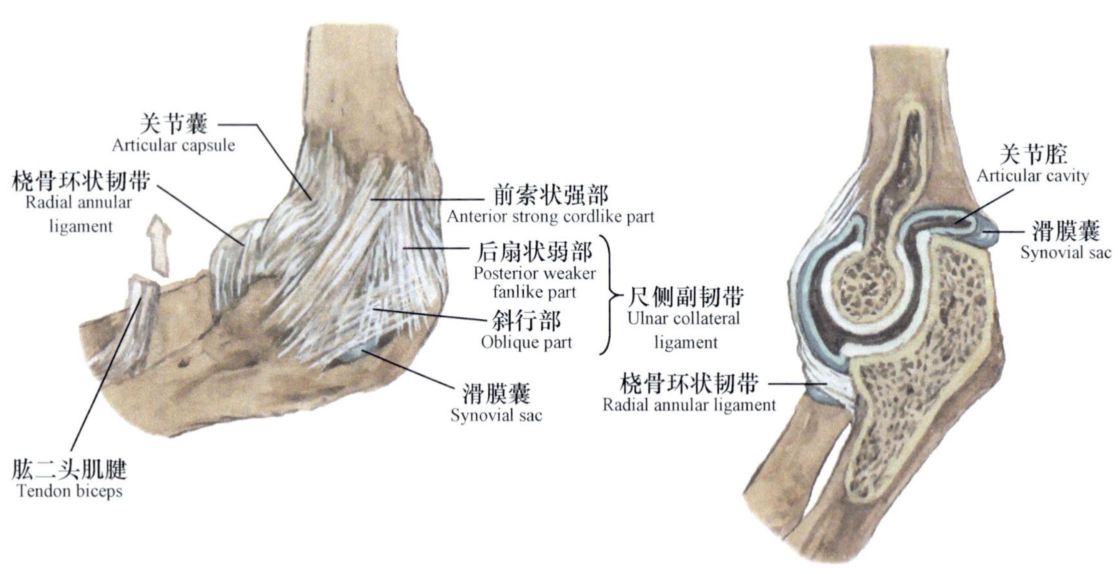

图 1-52 肘关节（2）
The elbow joint (2)

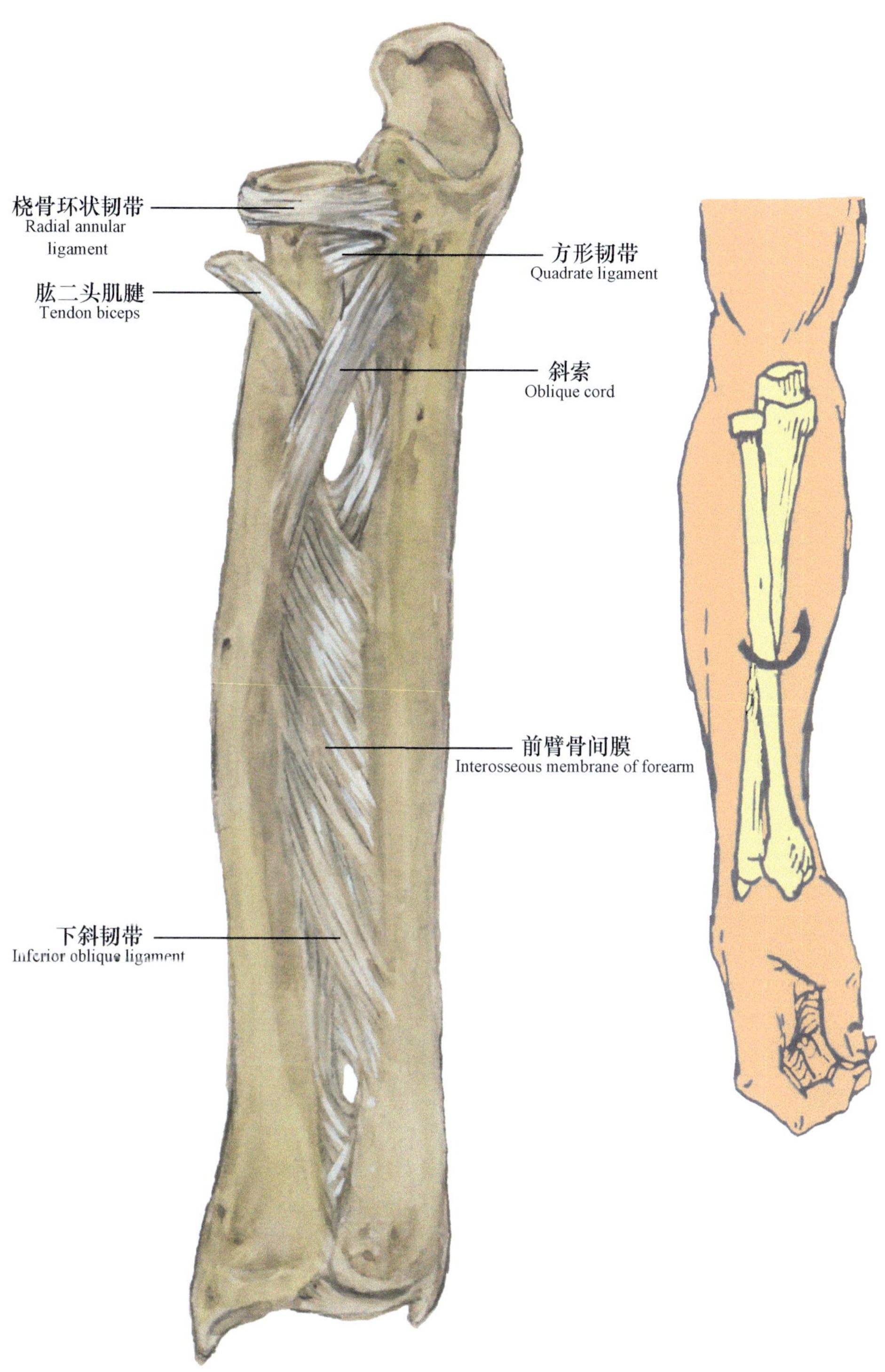

图 1-53 前臂骨间膜
Interosseous membrane of forearm

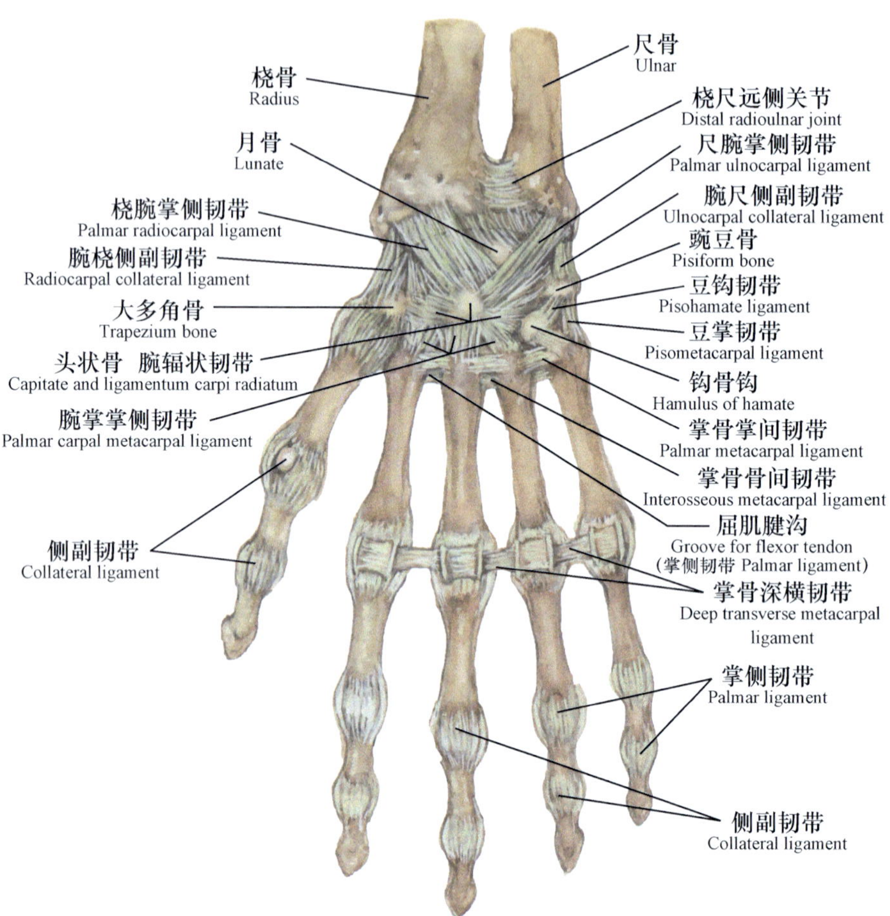

图 1-54 右手掌侧韧带
Ligaments of the right hand

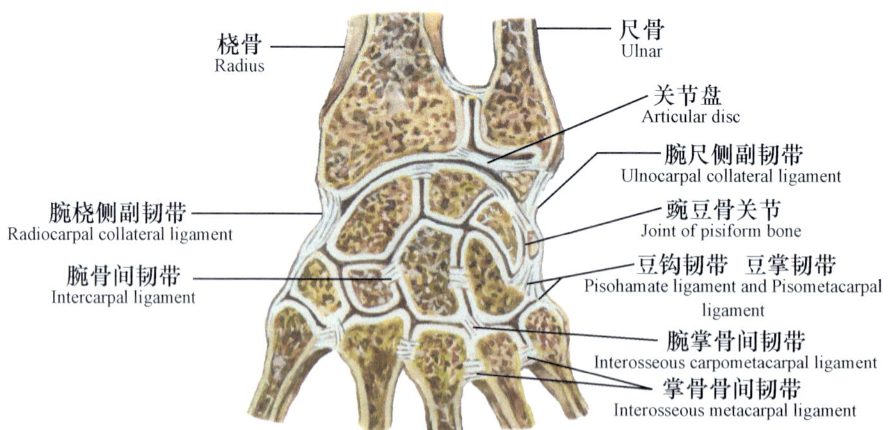

图 1-55 右手腕部冠状切面
Coronal section through the right wrist joint

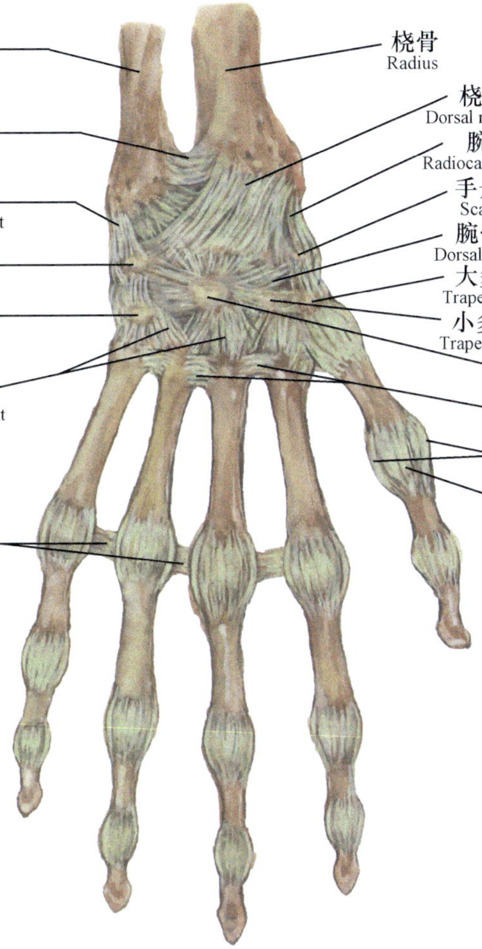

尺骨
Ulnar
桡骨
Radius
桡腕背侧韧带
Dorsal radiocarpal ligament
桡尺远侧关节
Distal radioulnar joint
腕桡侧副韧带
Radiocarpal collateral ligament
手舟骨
Scaphoid
腕尺侧副韧带
Ulnocarpal collateral ligament
腕骨间背侧韧带
Dorsal intercarpal ligaments
三角骨
Triquetrum
大多角骨
Trapezium bone
钩骨
Hamulus
小多角骨
Trapezoid bone
头状骨
Capitate
腕掌背侧韧带
Dorsal carpometacarpal ligament
掌骨背侧韧带
Dorsal metacarpal ligament
侧副韧带
Collateral ligament
背侧韧带
Dorsal ligament
掌骨深横韧带
Deep transverse metacarpal ligament

右手背侧韧带
Dosal ligaments of right hand

90°
展与收
Abductor and Adductor
伸与屈
Extensor and Flexsor
对掌
Oppenons

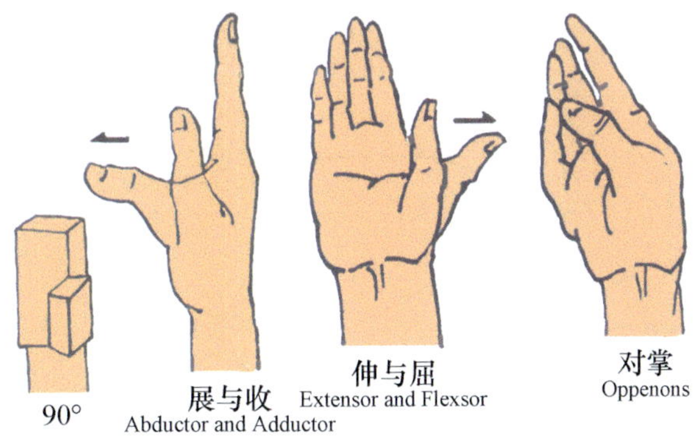

图 1-56　右手背侧韧带
Dosal ligaments of right hand

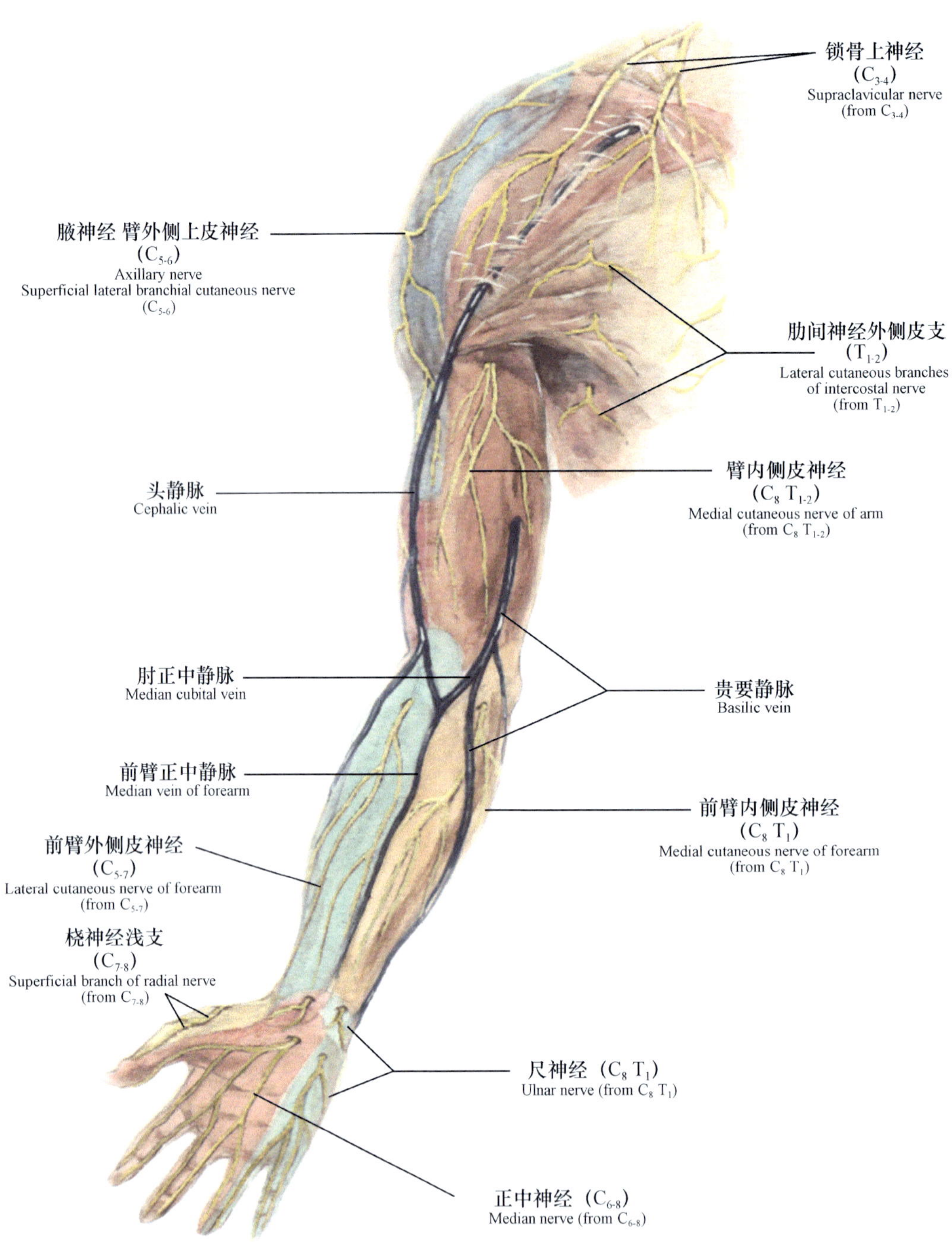

图 1-57　上肢皮神经与浅静脉（前面观）
Cutaneous nerves and superficial veins of the upper limb (Anterior aspect)

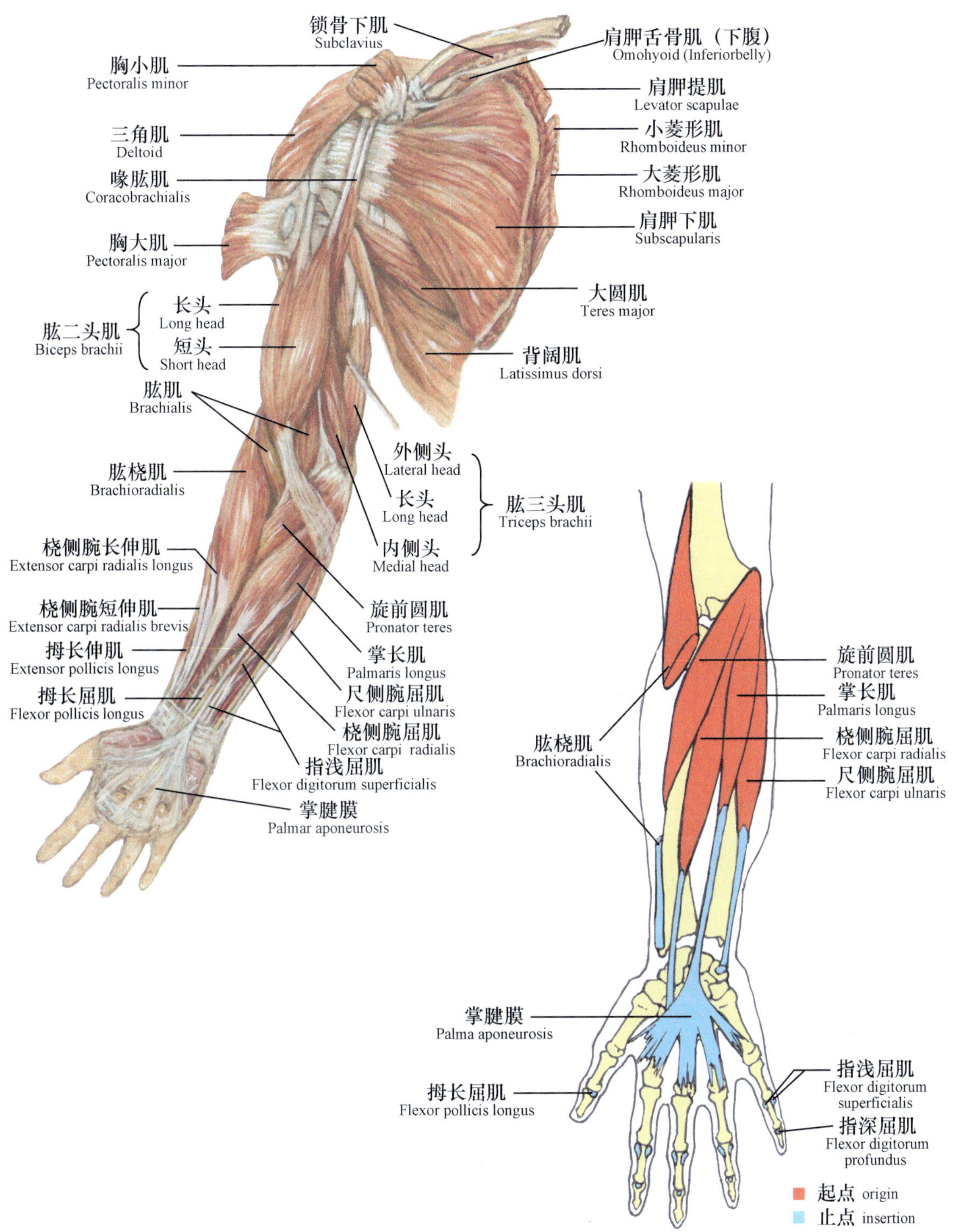

图 1-58 右侧上肢肌群（掌侧面观）
Muscles of the right upper limb (Anterior aspect)

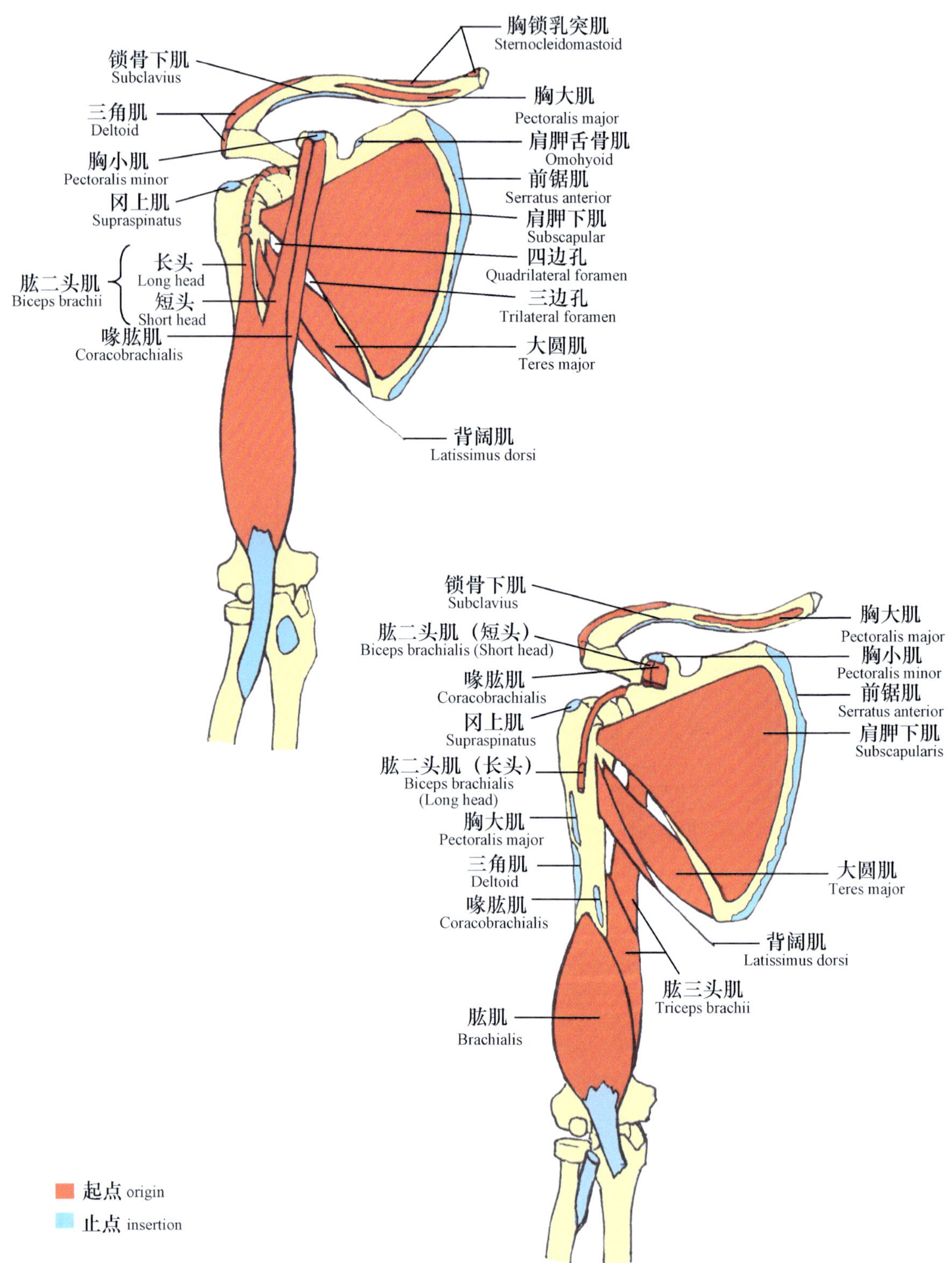

图 1-59 右侧肩锁肌、上臂肌（前面观）
Muscles of the right clavicle, shoulder and arm (Anterior aspect)

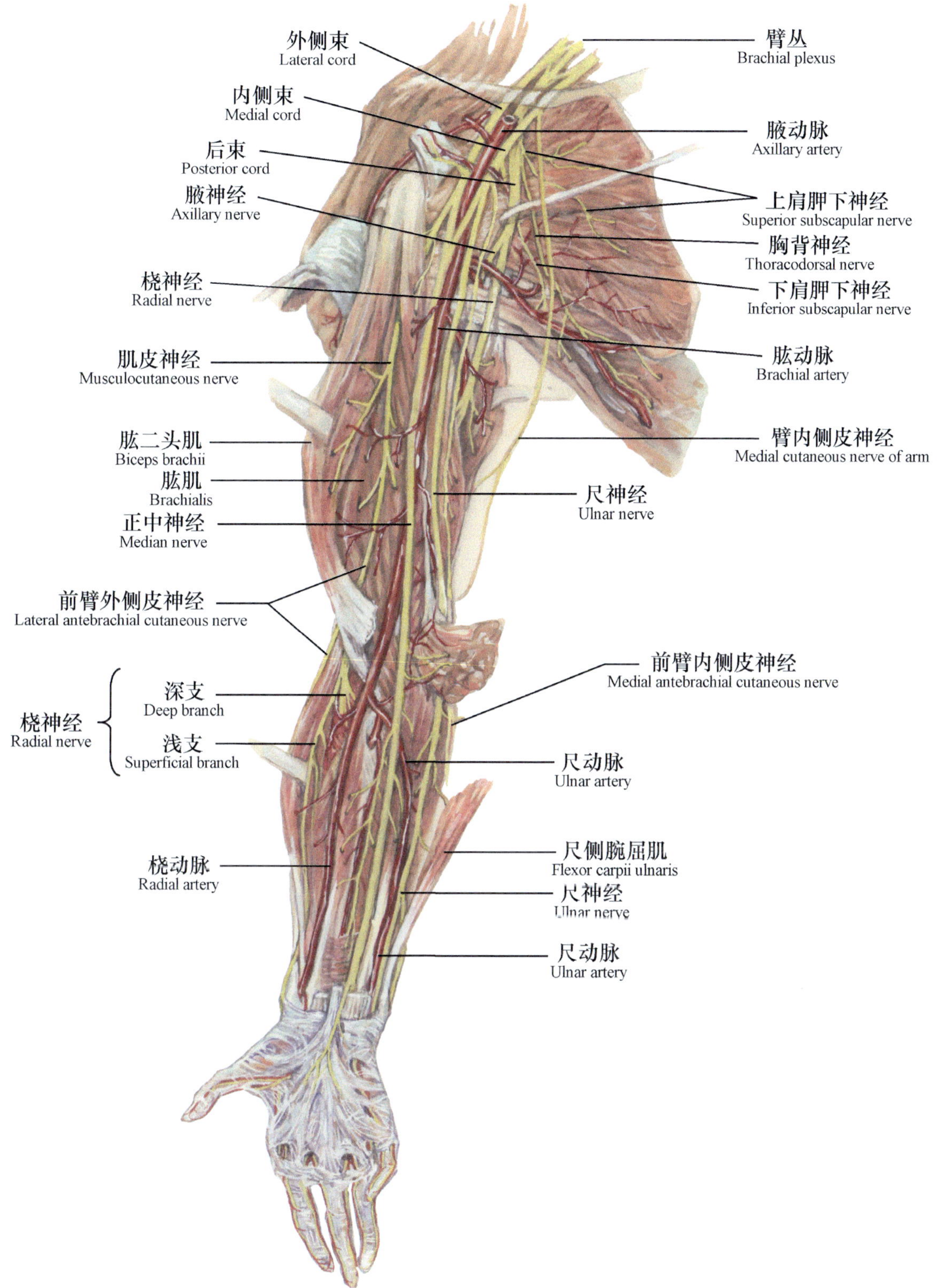

图 1-60 上肢神经及血管（前面观）
Nerves and arteries of the upper limb (Anterior aspect)

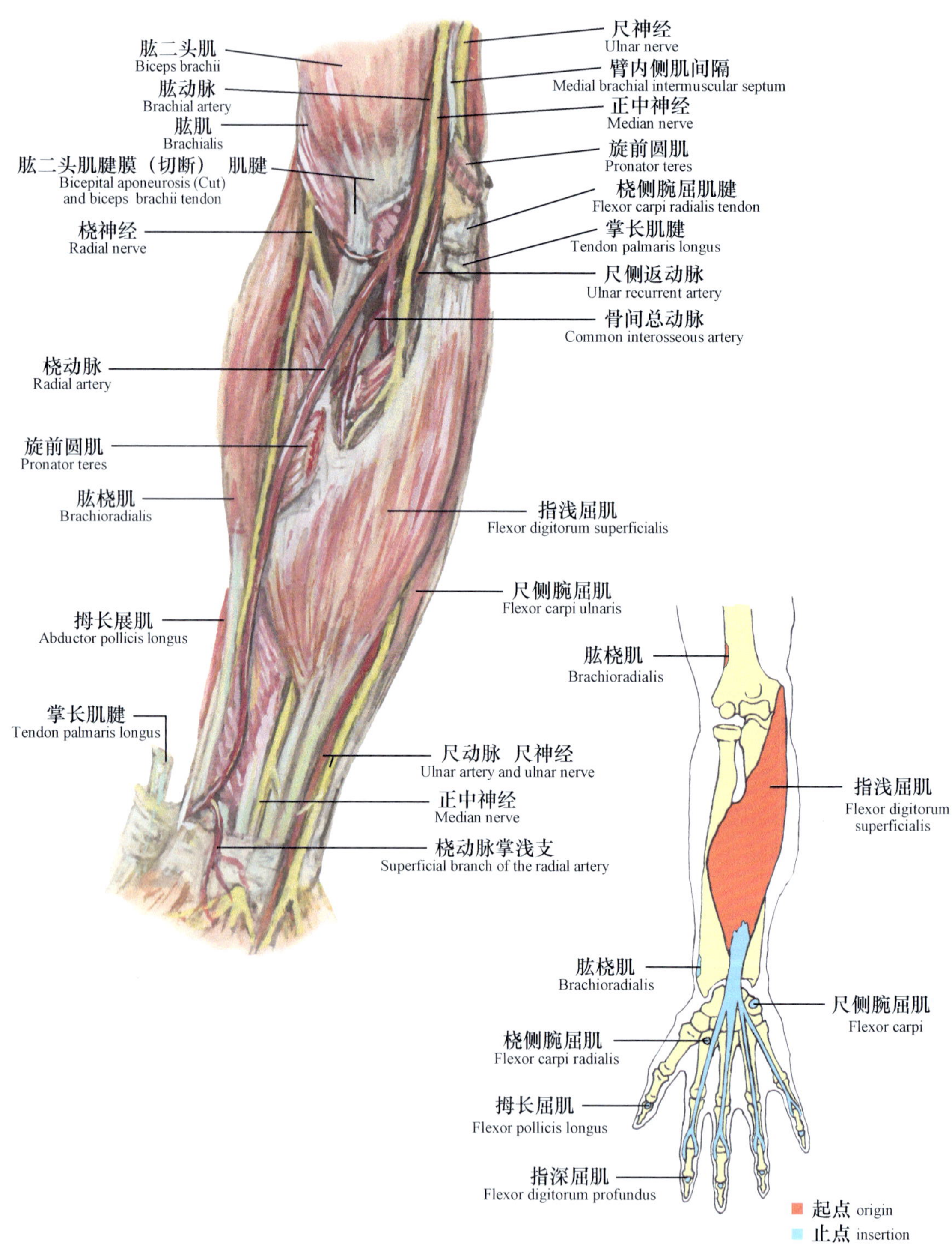

图 1-61 前臂第二层（前面观）
The second layer of the right forearm (Anterior aspect)

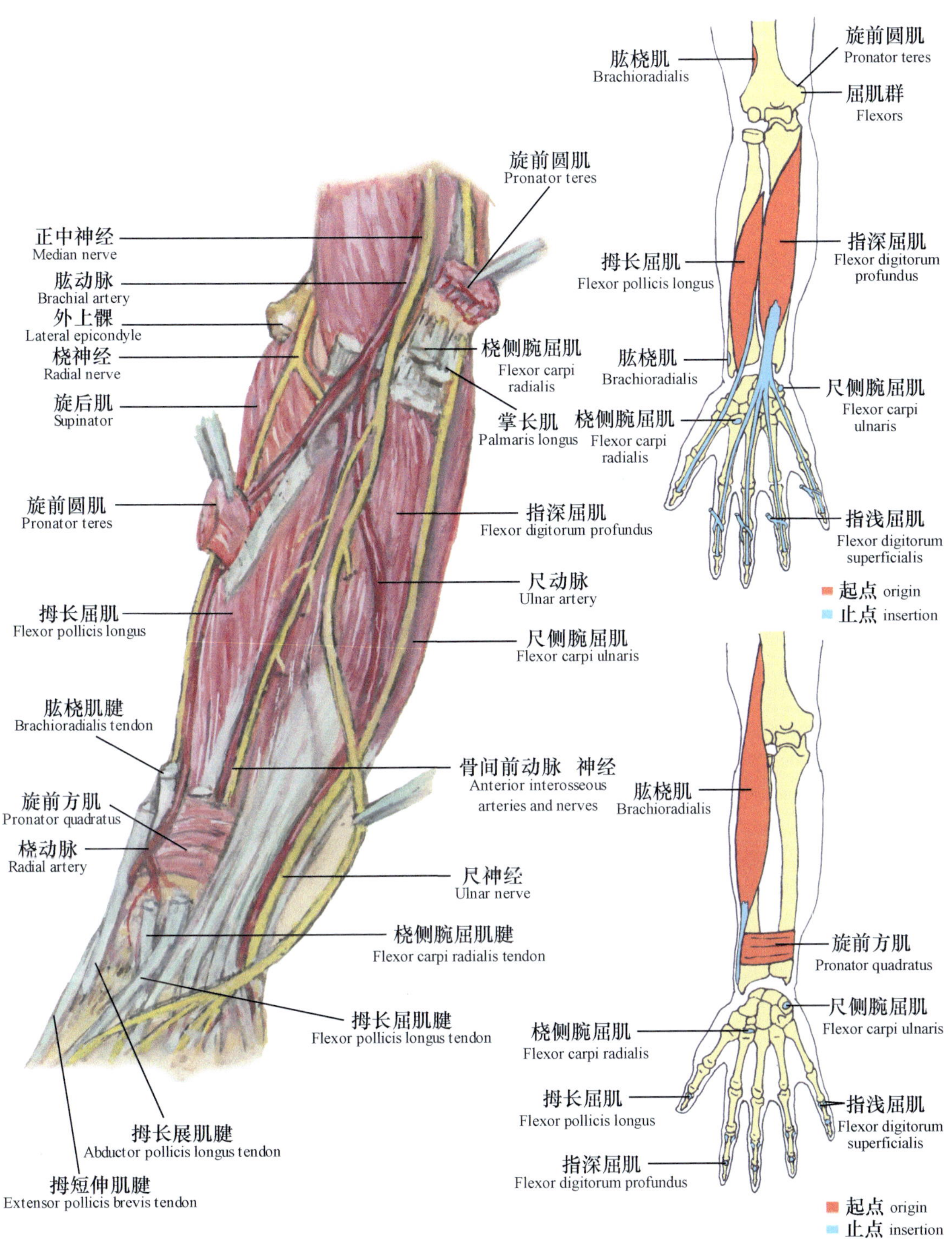

图 1-62 前臂深层（前面观）
Deep layer of the right forearm (Anterior aspect)

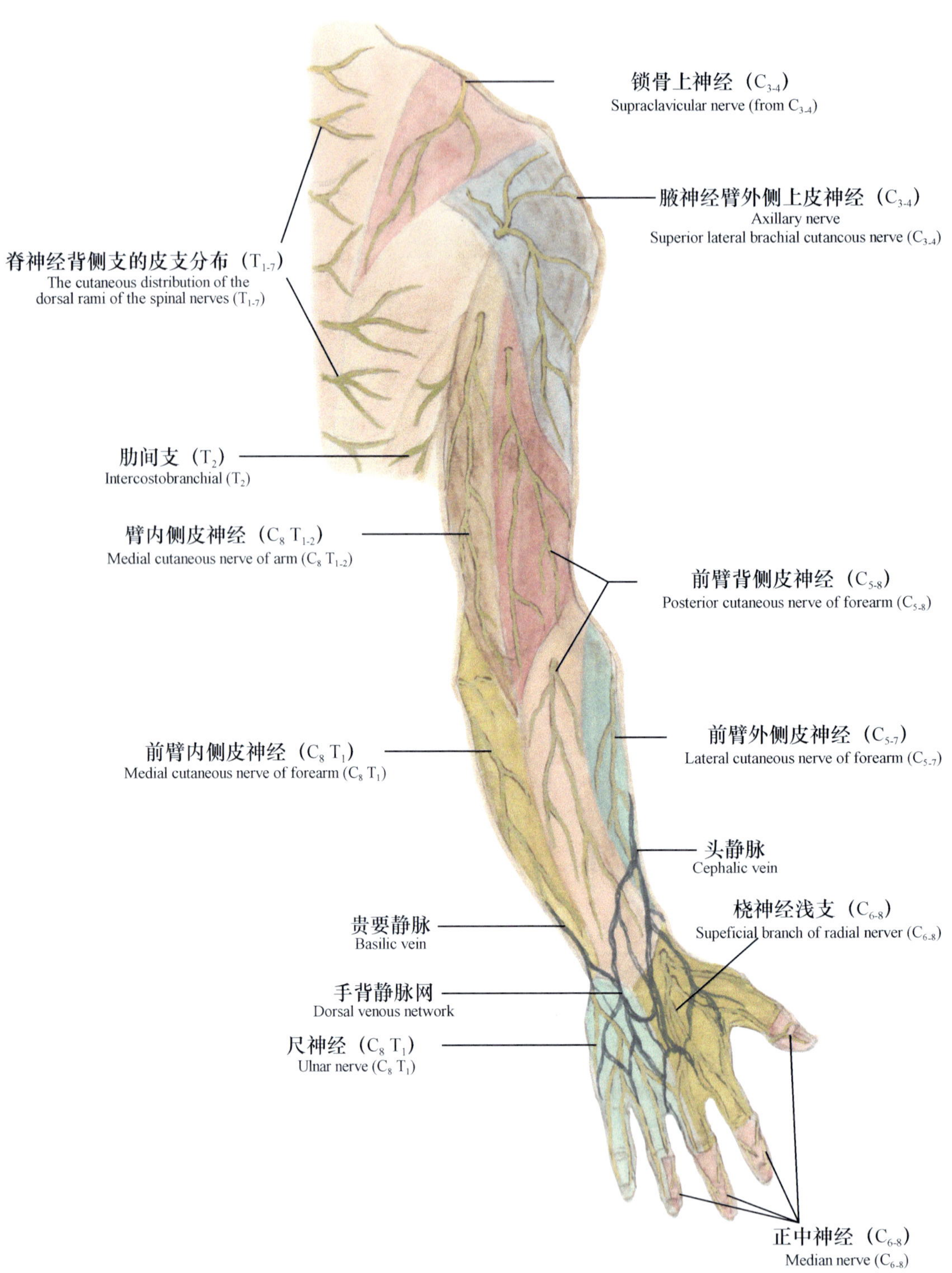

图 1-63　上肢皮神经与静脉（背侧观）
Cutaneous nerves and veins of the upper limb (Posterior aspect)

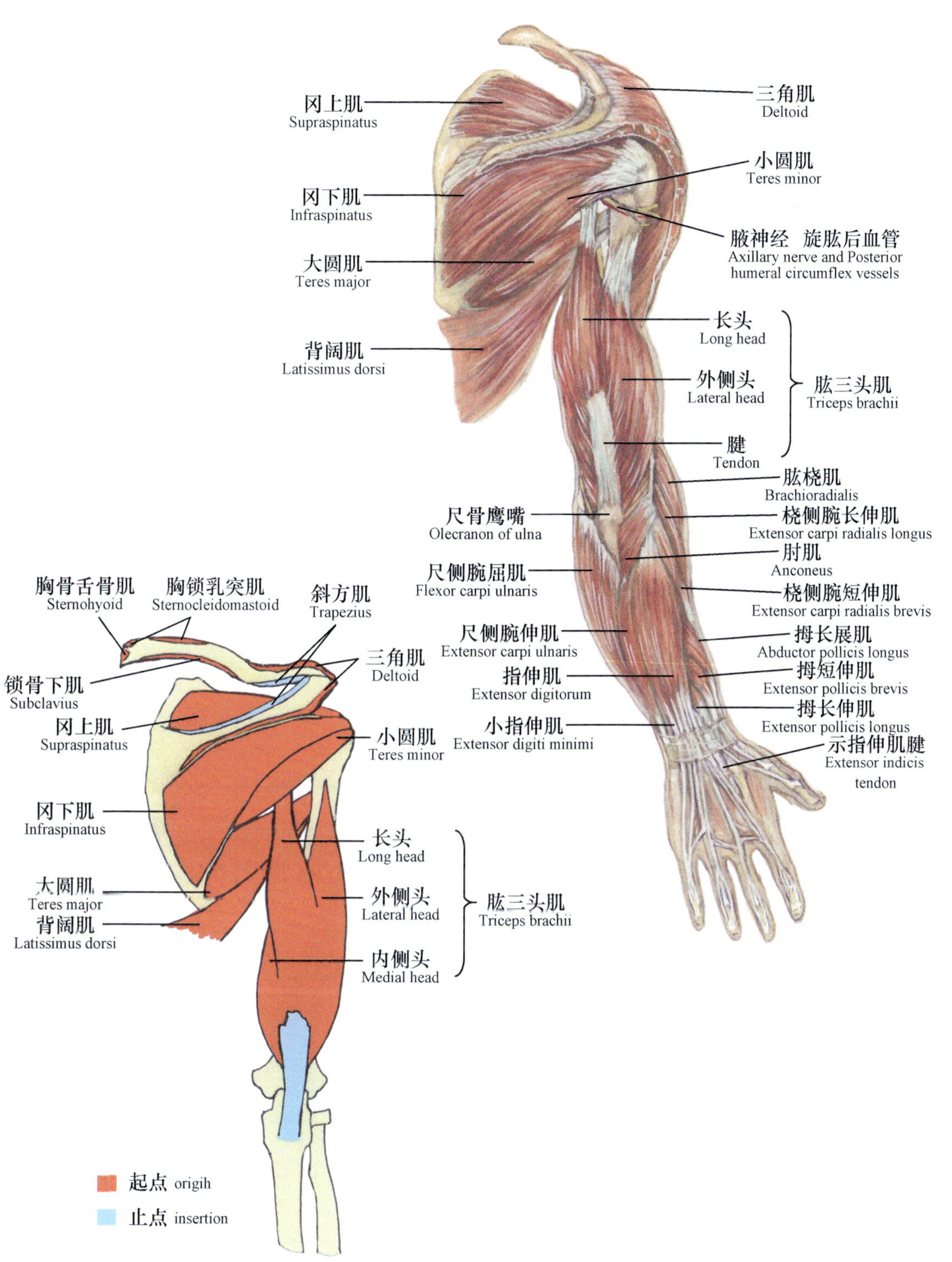

图 1-64 上肢肌群（背侧观）

Muscles of the upper limb (Posterior aspect)

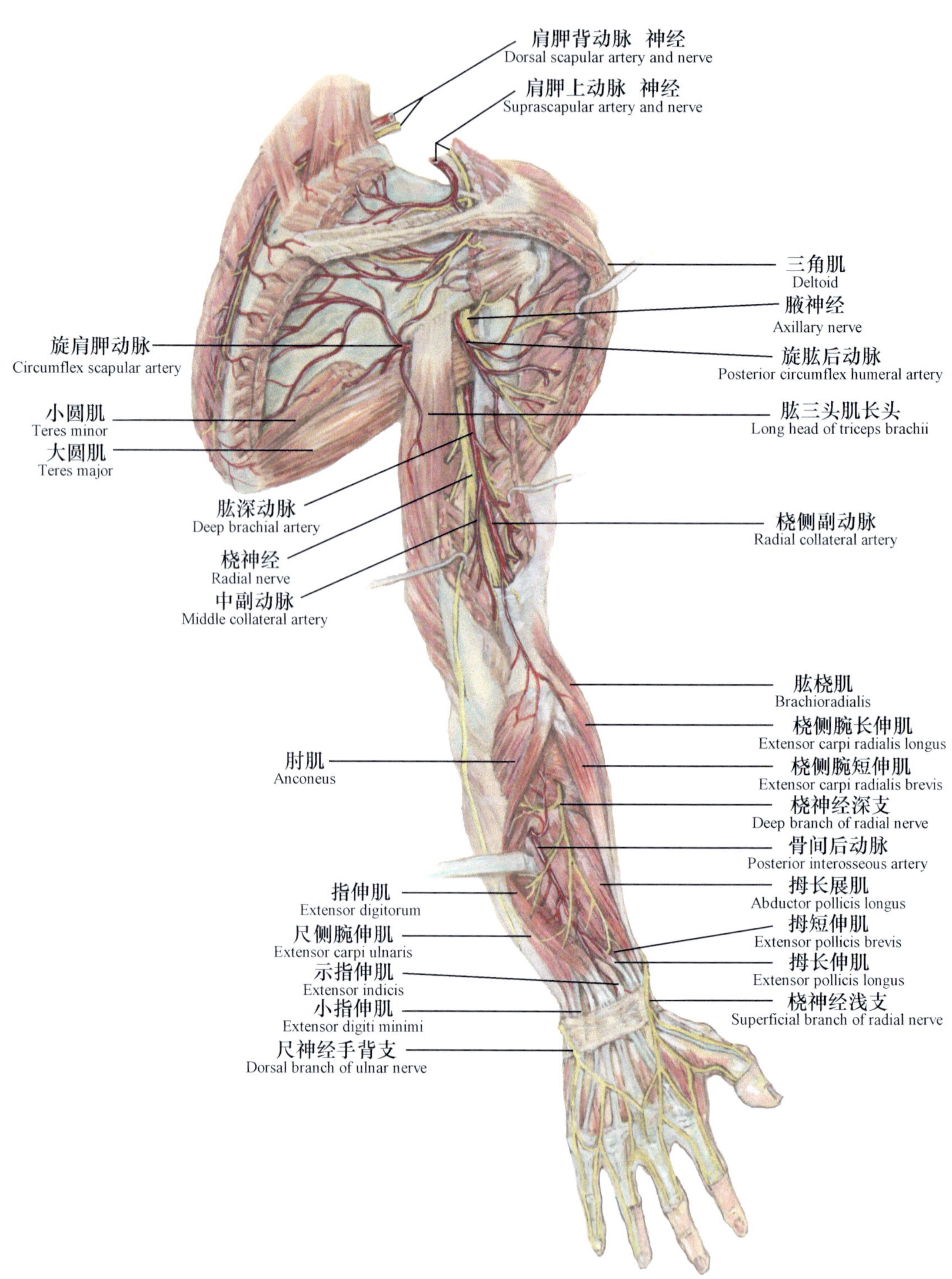

图 1-65 右侧上肢（后面观）
The right upper limb (Posterior aspect)

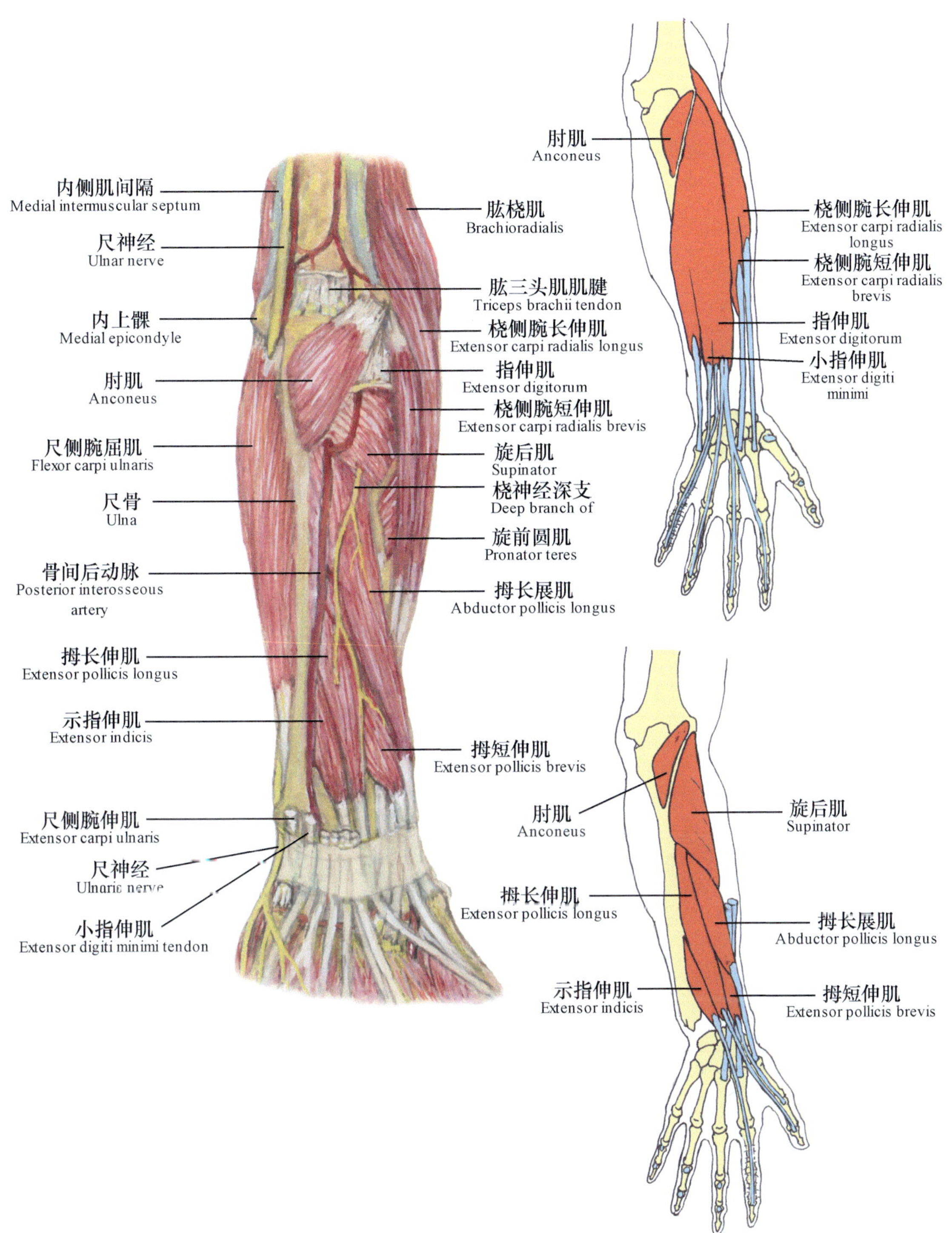

图 1-66 前臂深层（后面观）
Deep layer of forearm (Posterior aspect)

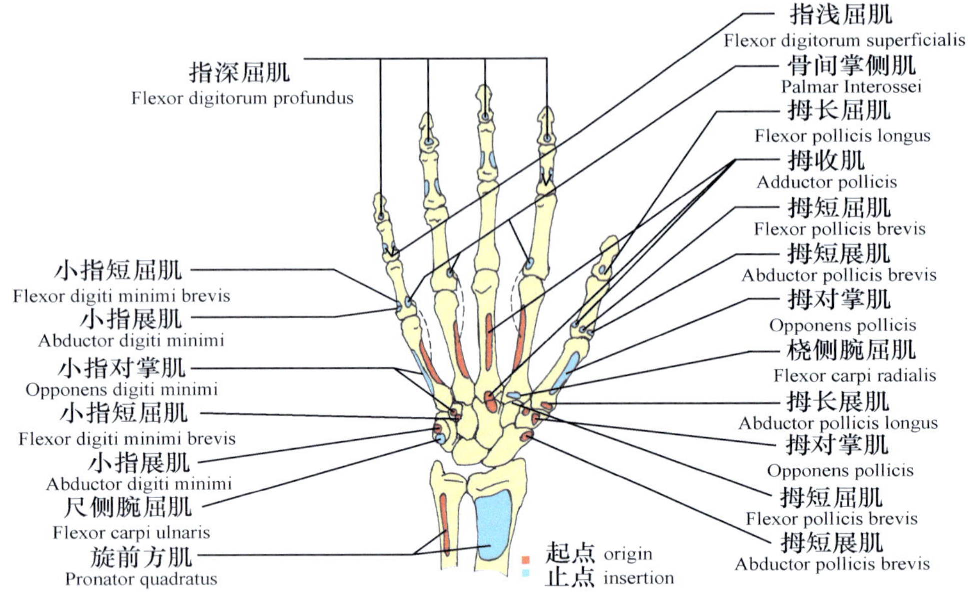

图 1-67　右侧掌侧肌的起止点

The attachments of muscles of the palmar aspect of the right hand

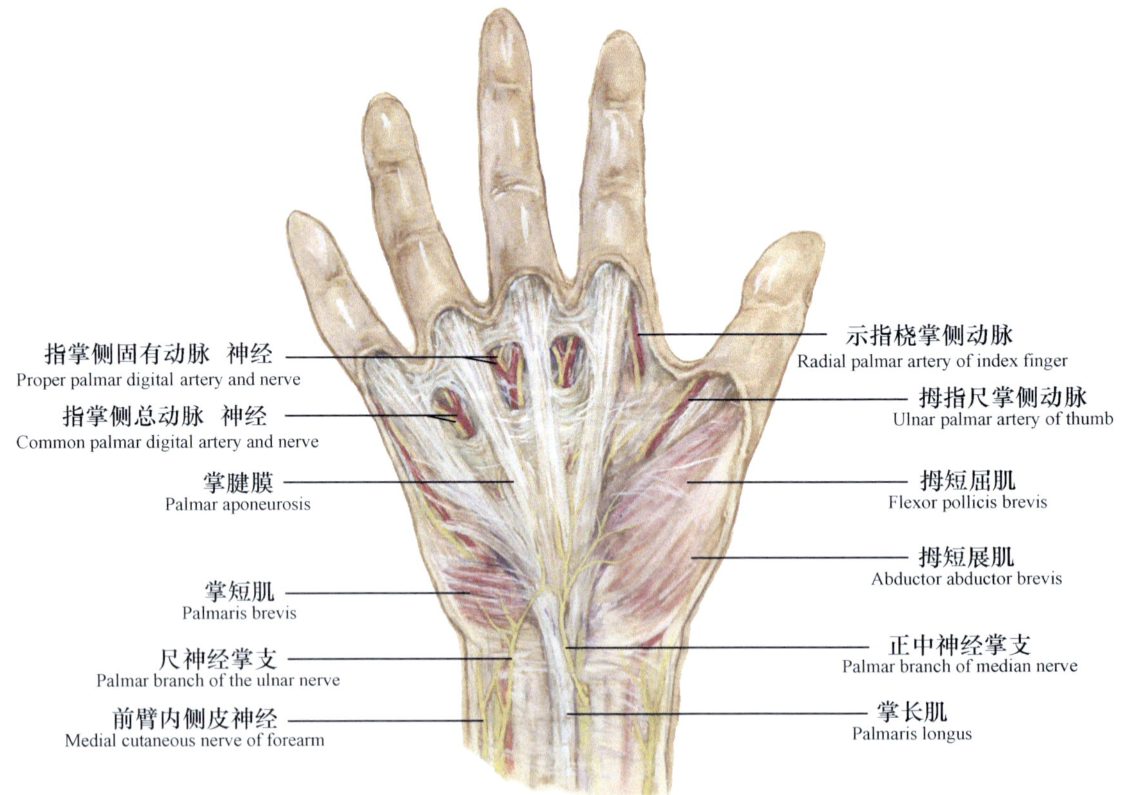

图 1-68　右手掌的肌肉、血管和神经（1）

The muscles, blood vessels and nerves of the right palm (1)

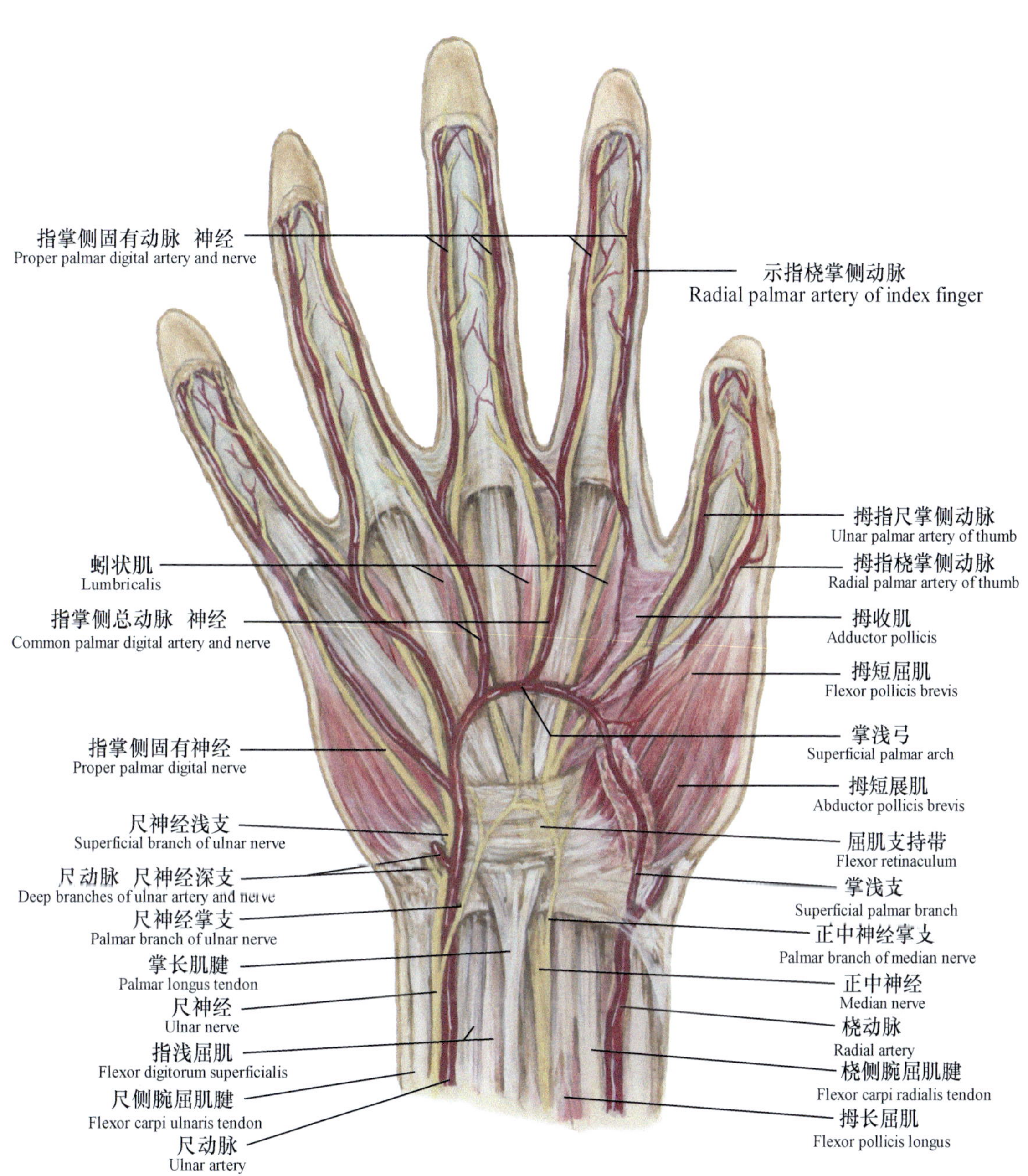

图 1-69 右手掌的肌肉、血管和神经（2）
The muscles, blood vessels and nerves of the right palm (2)

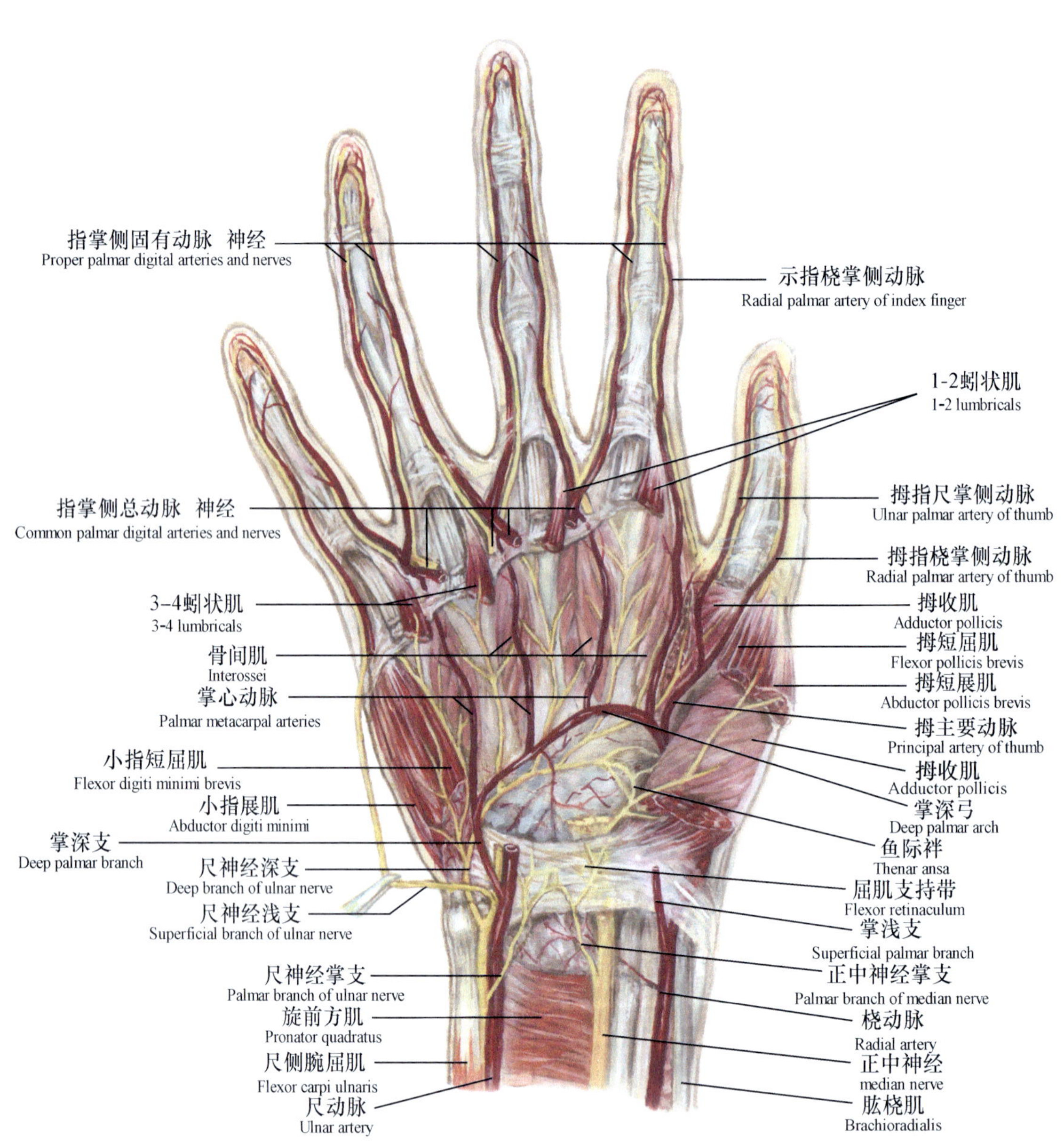

图 1-70 右手掌的肌肉、血管和神经（3）
The muscles, blood vessels and nerves of the right palm (3)

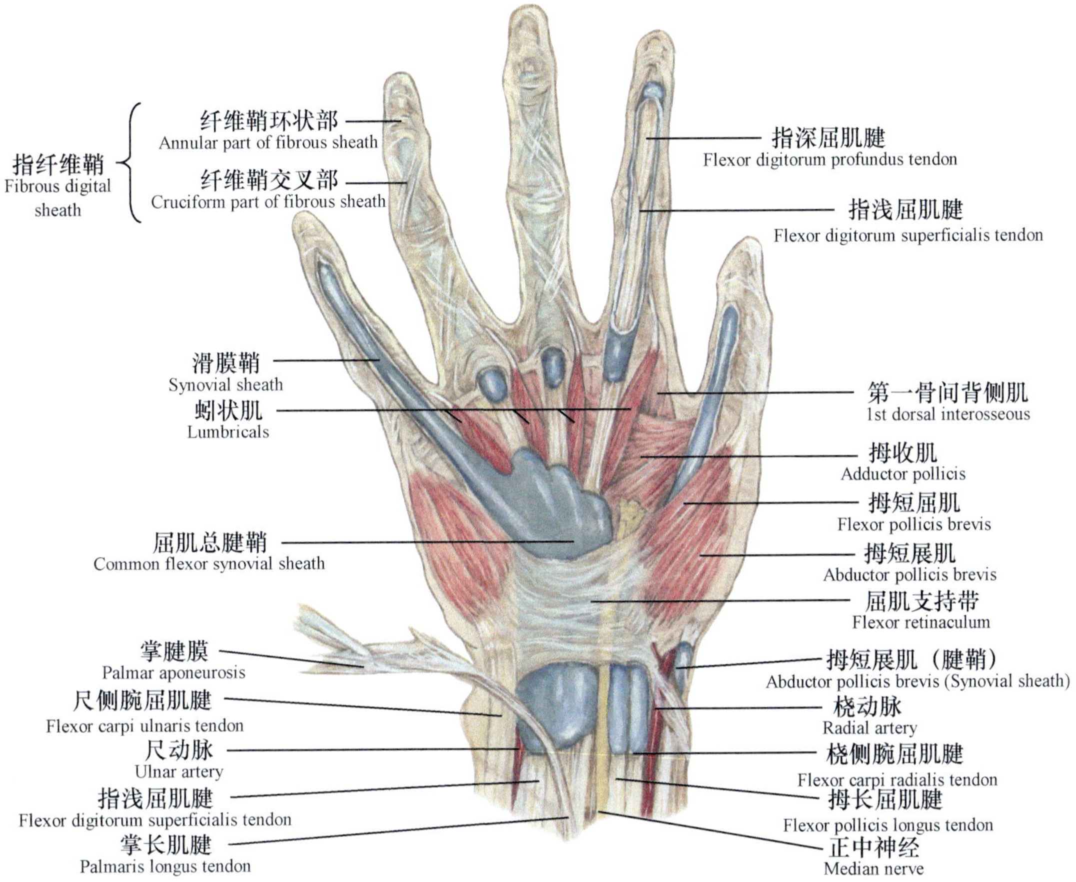

指纤维鞘
Fibrous digital sheath
纤维鞘环状部
Annular part of fibrous sheath
纤维鞘交叉部
Cruciform part of fibrous sheath
指深屈肌腱
Flexor digitorum profundus tendon
指浅屈肌腱
Flexor digitorum superficialis tendon
滑膜鞘
Synovial sheath
蚓状肌
Lumbricals
第一骨间背侧肌
1st dorsal interosseous
拇收肌
Adductor pollicis
拇短屈肌
Flexor pollicis brevis
屈肌总腱鞘
Common flexor synovial sheath
拇短展肌
Abductor pollicis brevis
屈肌支持带
Flexor retinaculum
掌腱膜
Palmar aponeurosis
拇短展肌（腱鞘）
Abductor pollicis brevis (Synovial sheath)
尺侧腕屈肌腱
Flexor carpi ulnaris tendon
桡动脉
Radial artery
尺动脉
Ulnar artery
桡侧腕屈肌腱
Flexor carpi radialis tendon
指浅屈肌腱
Flexor digitorum superficialis tendon
拇长屈肌腱
Flexor pollicis longus tendon
掌长肌腱
Palmaris longus tendon
正中神经
Median nerve

图 1-71　右手掌的屈肌腱滑膜鞘
Flexor synovial sheath of the right hand

拇长屈肌腱鞘
Synovial sheath
of flexor pollicis longus
屈肌支持带
Flexor retinaculum
屈肌总腱鞘
Common flexor synovial sheath
（包绕指浅屈肌与指深屈肌）
桡侧腕屈肌
Flexor carpi radialis

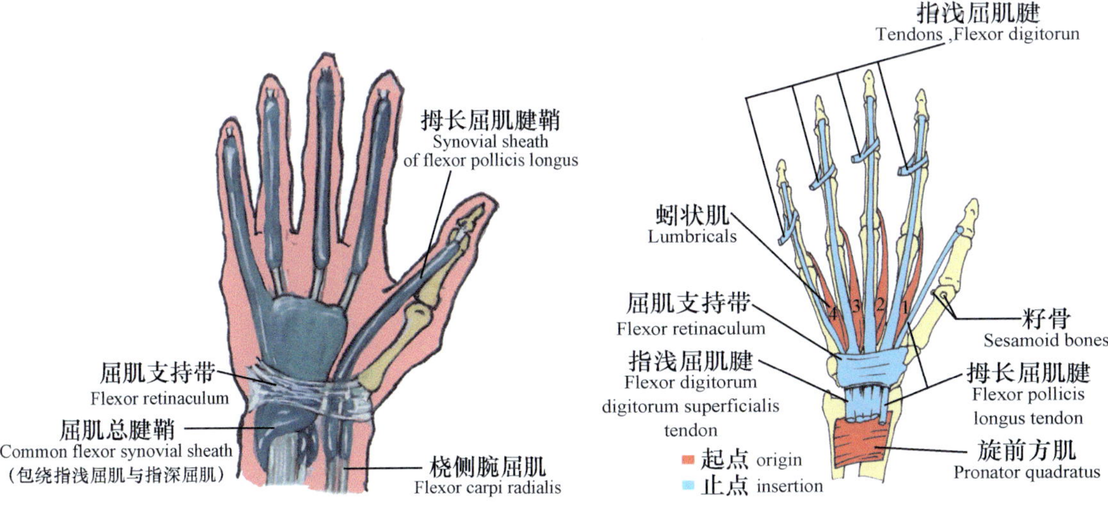

图 1-72　指屈肌腱滑膜鞘
Synovial sheaths of flexors of the right hand

指浅屈肌腱
Tendons ,Flexor digitorun
蚓状肌
Lumbricals
4 3 2 1
屈肌支持带
Flexor retinaculum
籽骨
Sesamoid bones
指浅屈肌腱
Flexor digitorum
digitorum superficialis
tendon
拇长屈肌腱
Flexor pollicis
longus tendon
旋前方肌
Pronator quadratus
起点 origin
止点 insertion

图 1-73　右手蚓状肌（掌侧观）
Lumbricals of the right hand (Palm aspect)

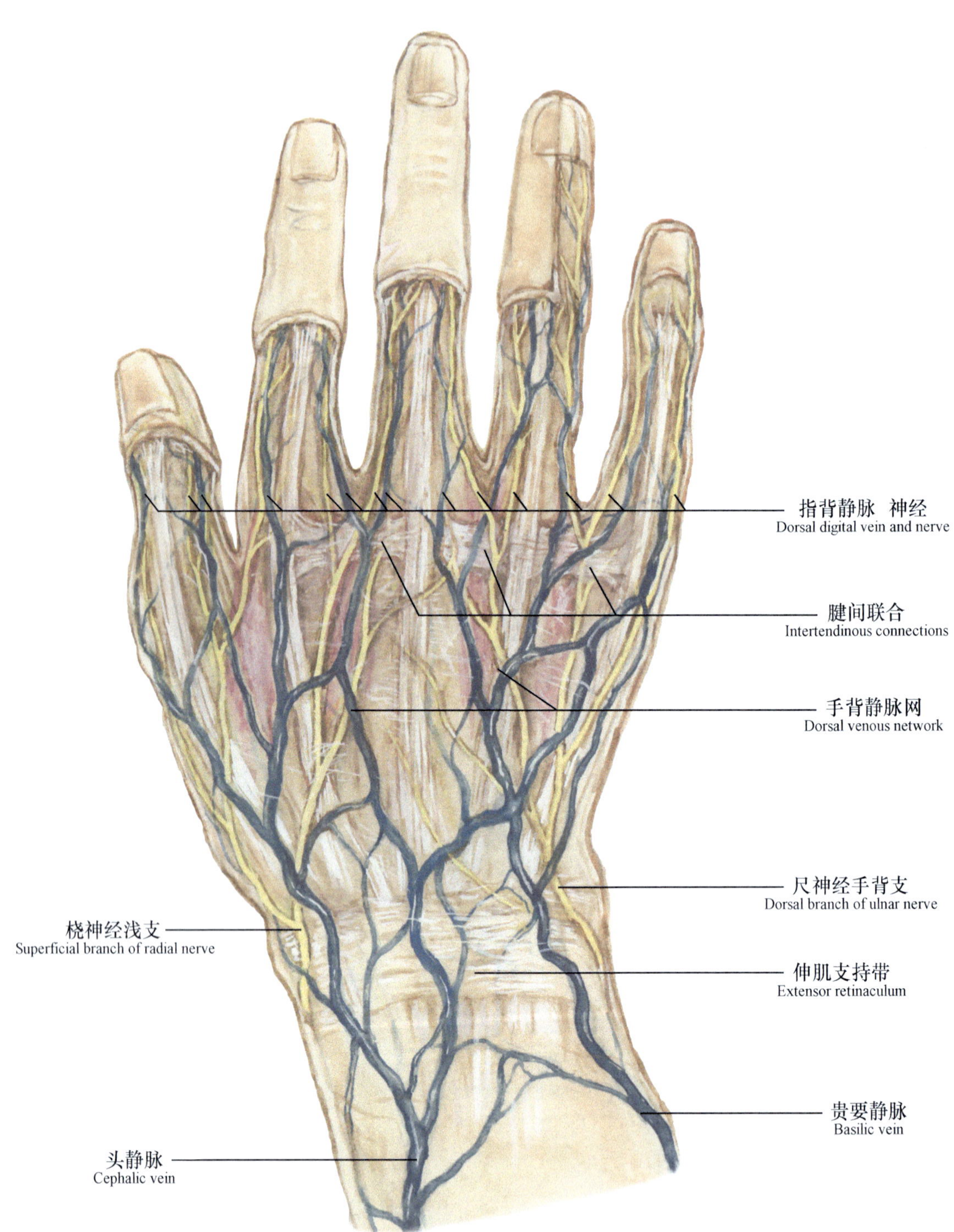

图 1-74 右手背的肌肉、血管和神经（1）
The muscles, blood vessels and nerves of the right hand (1)

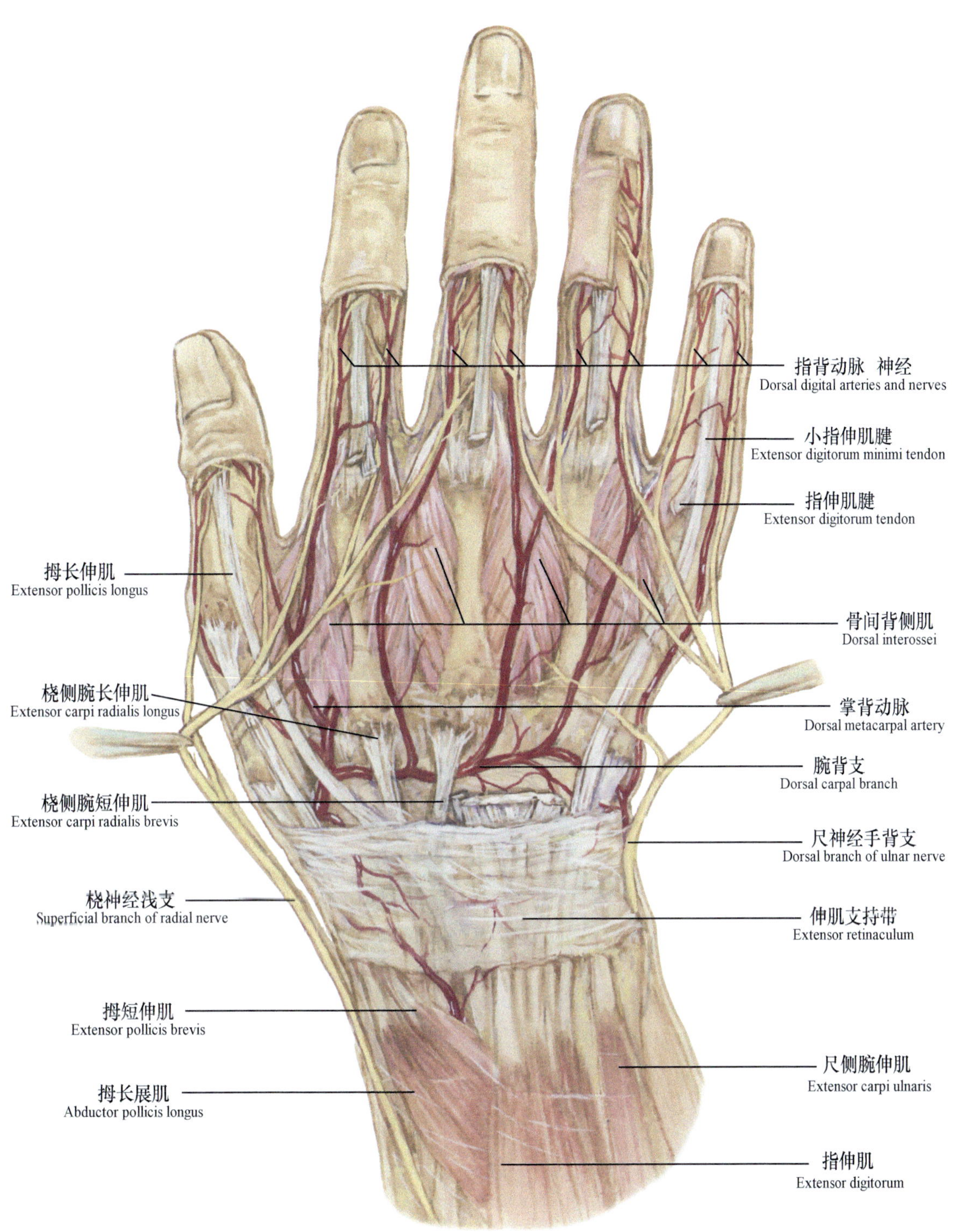

图 1-75 右手背的肌肉、血管和神经（2）
The muscles, blood vessels and nerves of the right hand (2)

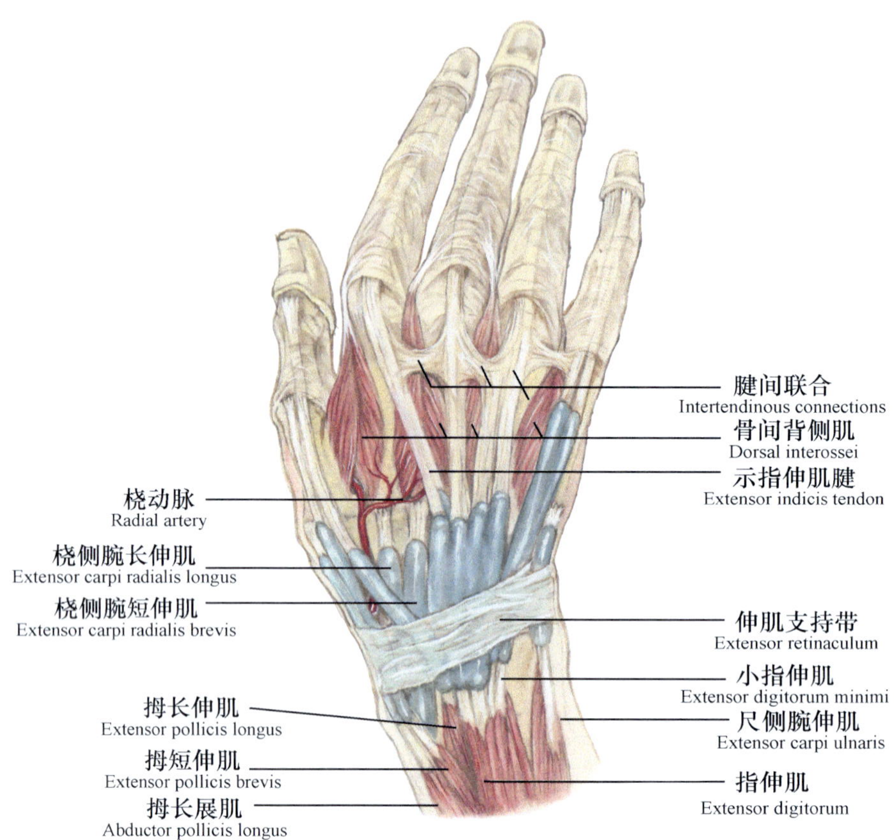

图 1-76 右手手背的伸肌腱滑膜鞘
Extensor tendon synovial sheath of the dorsum of the right hand

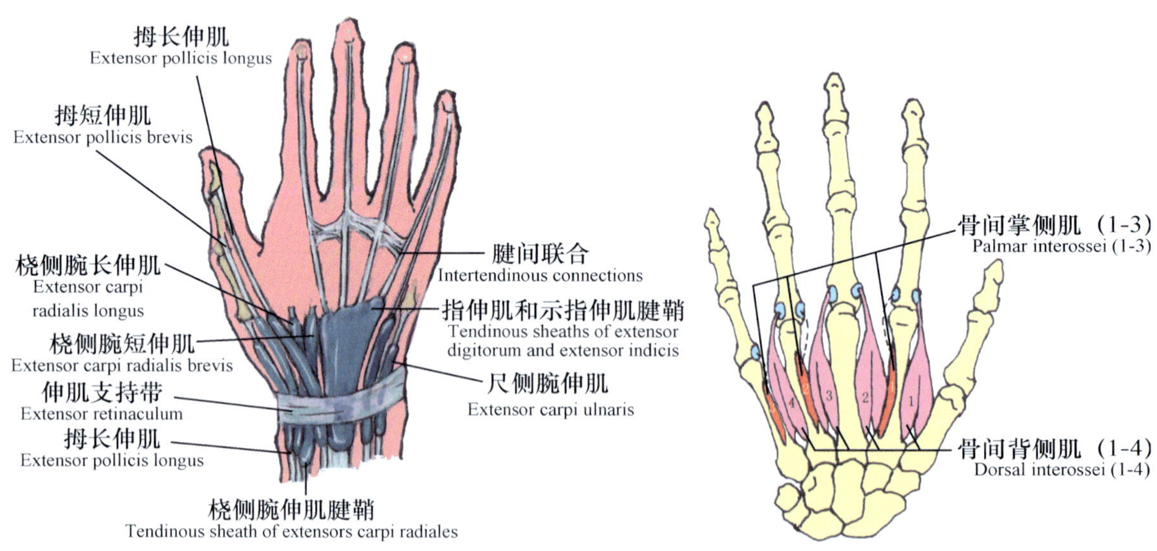

图 1-77 指伸肌腱滑膜鞘
Synovial sheaths of extensors of the right hand

图 1-78 右手骨间肌
Interossei of the right hand

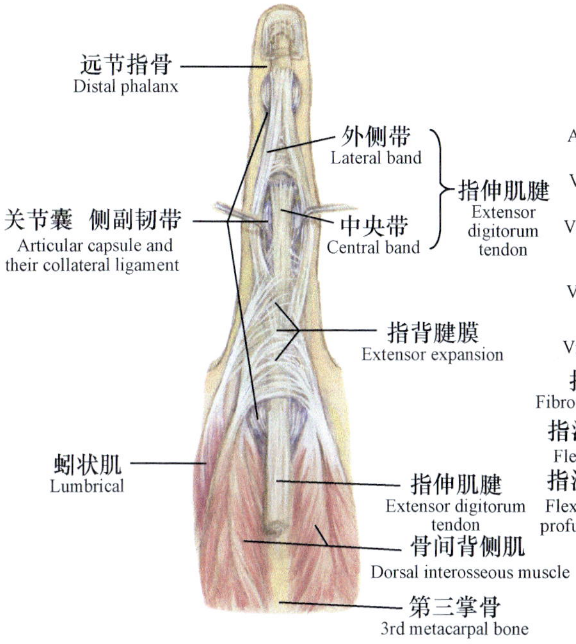

远节指骨
Distal phalanx
外侧带
Lateral band
关节囊 侧副韧带
Articular capsule and
their collateral ligament
中央带
Central band
指伸肌腱
Extensor
digitorum
tendon
指背腱膜
Extensor expansion
蚓状肌
Lumbrical
指伸肌腱
Extensor digitorum
tendon
骨间背侧肌
Dorsal interosseous muscle
第三掌骨
3rd metacarpal bone

A. 右手中指肌腱止点（背侧观）
Tendon insertion of the middle finger of the right hand (Dorsal aspect)

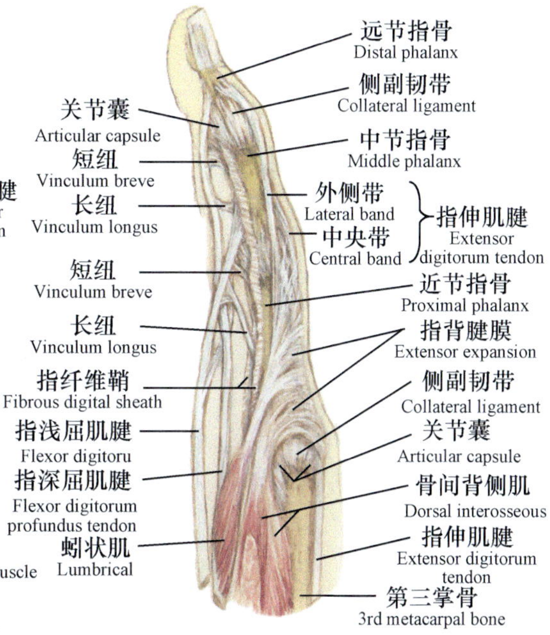

远节指骨
Distal phalanx
侧副韧带
Collateral ligament
关节囊
Articular capsule
中节指骨
Middle phalanx
短纽
Vinculum breve
长纽
Vinculum longus
外侧带
Lateral band
中央带
Central band
指伸肌腱
Extensor
digitorum tendon
短纽
Vinculum breve
近节指骨
Proximal phalanx
长纽
Vinculum longus
指背腱膜
Extensor expansion
指纤维鞘
Fibrous digital sheath
侧副韧带
Collateral ligament
指浅屈肌腱
Flexor digitoru
关节囊
Articular capsule
指深屈肌腱
Flexor digitorum
profundus tendon
骨间背侧肌
Dorsal interosseous
蚓状肌
Lumbrical
指伸肌腱
Extensor digitorum
tendon
第三掌骨
3rd metacarpal bone

B. 右手中指肌腱止点（侧面观）
Tendon insertion of the middle finger of the right hand (Lateral aspect)

远节指骨
Distal phalanx
指深屈肌腱
Flexor digitorum profundus tendon
指掌侧固有动脉 神经
Proper palmar digital artery and nerve
纤维鞘环状部
Annular part of fibrous sheath
指纤维鞘
Fibrous digital
sheath
纤维鞘交叉部
Cruciform part of fibrous sheath
壁层
Parietal layer
指浅屈肌腱
Flexor digitorum superficialis tendon
脏层
Visceral layer
指滑膜鞘
Synovial sheath
of fingers
指深屈肌腱
Flexor digitorum profundus tendon
腱系膜
Mesotendon
指背动脉 神经
Dorsal digital artery and nerve
近节指骨
Proximal phalanx
指伸肌腱
Extensor digitorum tendon

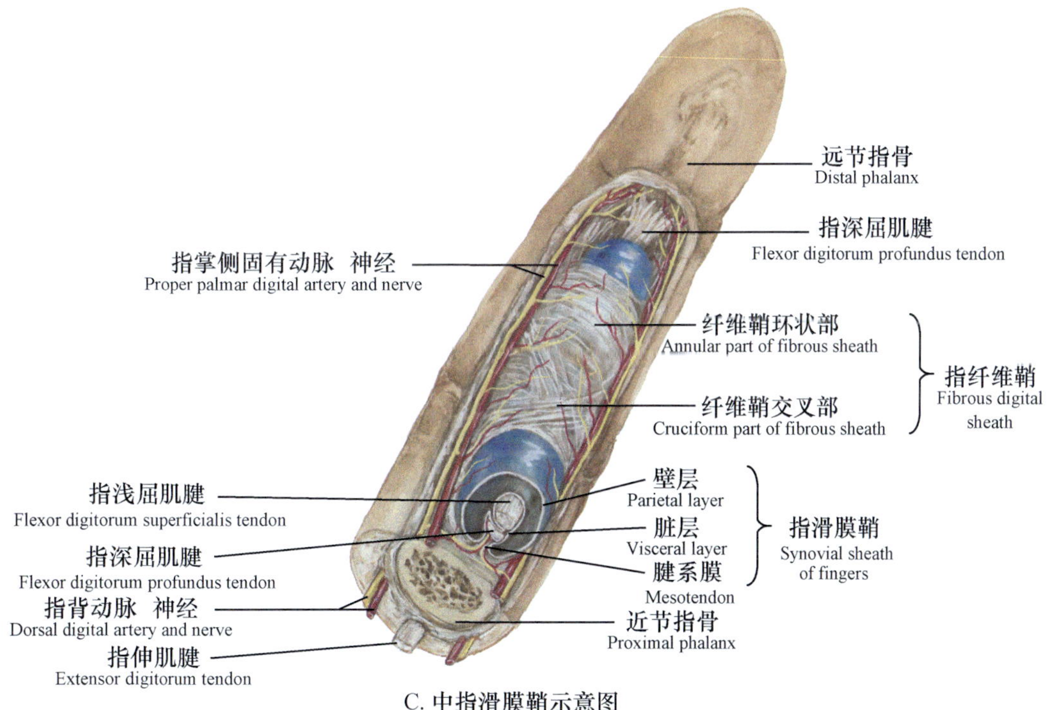

C. 中指滑膜鞘示意图
Diagram of synovial sheath of the middle finger

图 1-79 右手中指
Middle finger of the right hand

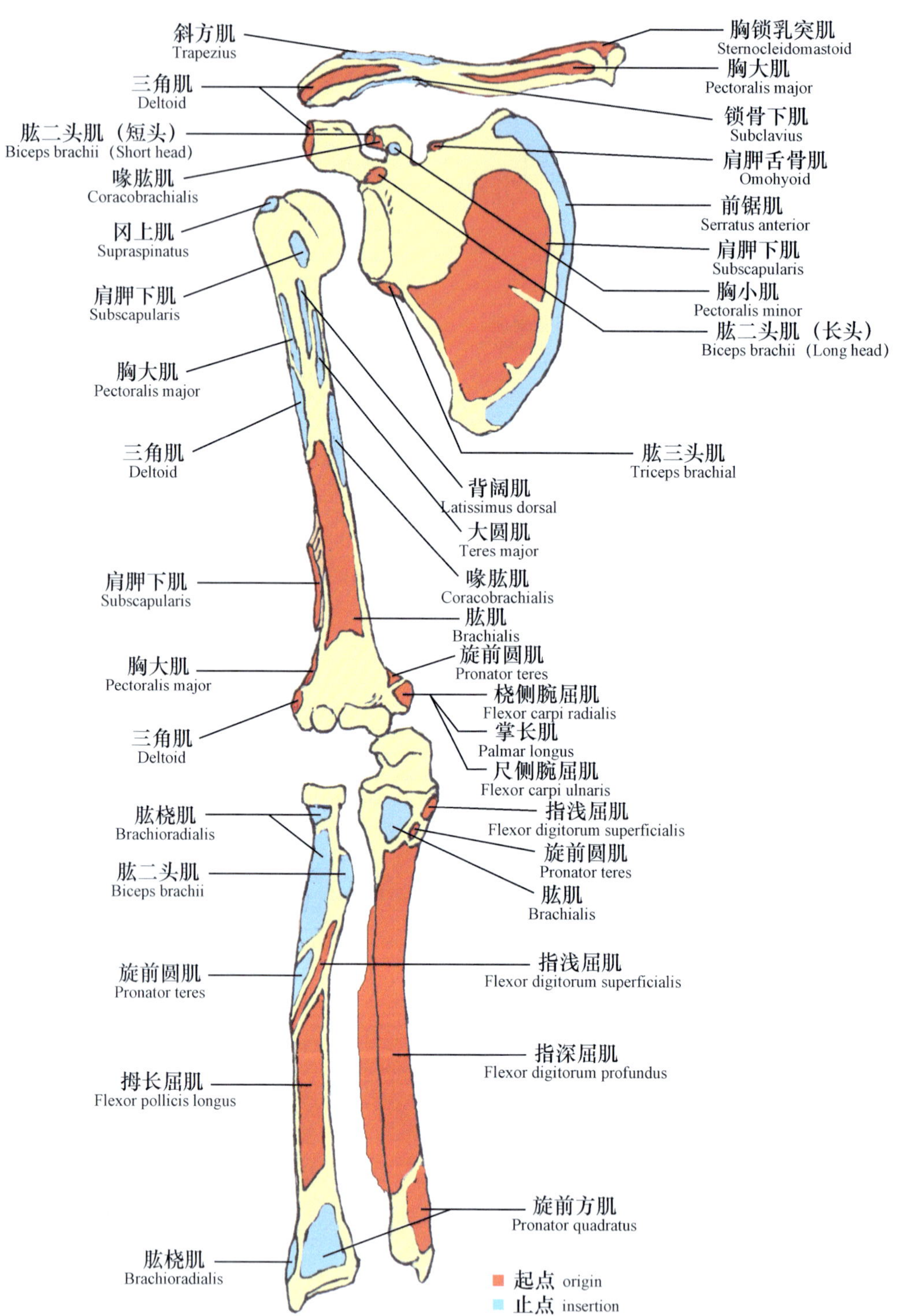

图 1-80　右侧上肢肌起止点示意图（前面观）
Diagram of the attachments of muscles of the upper limb (Anterior aspect)

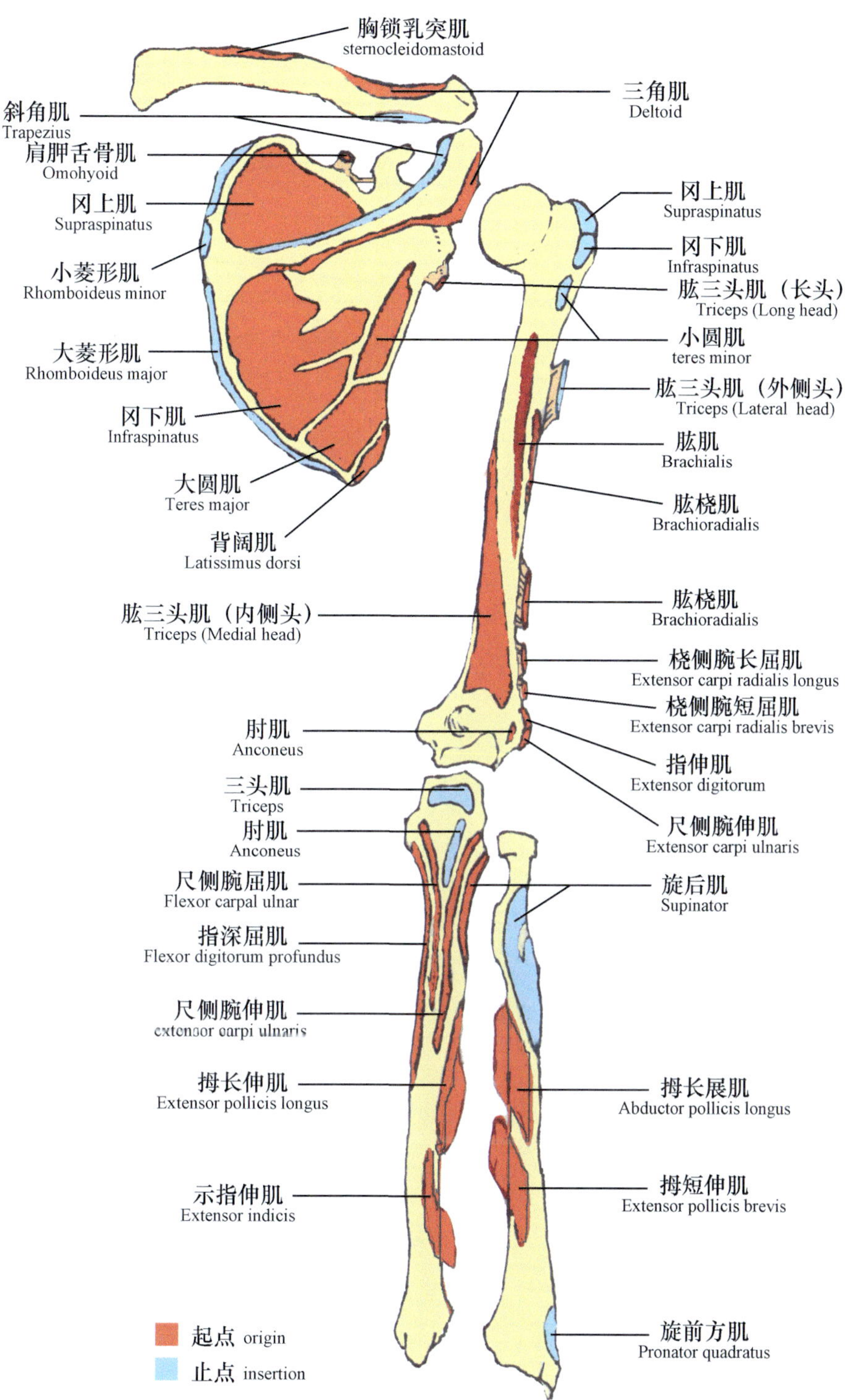

图 1-81　右侧上肢肌起止点示意图（后面观）
Diagram of the attachments of muscles of the right upper limb (Posterior aspect)

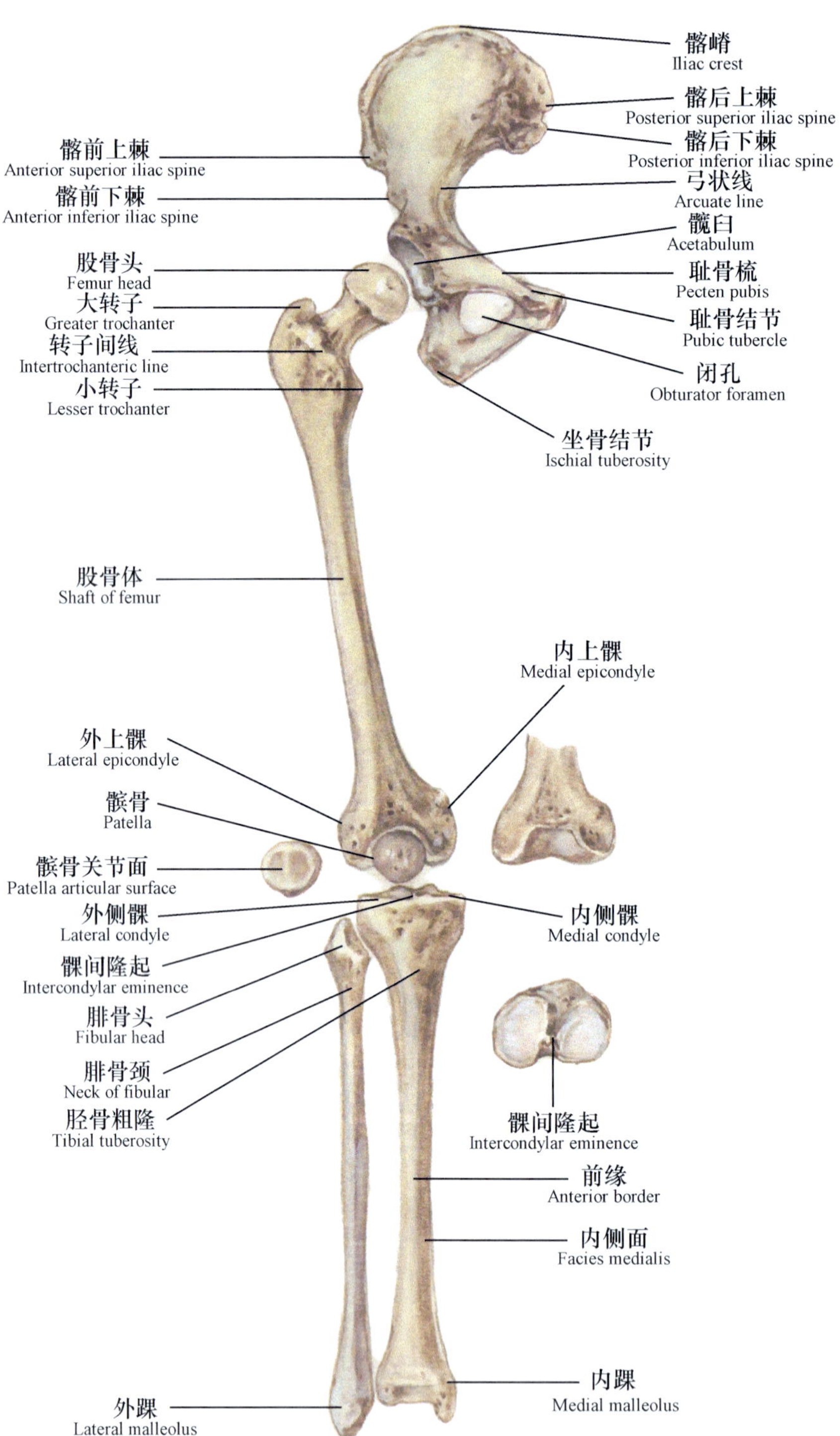

图 1-82 下肢骨（前面观）
Bone of lower limb (Anterior aspect)

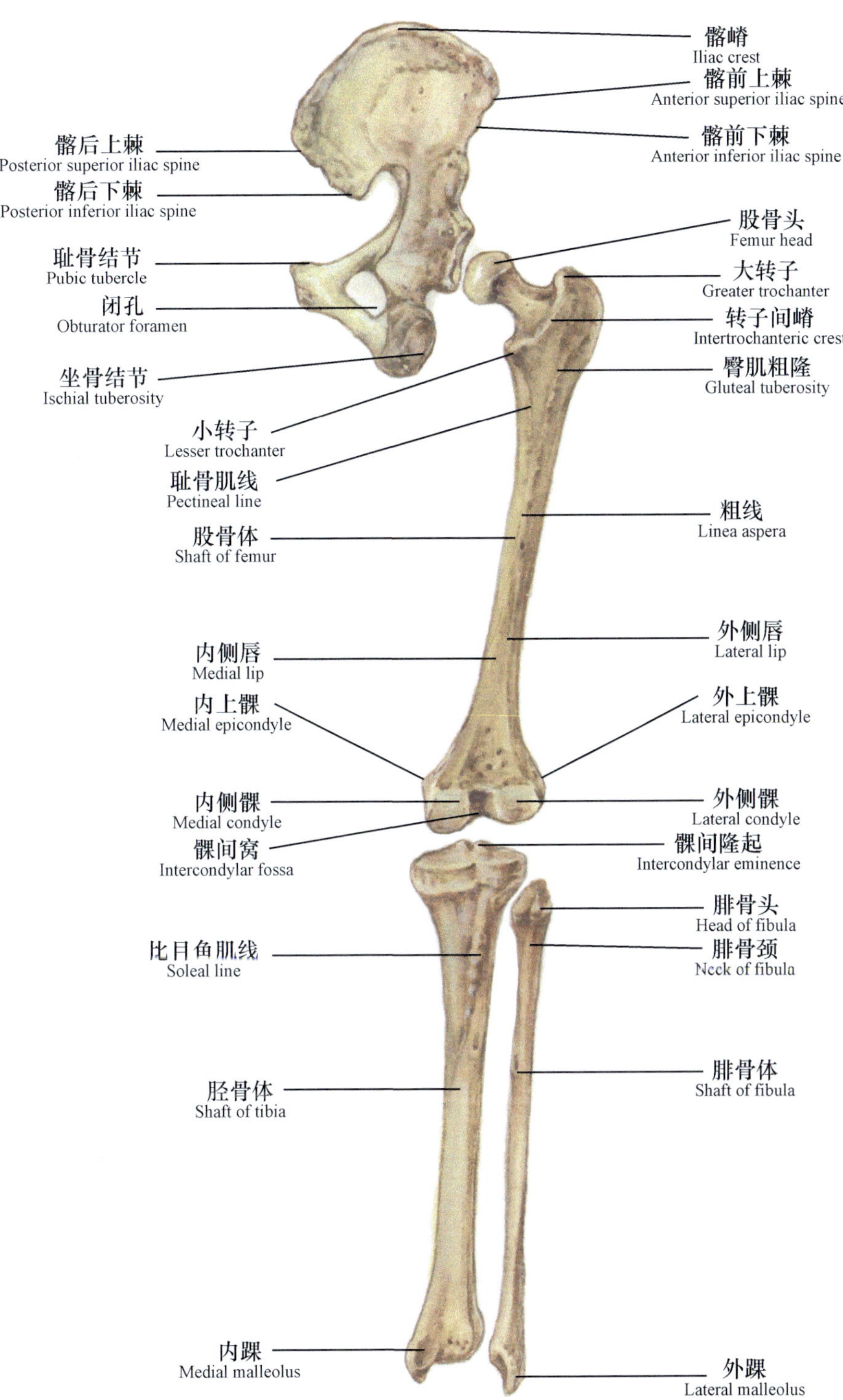

图 1-83 下肢骨（后面观）
Bone of lower limb (Posterior aspect)

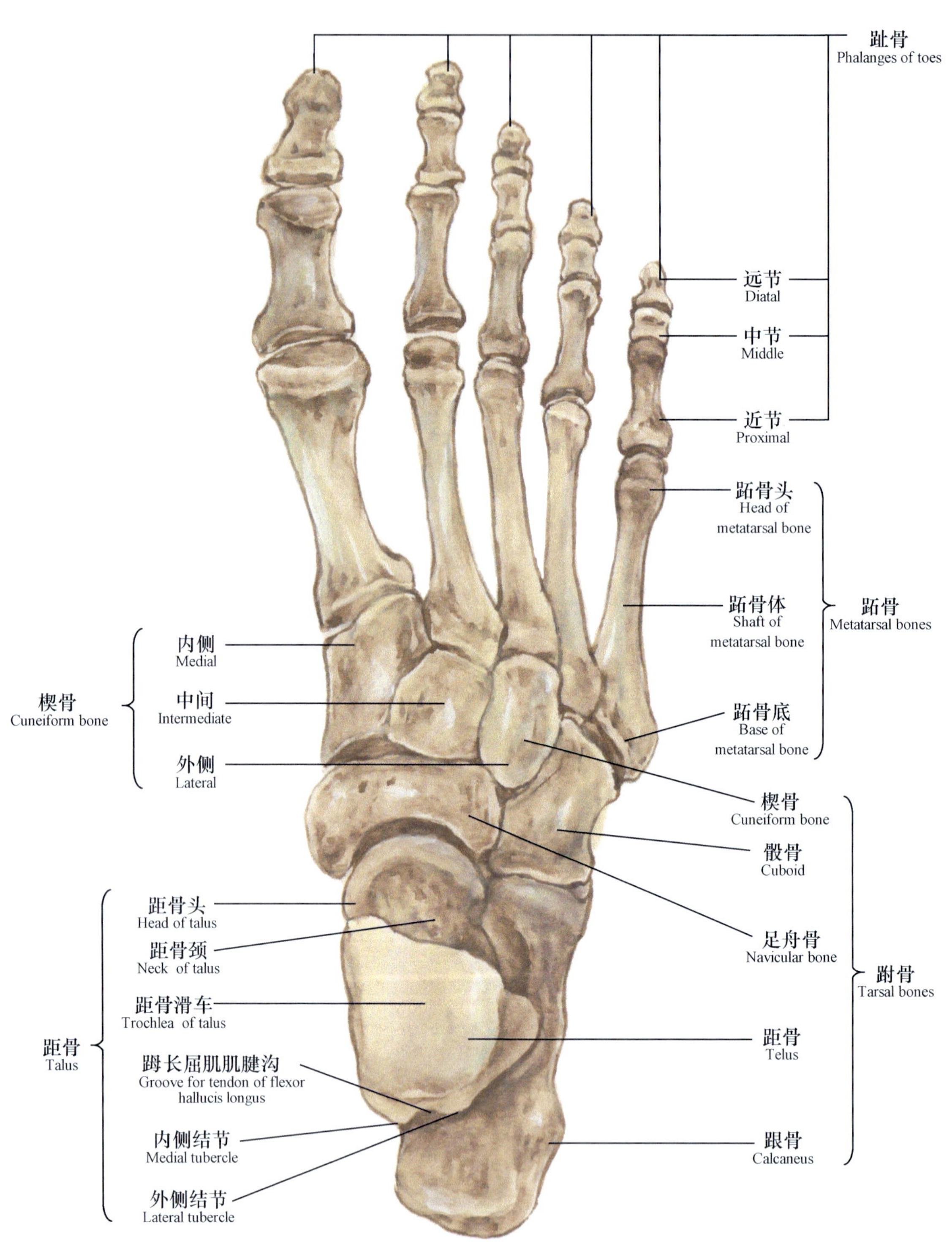

图 1-84 足骨（上面观）
Bones of foot (Superior aspect)

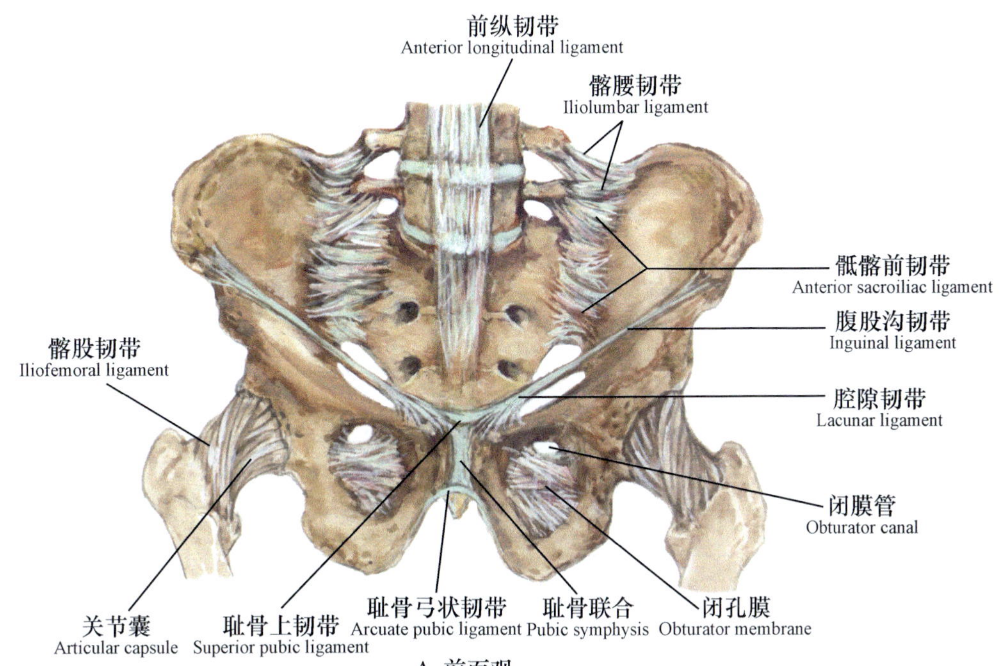

A. 前面观
Anterior aspect

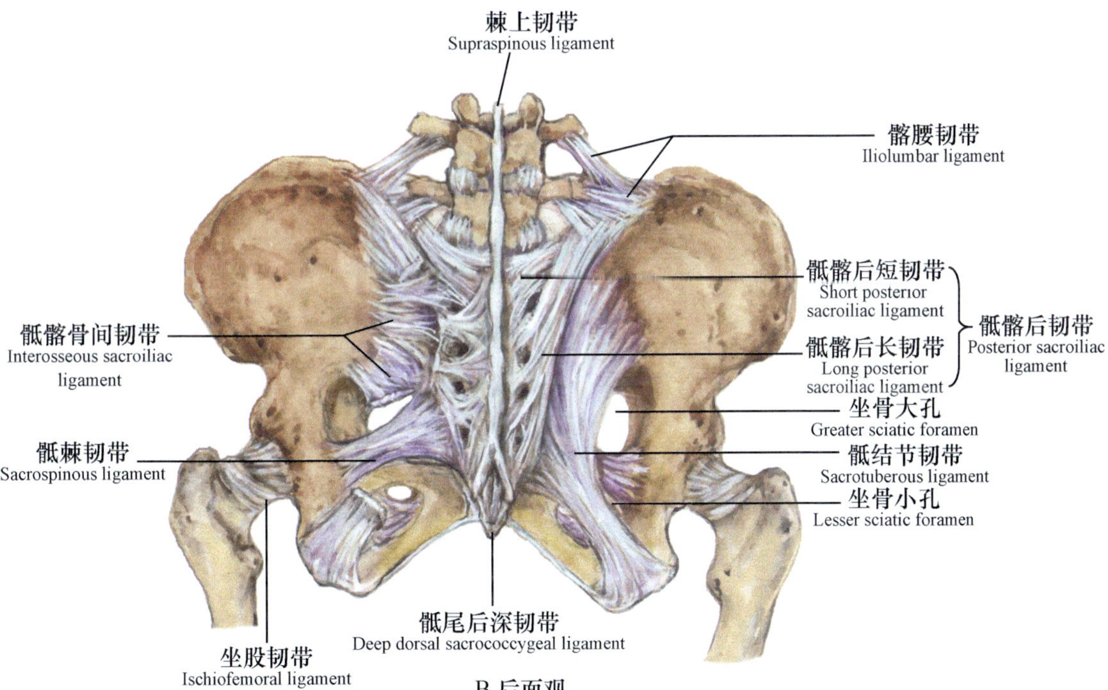

B.后面观
Posterior aspect

图 1-85 骨盆韧带
The ligaments of the pelvis

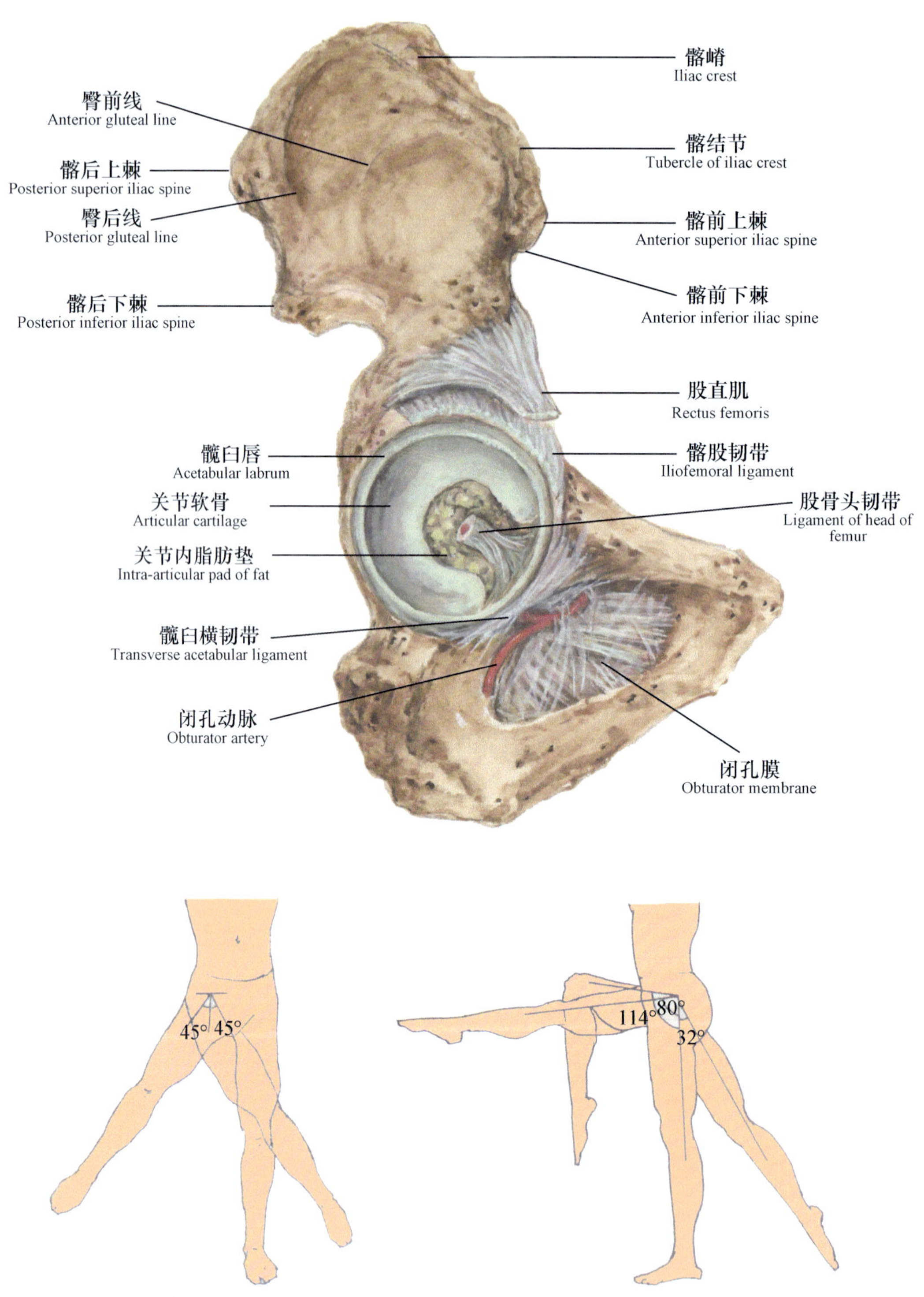

图 1-86 髋臼 - 股骨头窝
Acetabulum-Socket for the head of the femur

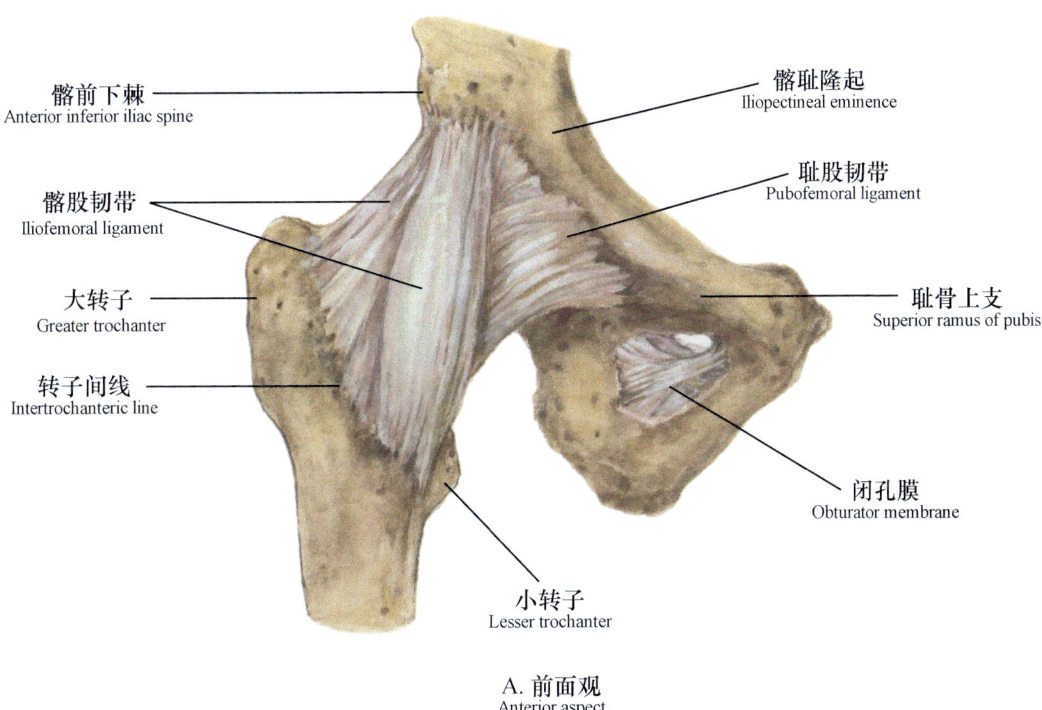

A. 前面观
Anterior aspect

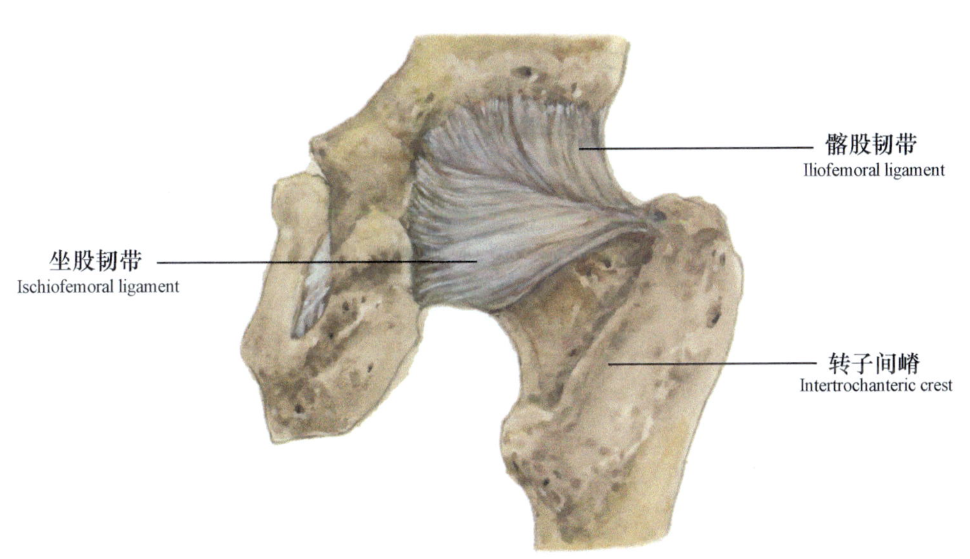

B. 后面观
Posterior aspect

图 1-87　右侧髋关节
The right hip joint

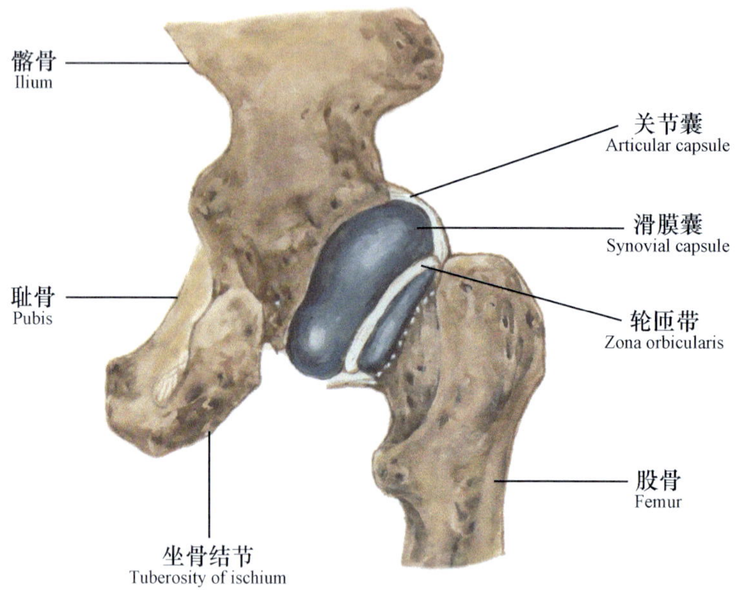

A. 冠状切面（背侧观）
A coronal section (Dorsal aspect)

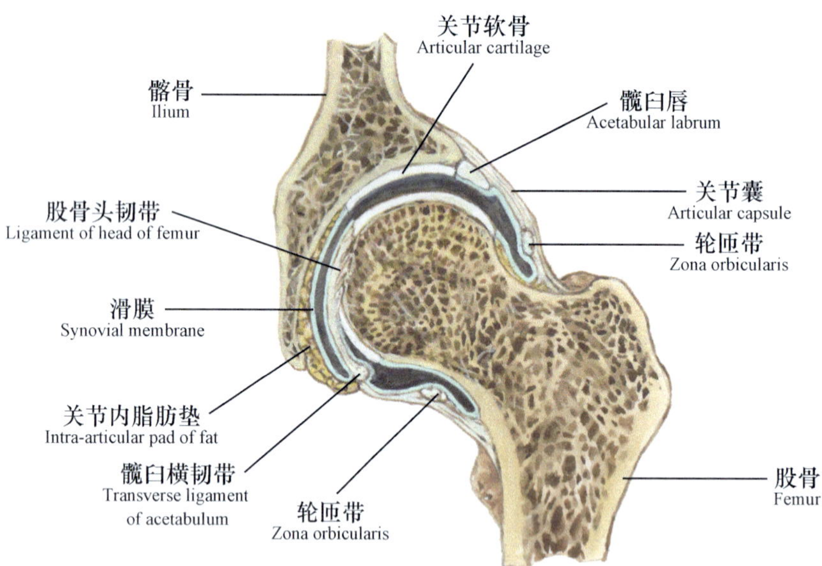

B. 冠状切面（前面观）
A coronal section (Anterior aspect)

图 1-88　右髋关节冠状切面
A coronal section through the right hip joint

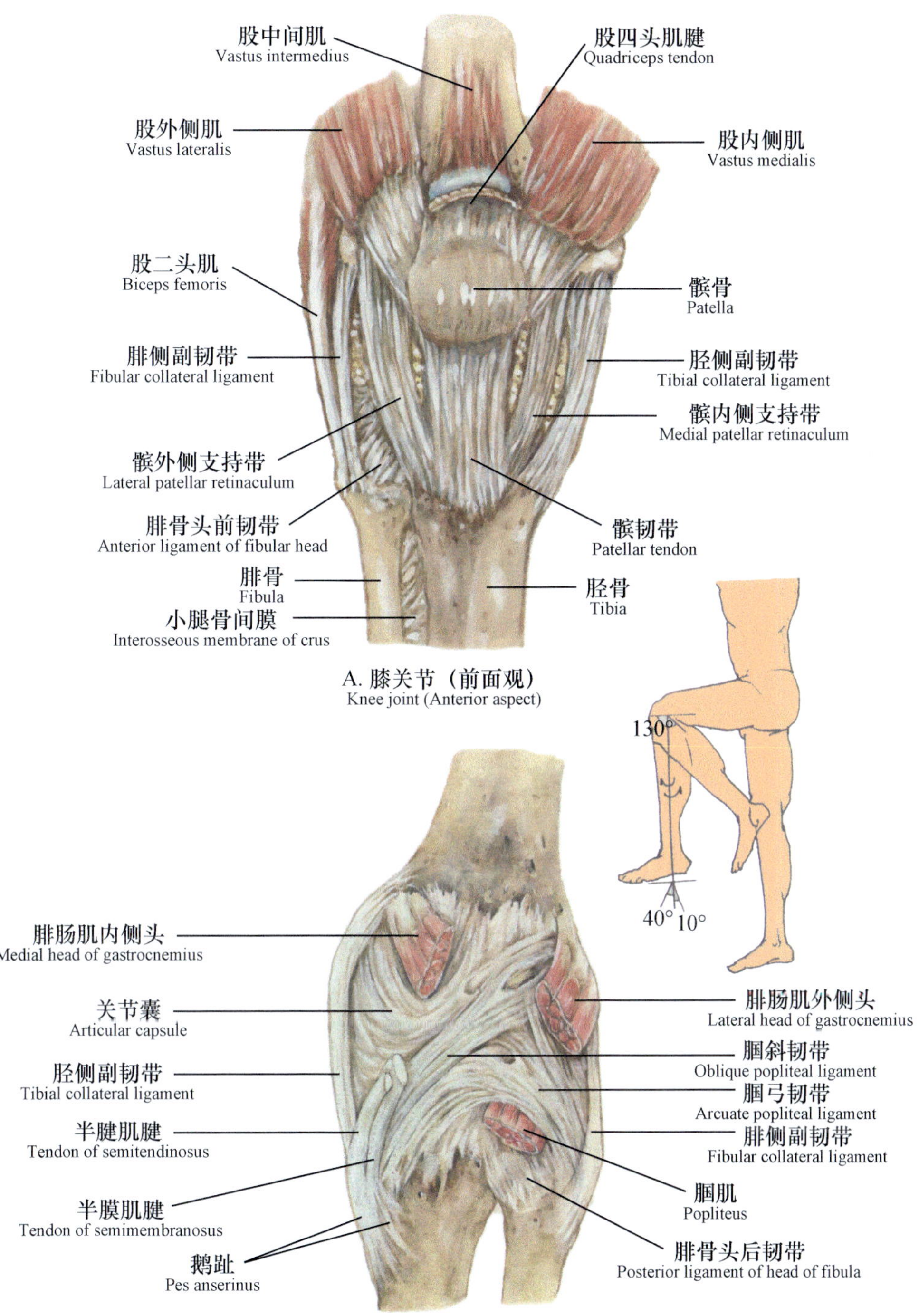

图 1-89　膝关节
Knee joint

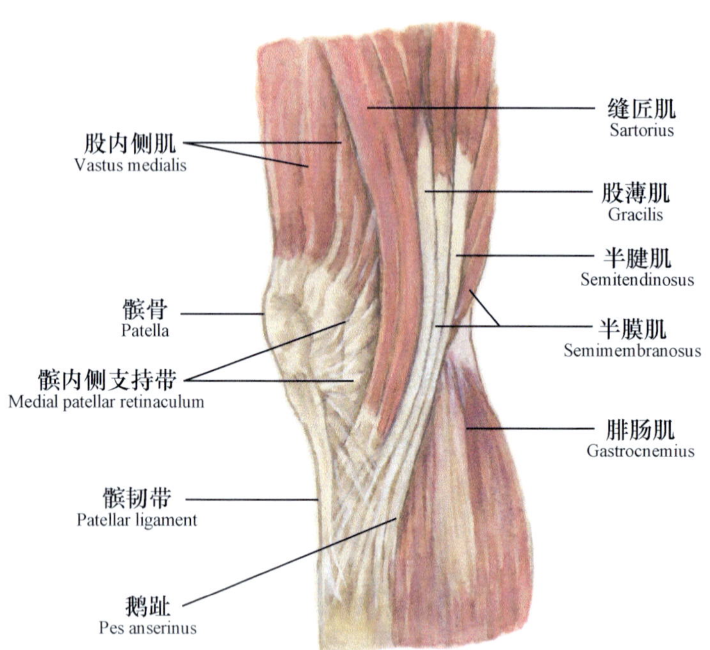

A. 浅层内侧观
Superficial medial aspect

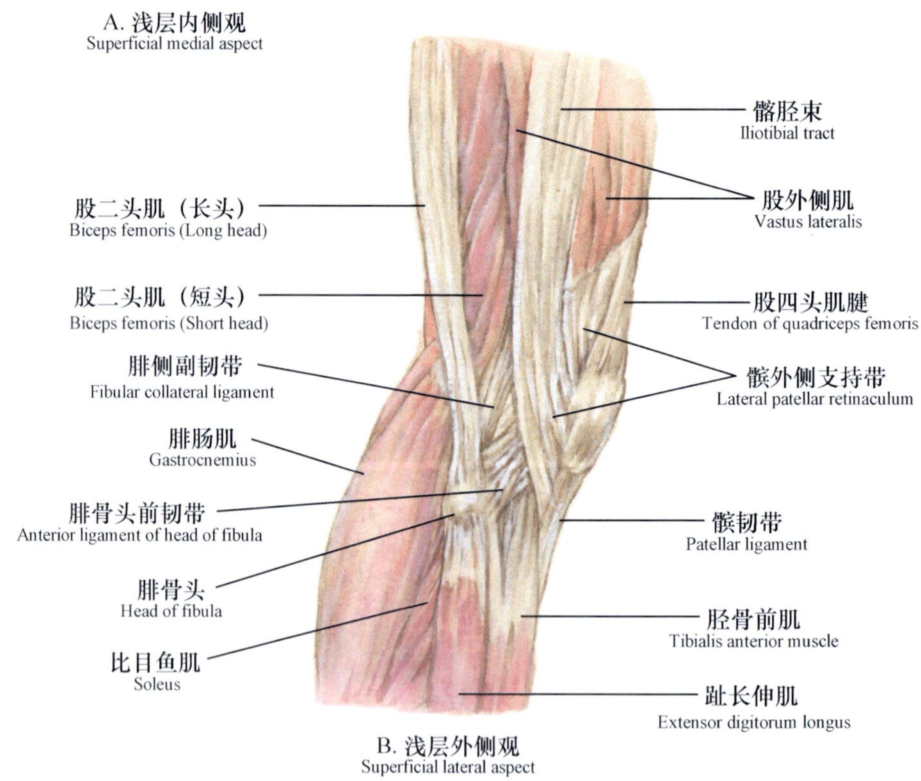

B. 浅层外侧观
Superficial lateral aspect

图 1-90 右侧膝关节（浅层）
Right knee joint (Superficial)

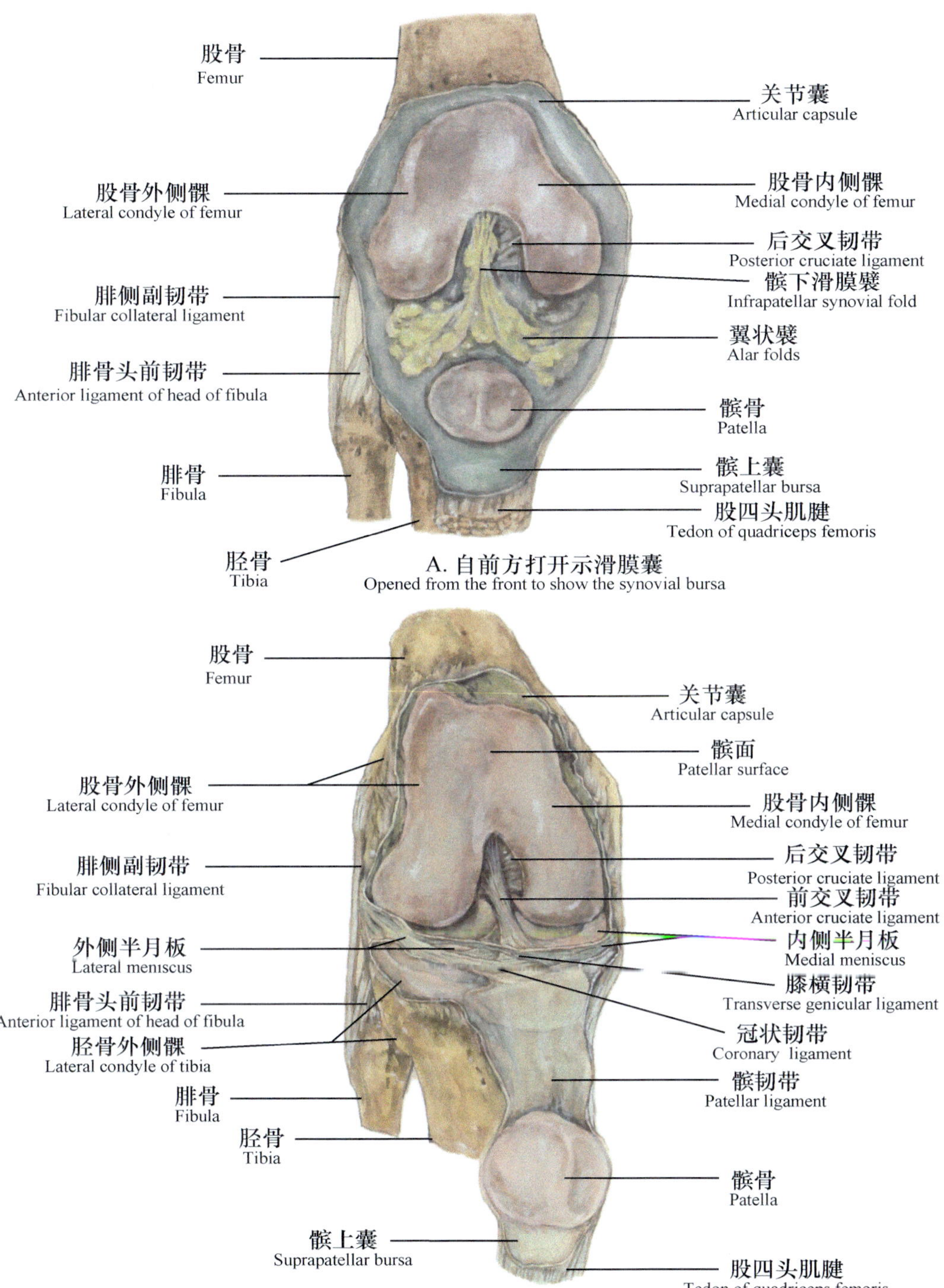

图 1-91 右侧膝关节（1）
The right knee joint (1)

髌韧带
Patellar ligament
膝横韧带
Transverse genicular ligament
髌下深囊
Deep infrapatellar bursa
冠状韧带
Coronary ligament
内侧半月板
Medial meniscus
前交叉韧带
Anterior cruciate ligament
外侧半月板
Lateral meniscus
后交叉韧带
Posterior cruciate ligament
腘肌腱
Popliteus tendon
板股后韧带
Posterior meniscofemoral ligament
冠状韧带
Coronary ligament

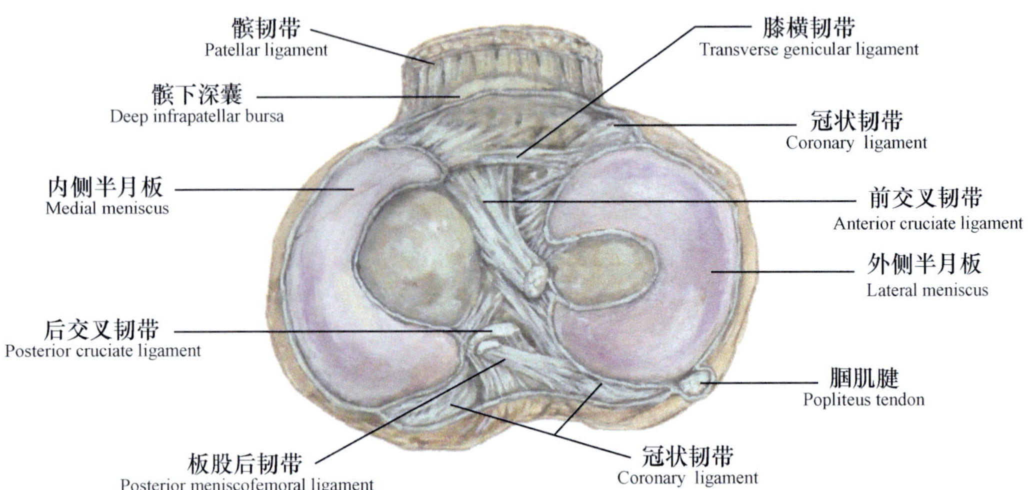

A.自上方示胫骨髁上面的交叉韧带与半月板
From above showing the cruciate ligaments on the condyles of the tibia and meniscus

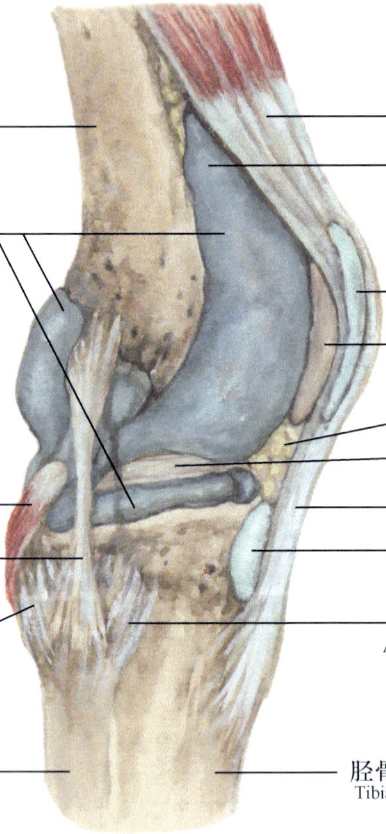

股骨
Femur
股四头肌腱
Tendon of quadriceps femoris
髌上囊
Suprapatellar bursa
滑膜囊
Synovial capsule
髌前皮下囊
Subcutaneous prepatellar bursa
髌骨
Patella
髌下脂体
Infrapatellar fat pad
外侧半月板
Lateral meniscus
腘肌腱
Popliteus tendon
髌韧带
Patellar ligament
腓侧副韧带
Fibular collateral ligament
髌下深囊
Deep infrapatellar bursa
腓骨头前韧带
Anterior ligament of head of fibula
腓骨头后韧带
Posterior ligament of head of fibula
腓骨
Fibula
胫骨
Tibia

B.外侧观
Lateral aspect

图 1-92 右侧膝关节（2）
The right knee joint (2)

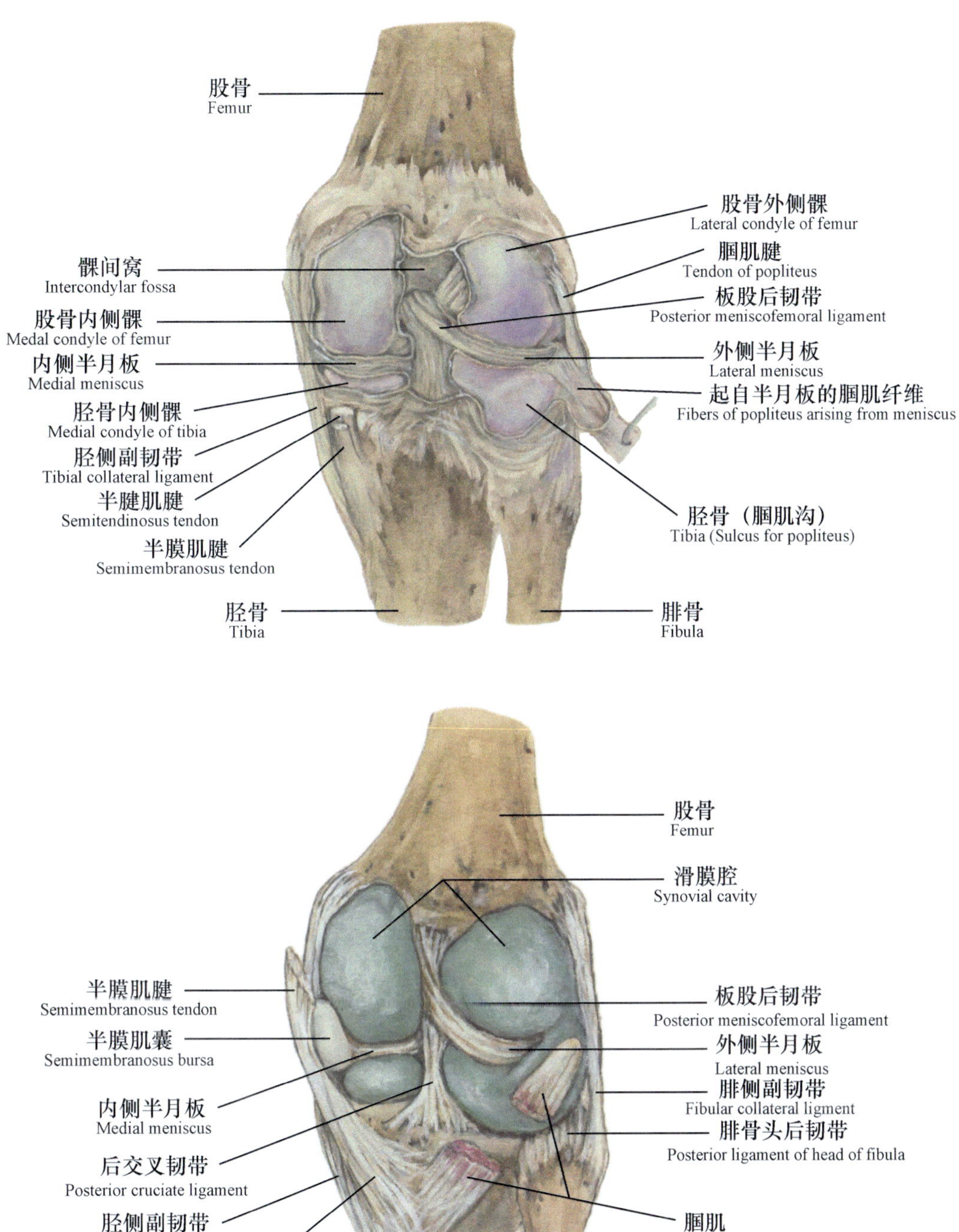

图 1-93　右膝关节铸型（背侧观）
The right knee joint (Posterior aspect)

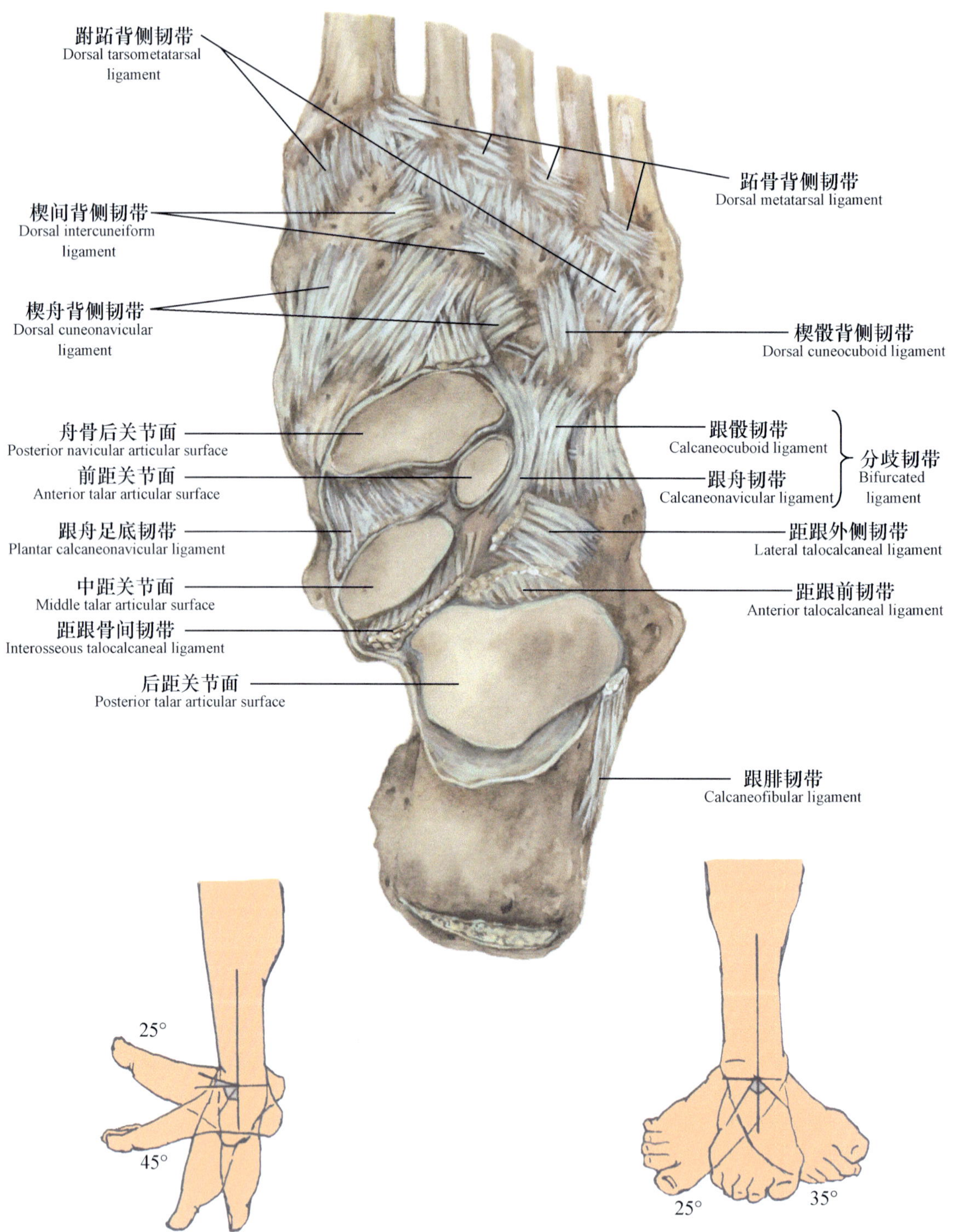

图 1-94 右侧踝关节与跗跖关节韧带（上面观）

The ligaments of the right ankle and tarsometatarsal joints (Superior aspect)

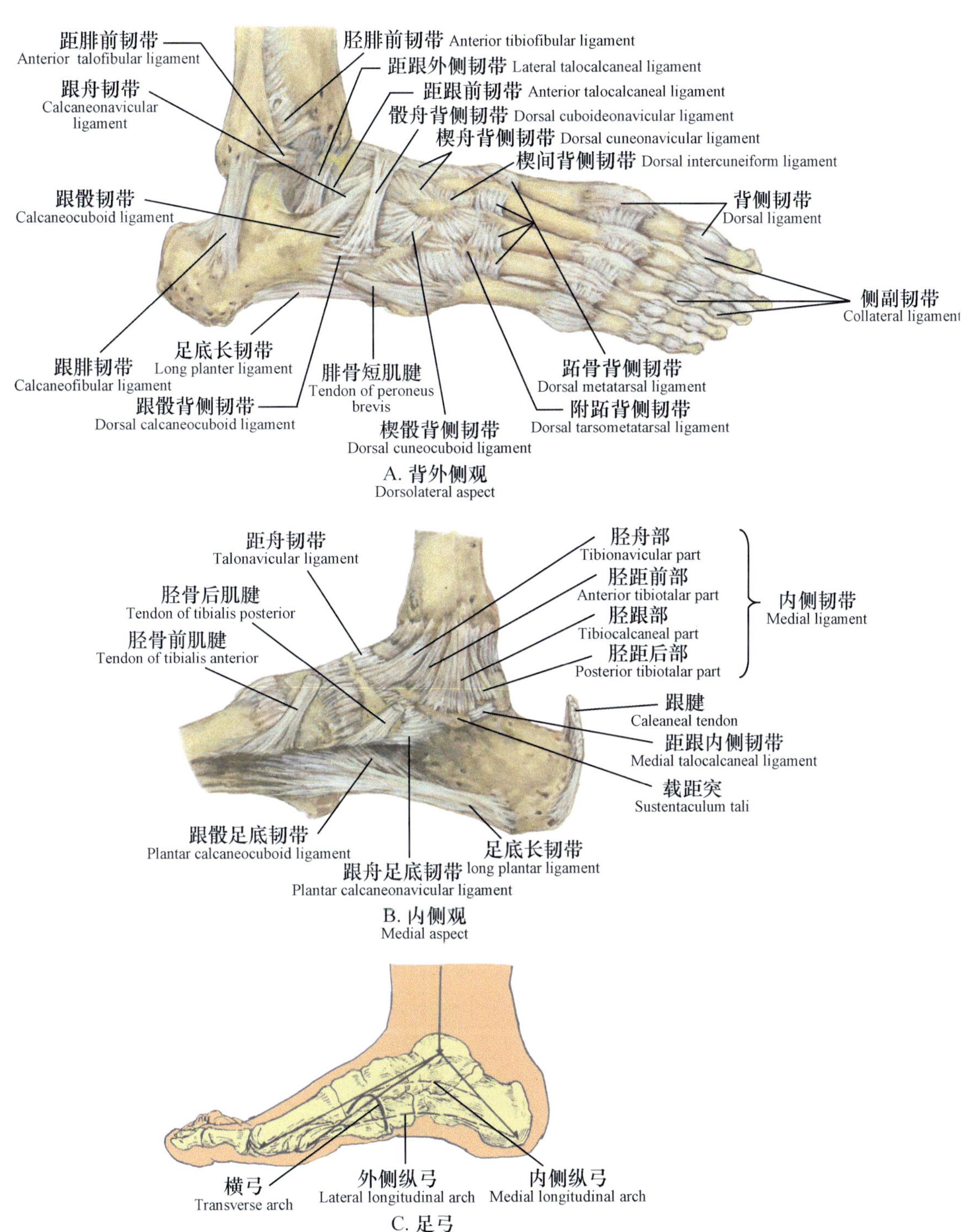

图 1-95 右踝关节与足关节韧带
Ligaments of the right ankle and feet joints

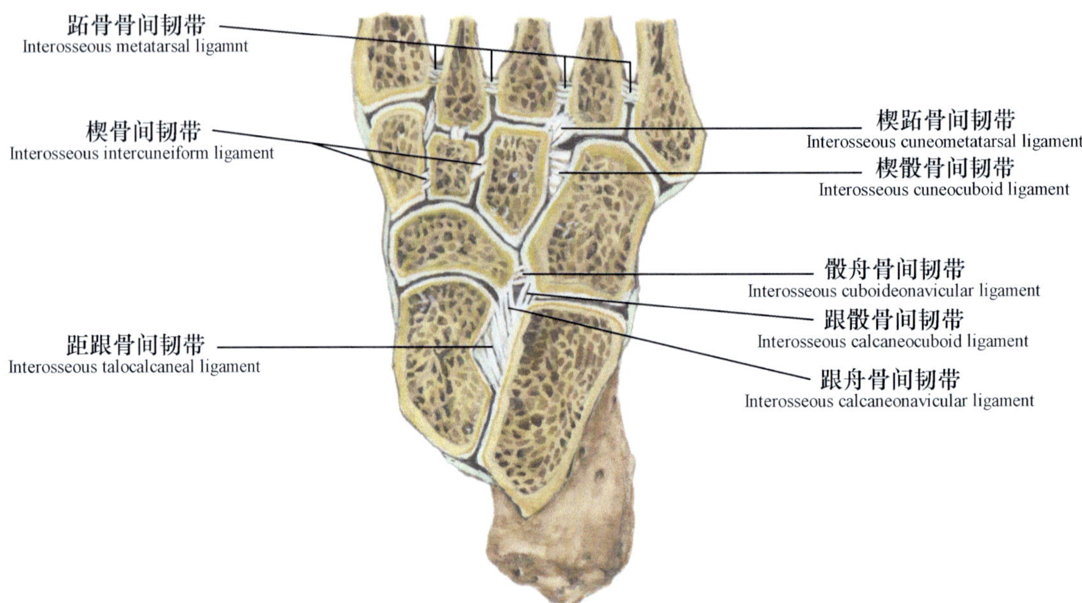

图 1-96　右侧足关节水平断面（上面观）
Horizontal section of the right foot (Superior aspect)

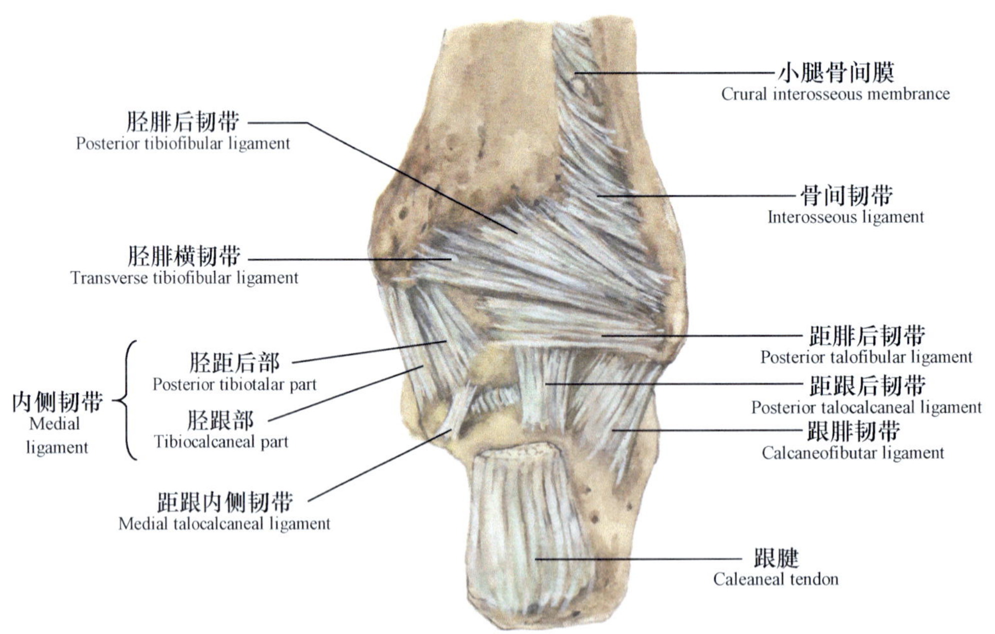

图 1-97　右侧踝关节韧带（背侧观）
Ligaments of the right ankle joint (Posterior aspect)

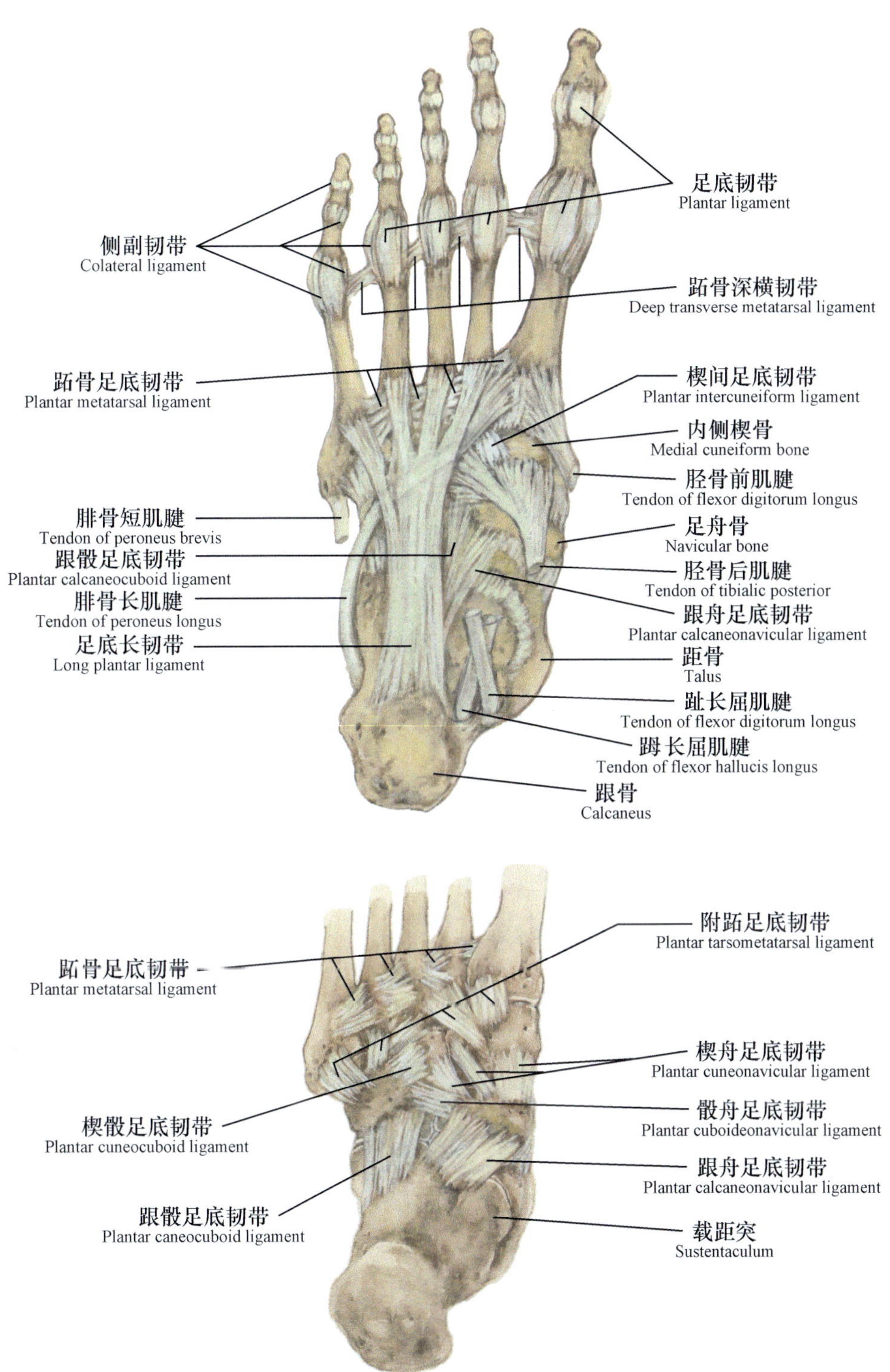

图 1-98 右侧足底韧带
Plantar ligament of the right foot

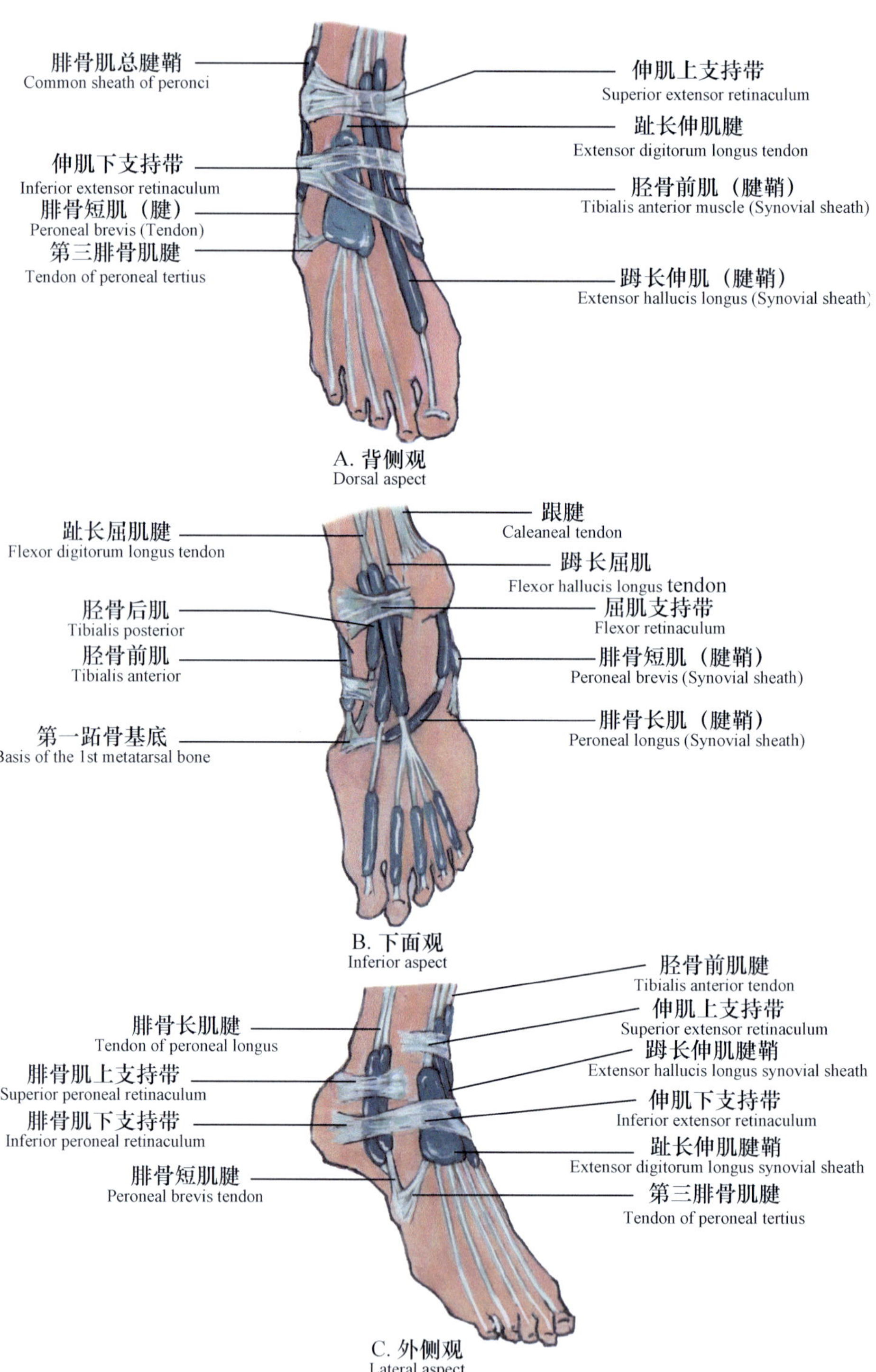

图 1-99 踝部腱鞘
Synovial sheathes of malleolus of the right foot

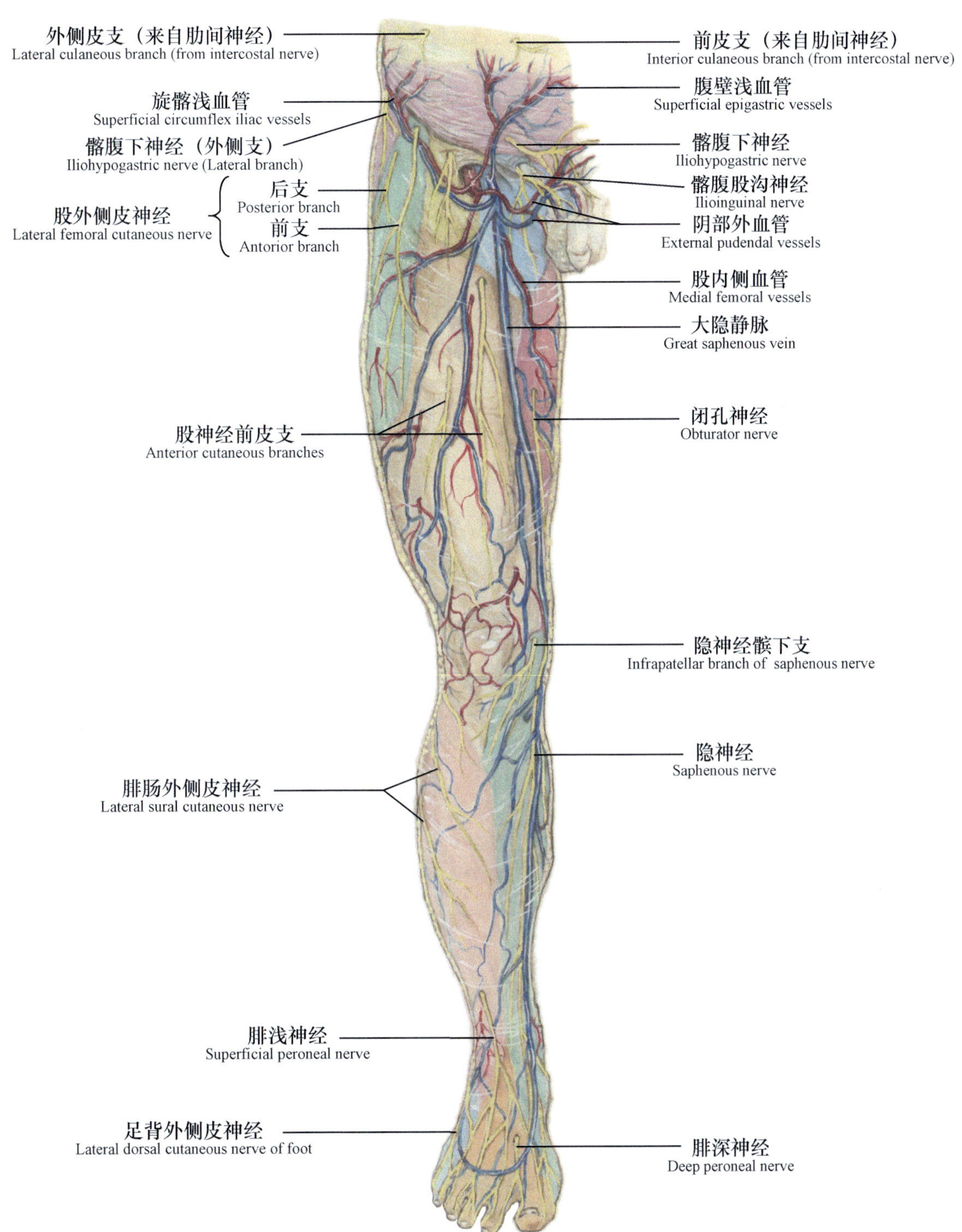

图 1-100 右下肢皮下神经和血管分布区（前面观）
The culenous innervation and blood vessels of the right lower limb (Anterior aspect)

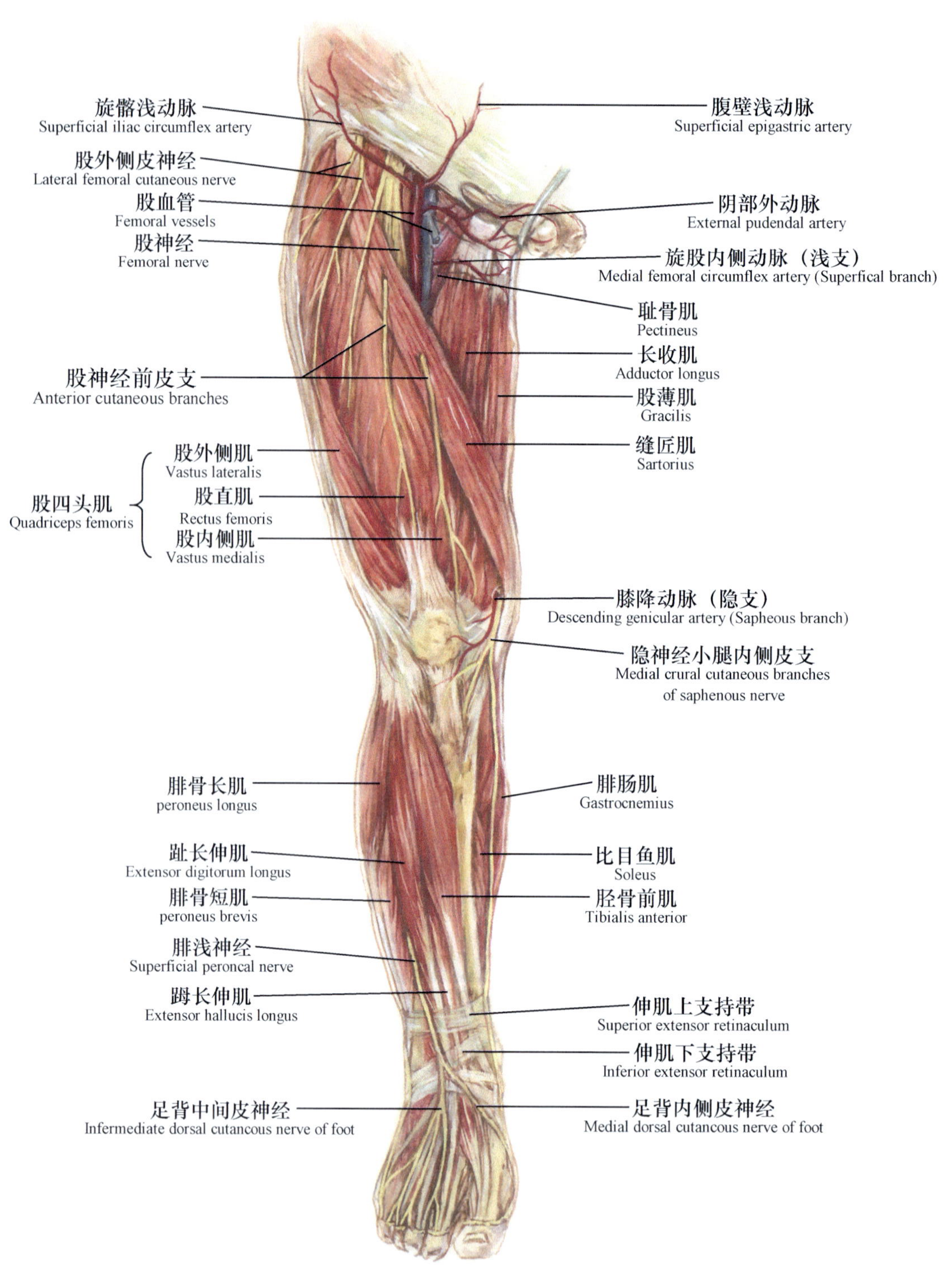

图 1-101 右下肢浅层神经和血管（前面观）
The superficial part nervation and blood vessels of the right lower limb (Anterior aspect)

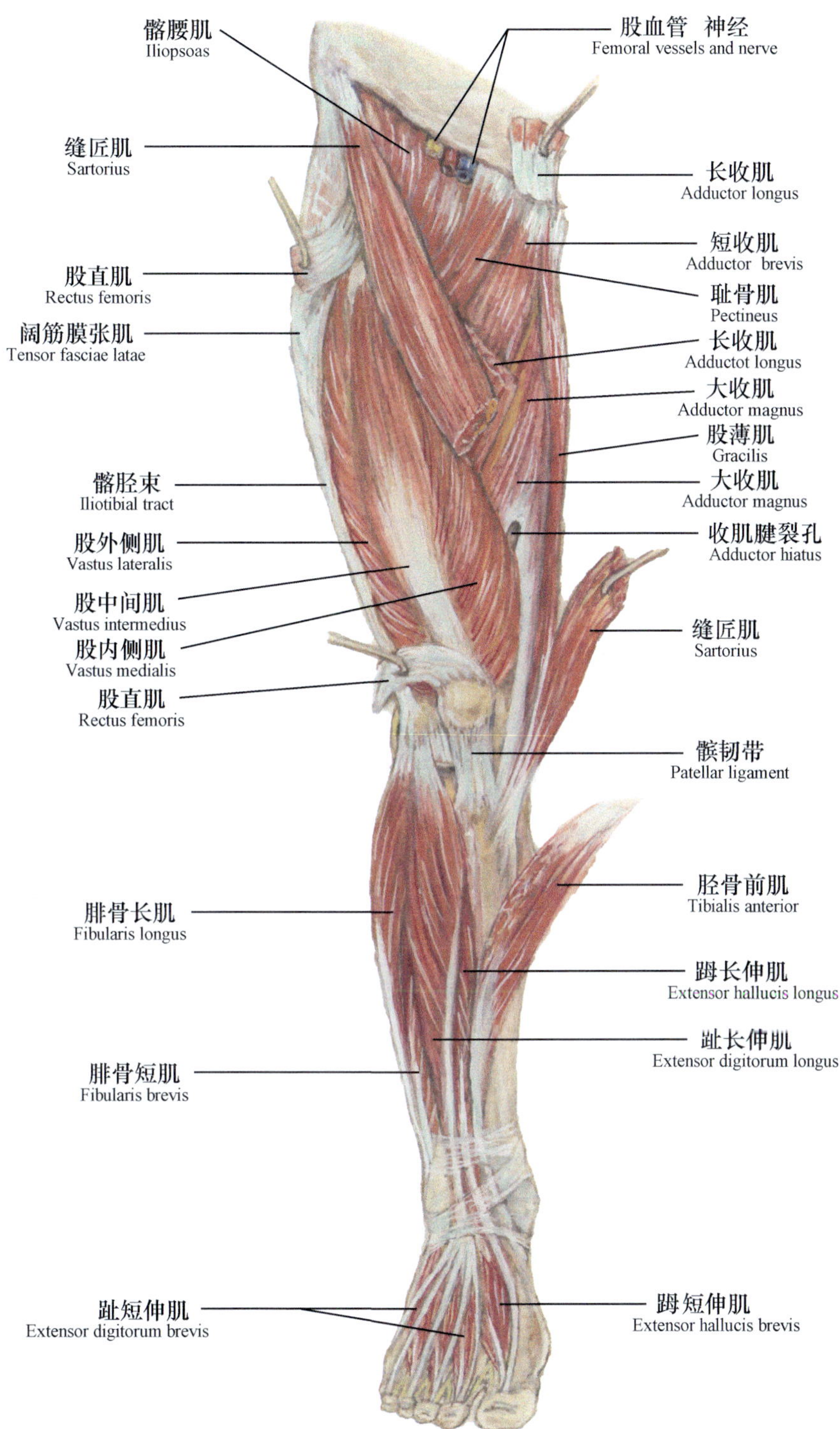

图 1-102 下肢肌（前面观）
Muscles of lower limb (Anterior aspect)

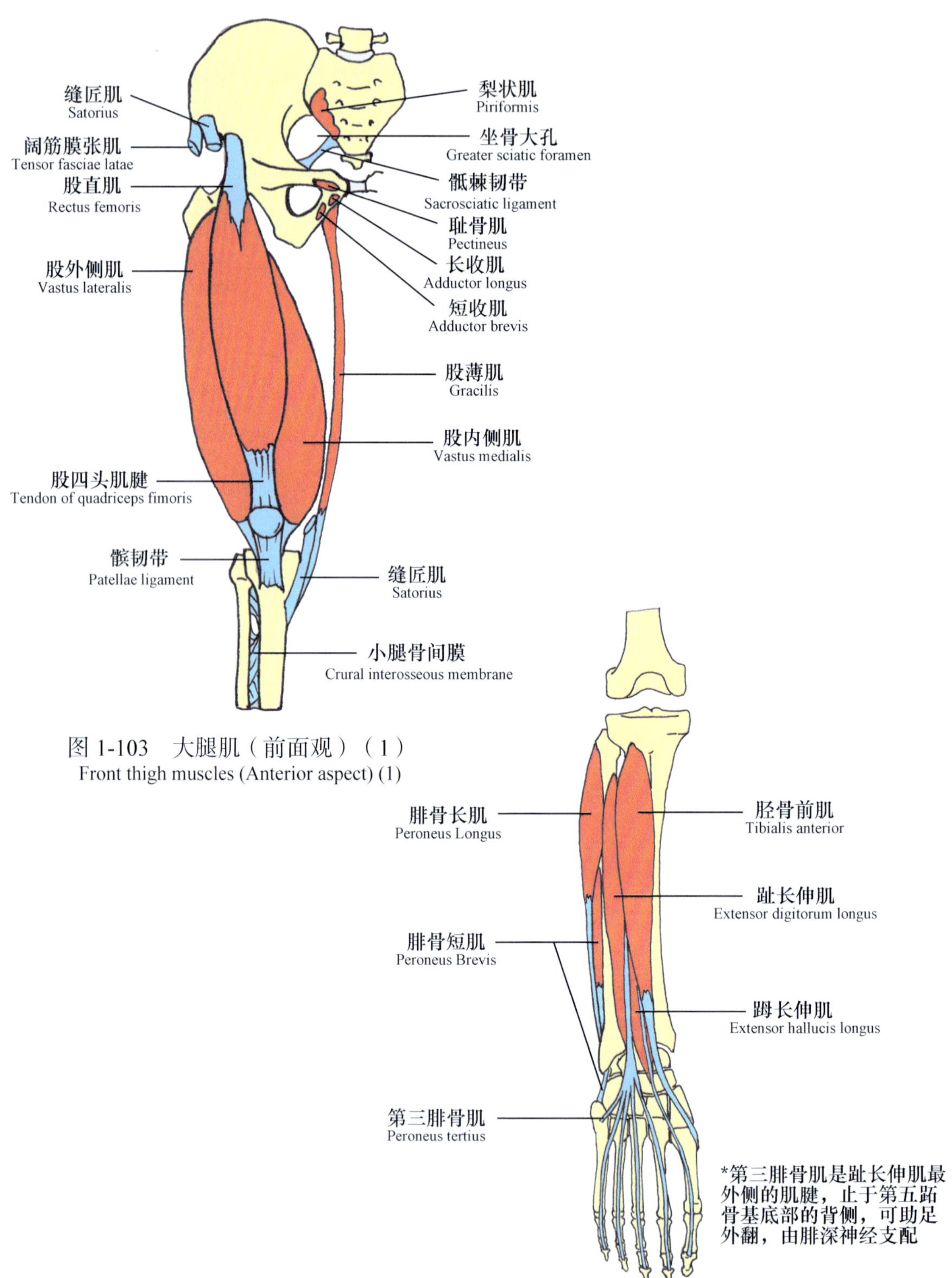

图 1-104 小腿肌（前面观）

Crus muscles (Anterior aspect)

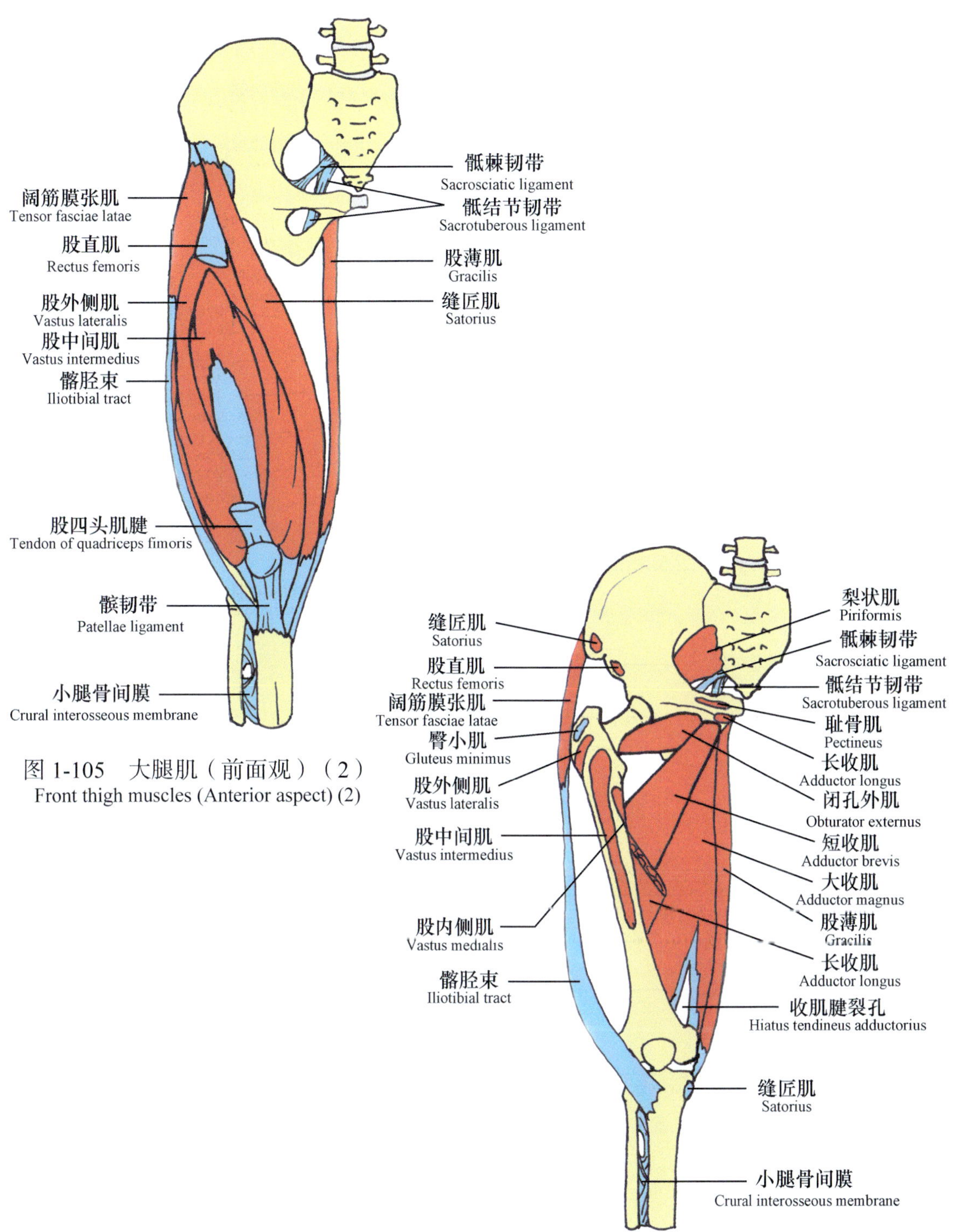

图 1-105　大腿肌（前面观）（2）
Front thigh muscles (Anterior aspect) (2)

图 1-106　大腿肌（前面观）（3）
Front thigh muscles (Anterior aspect) (3)

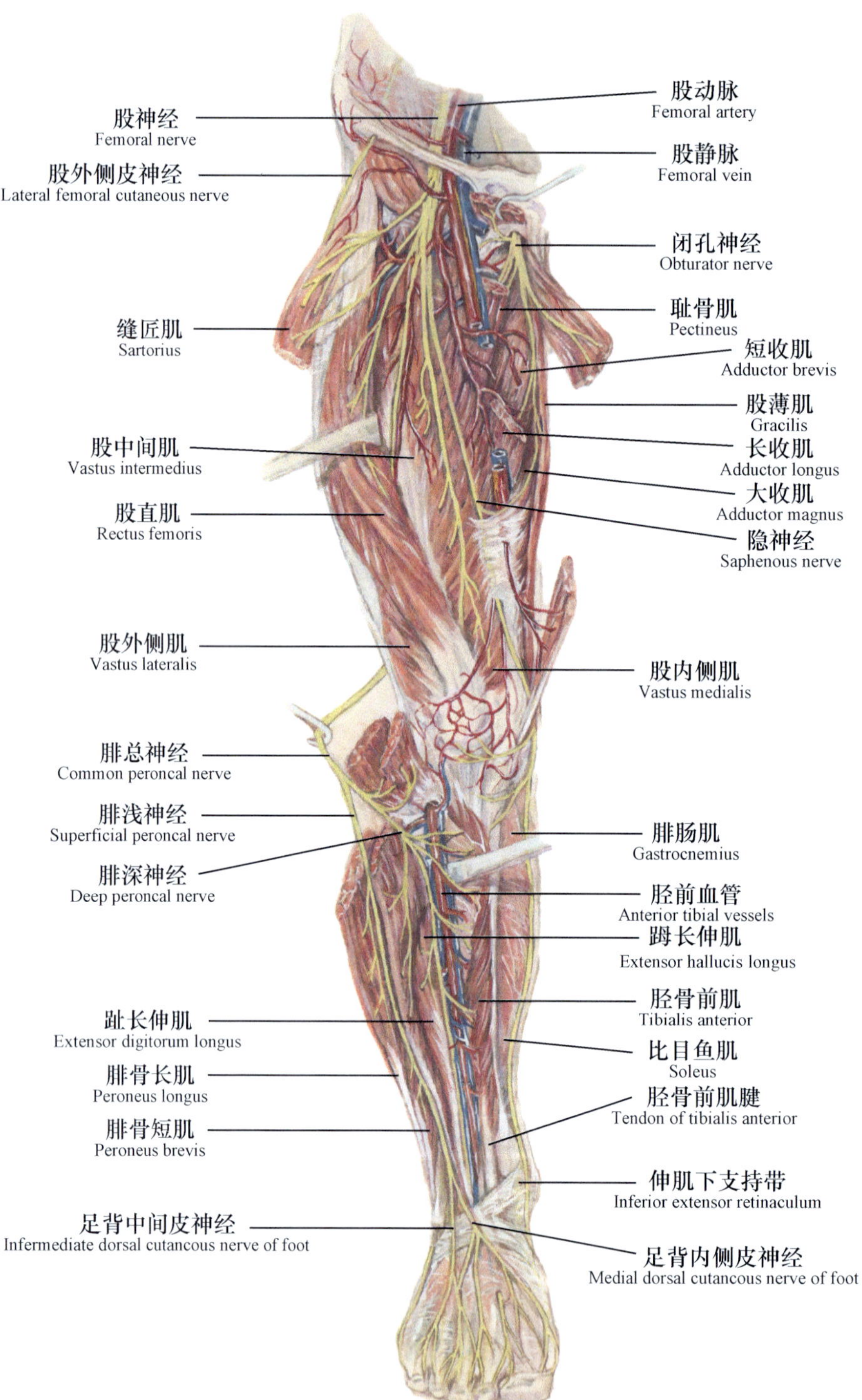

图 1-107 右下肢深层神经和血管（前面观）
The deep part innervation and blood vessels of the right lower limb (Anterior aspect)

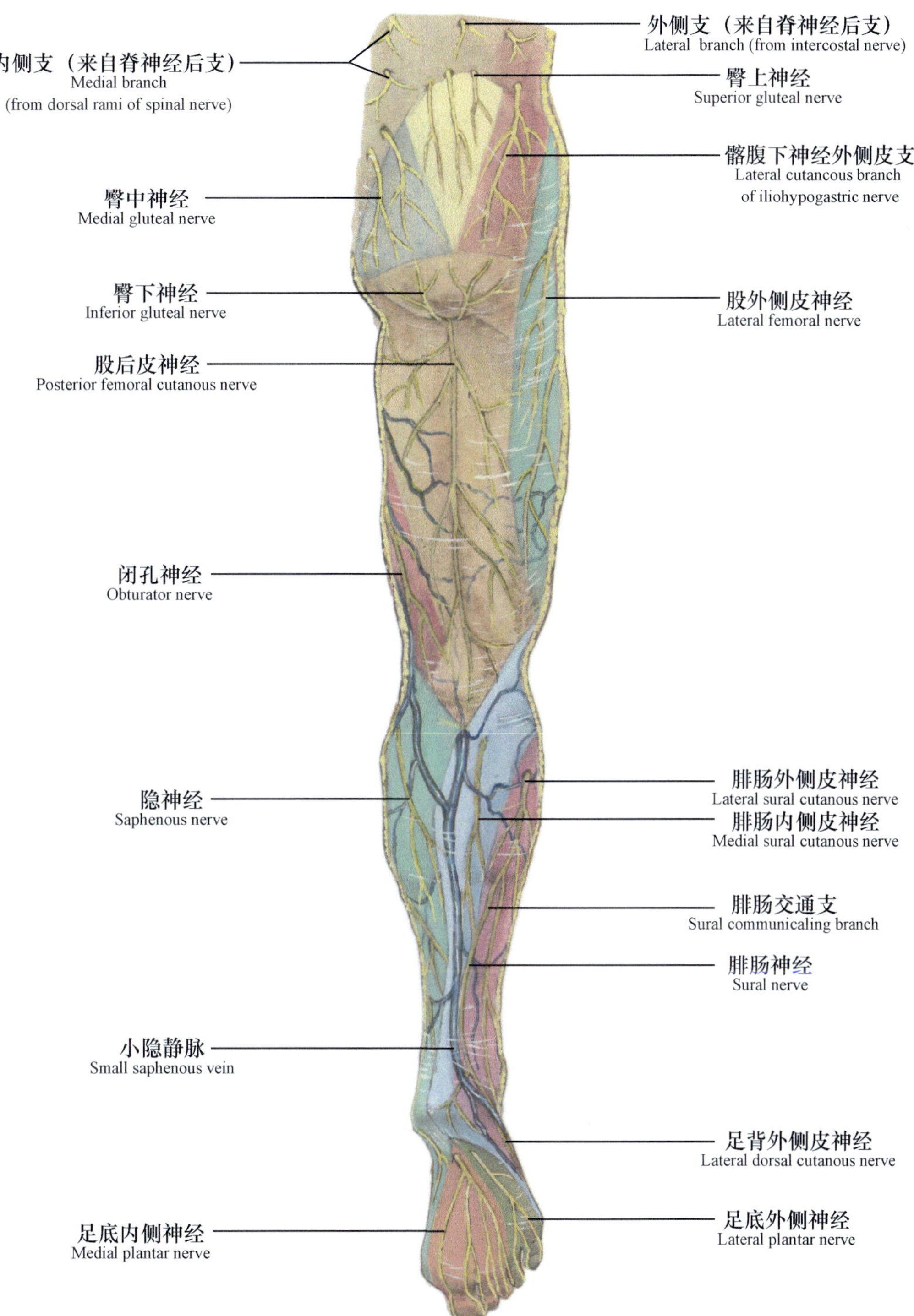

图 1-108 右下肢皮神经和血管分布区（后面观）
The cutanous innervation and blood vessels of the right lower limb (Posterior aspect)

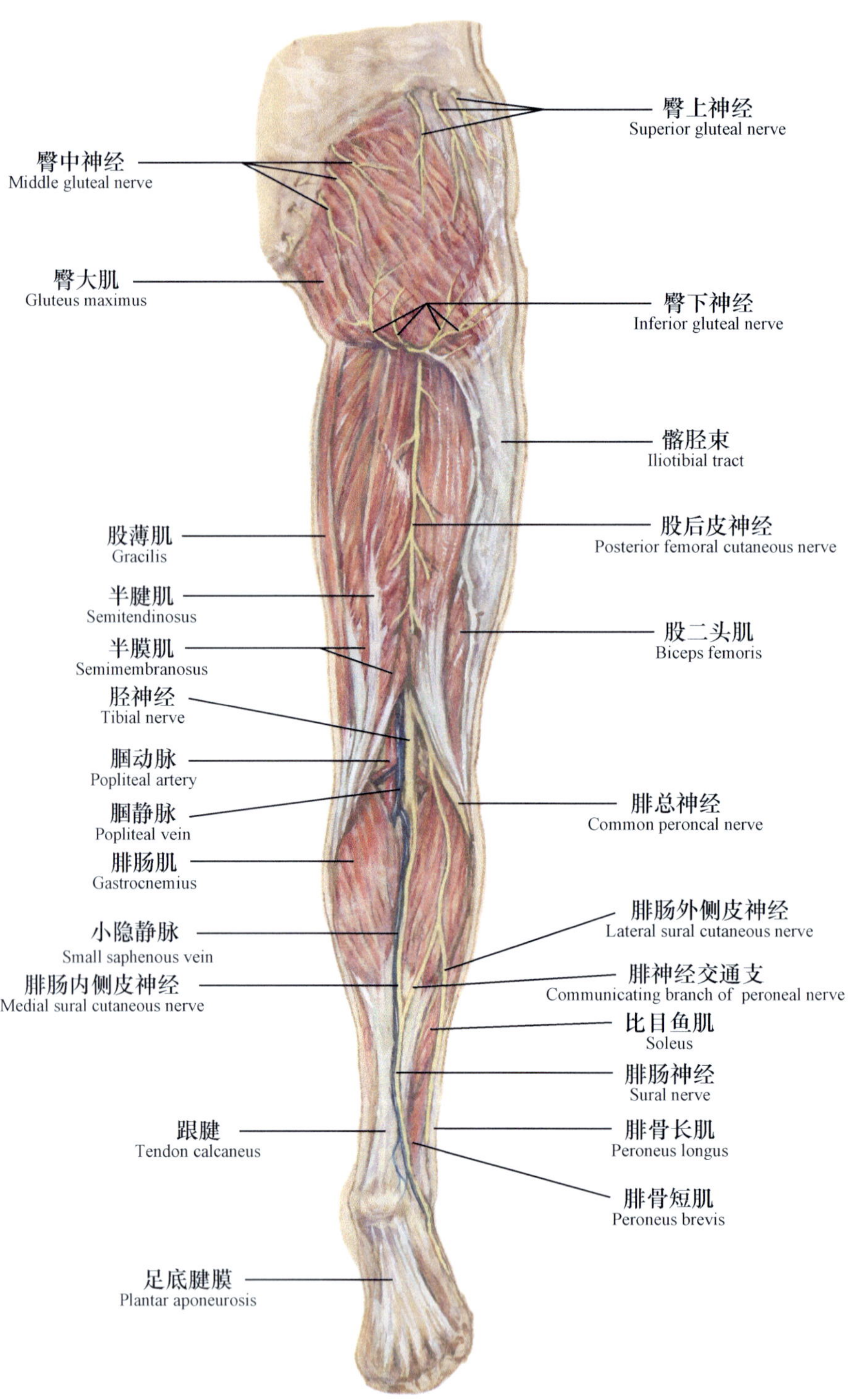

图 1-109 右下肢浅层神经和血管（后面观）
The superficial part innervation and blood vessels of the right lower limb (Posterior aspect)

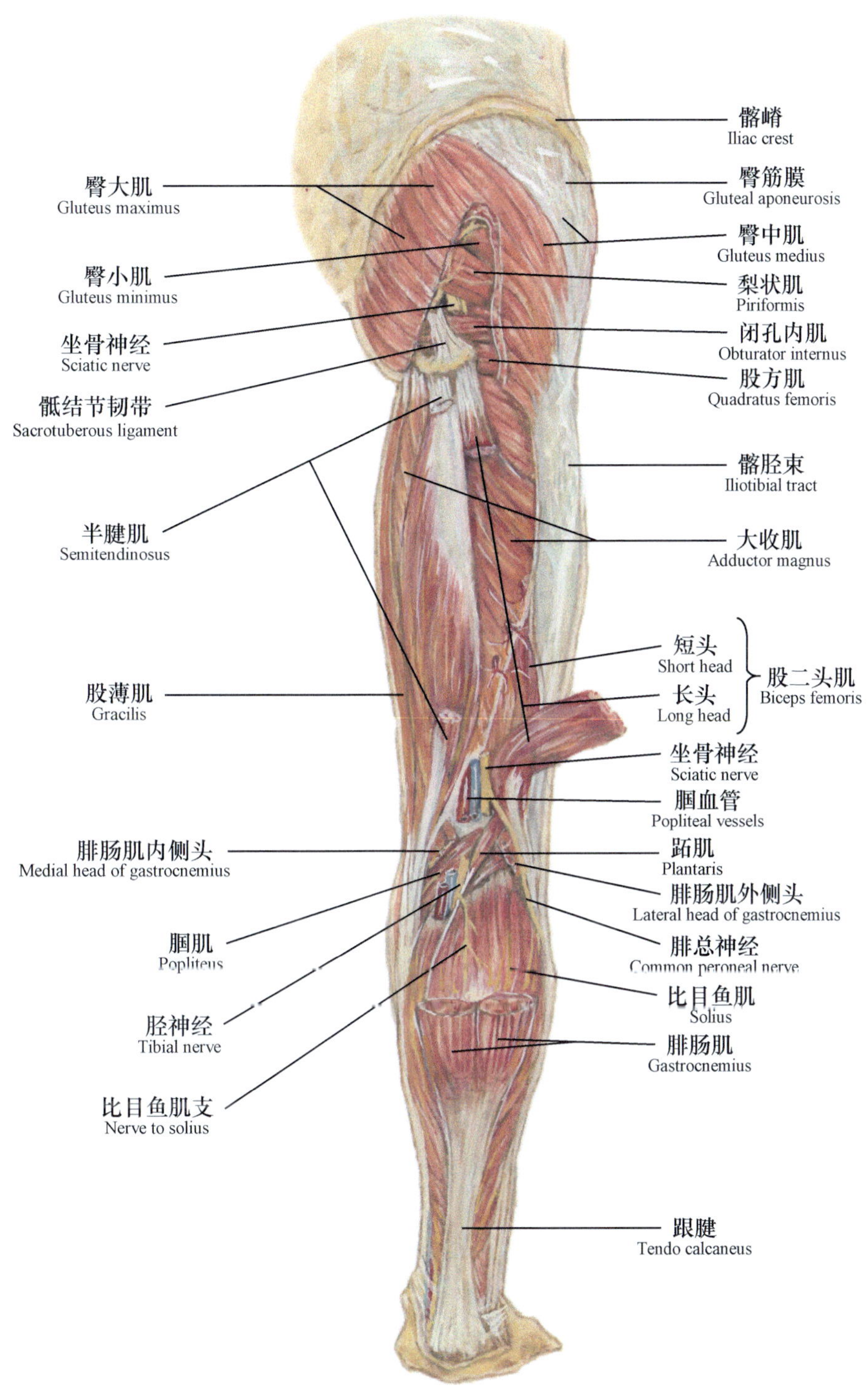

图 1-110 下肢背侧肌
Muscles of lower limb posterior aspect

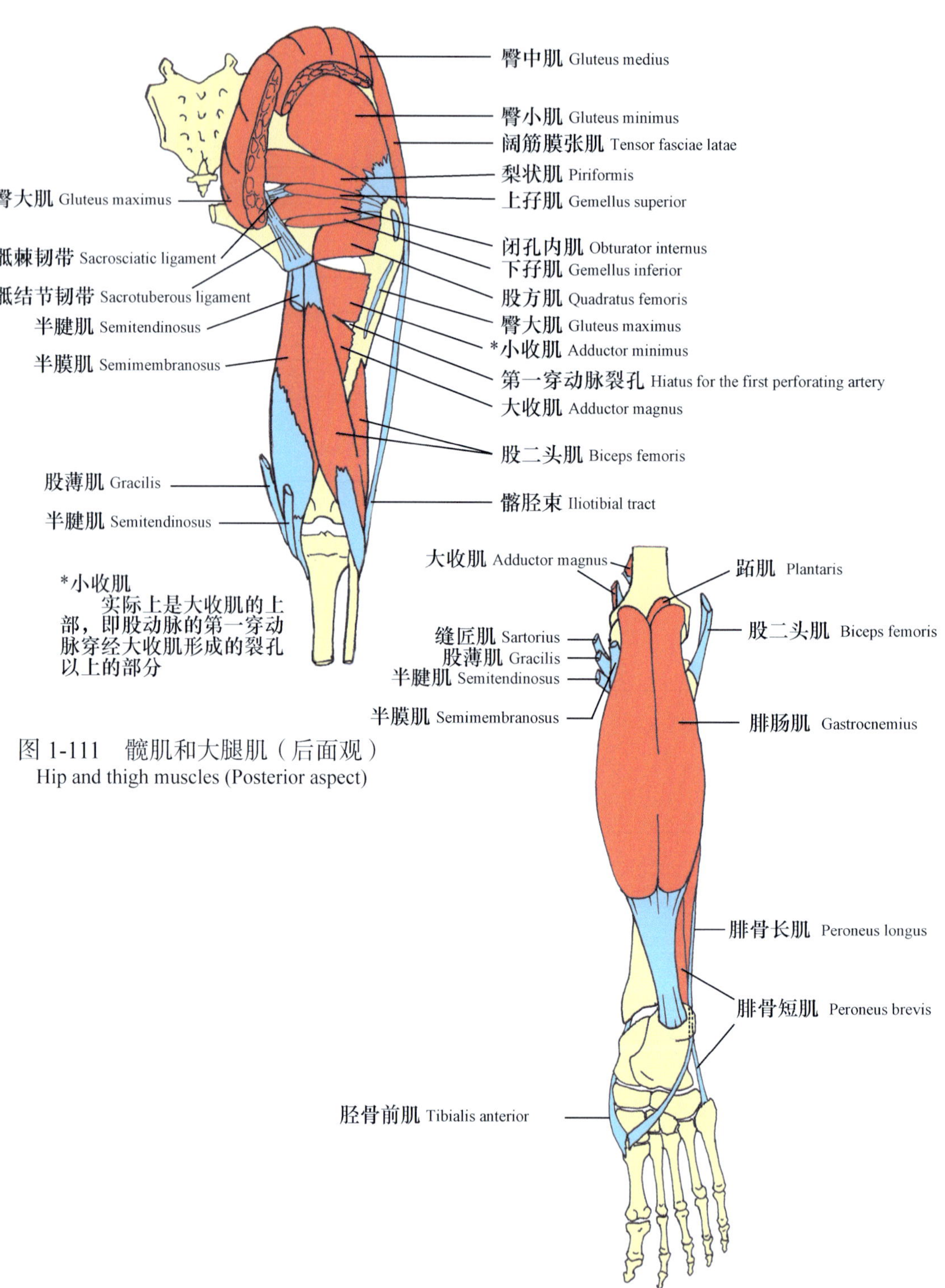

图 1-111 髋肌和大腿肌（后面观）
Hip and thigh muscles (Posterior aspect)

图 1-112 小腿肌（后面观）（1）
Crus muscles (Posterior aspect) (1)

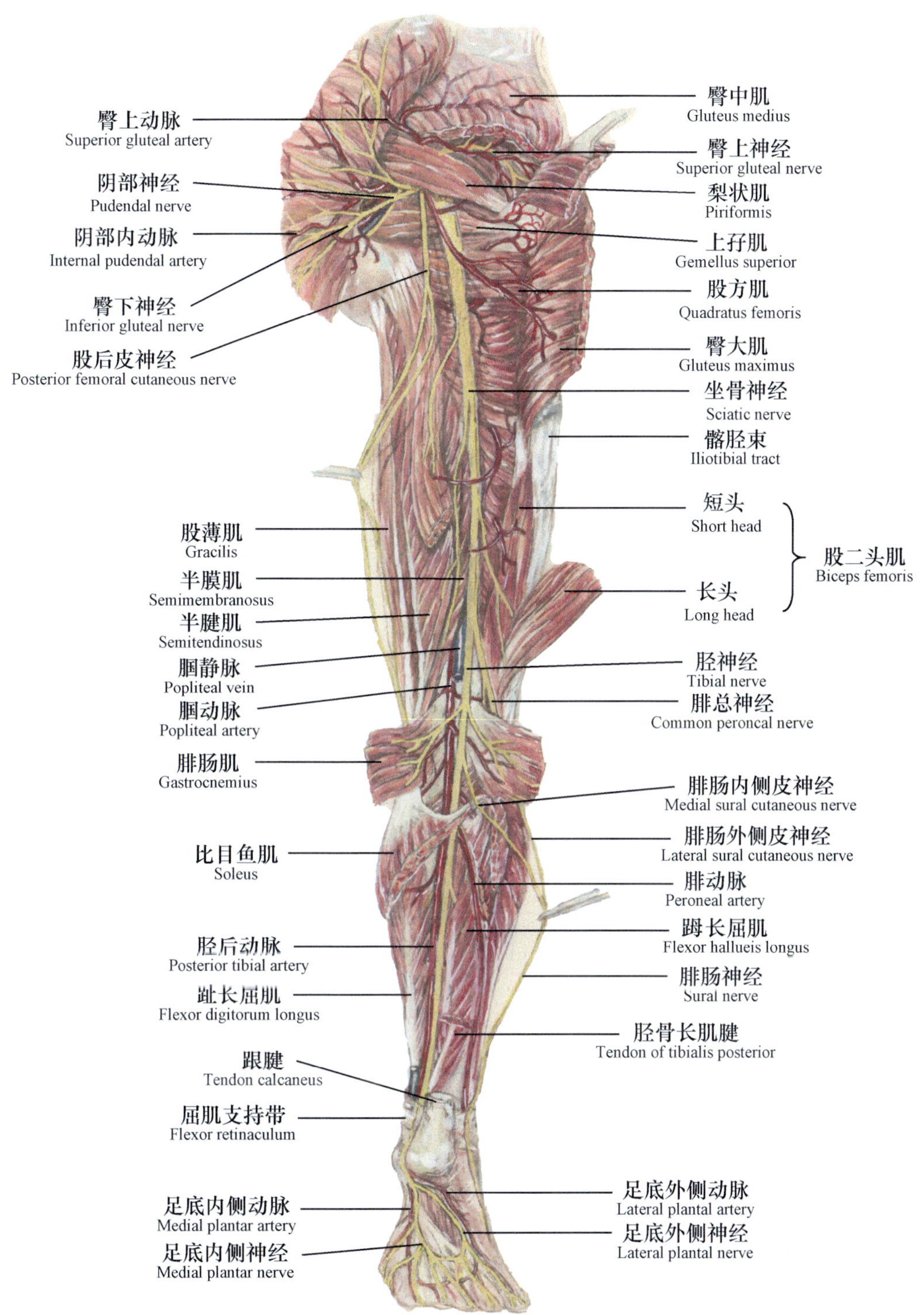

图 1-113　右下肢深层神经和血管（后面观）
The deep part innervation and blood vessels of the right lower limb (Posterior aspect)

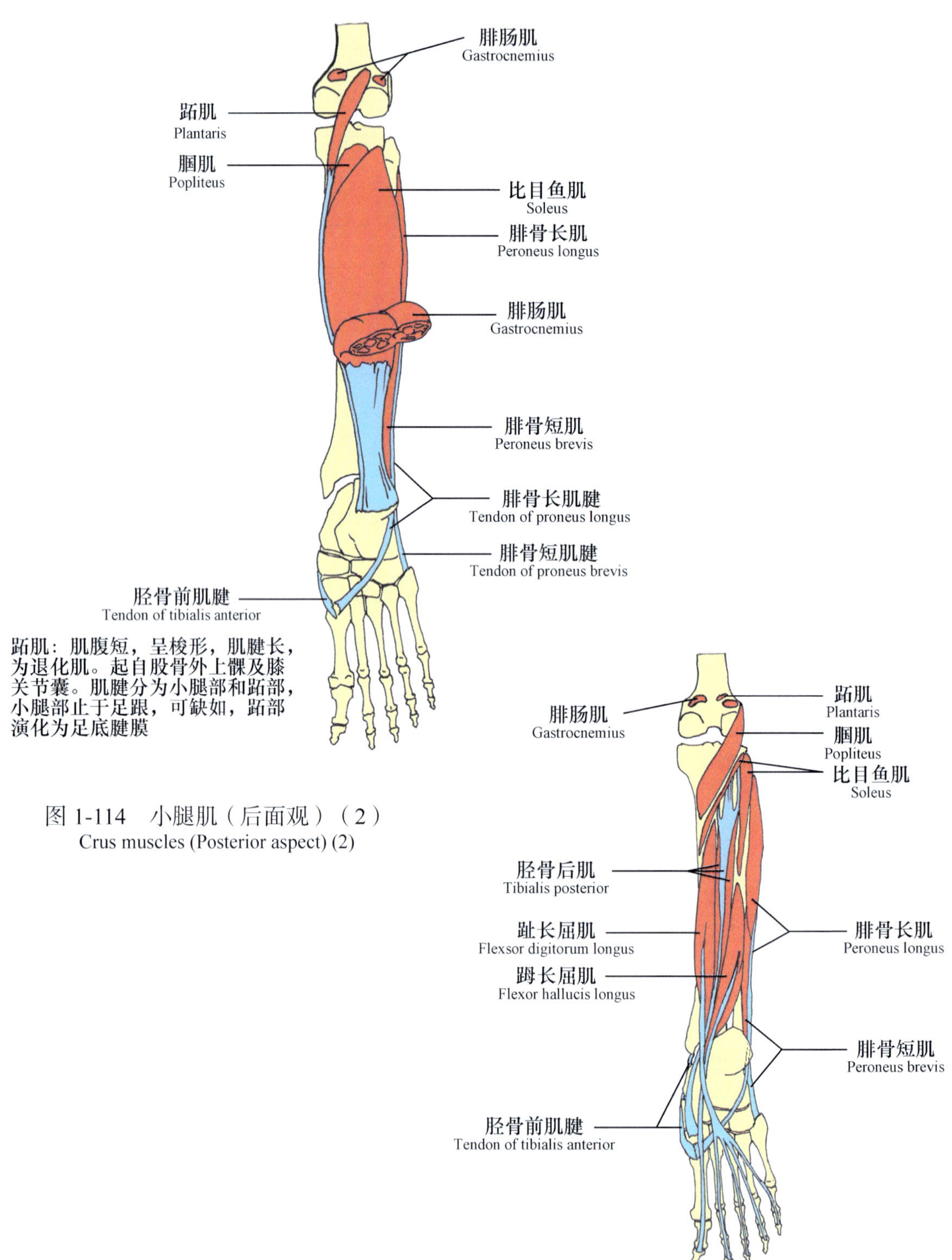

跖肌：肌腹短，呈梭形，肌腱长，为退化肌。起自股骨外上髁及膝关节囊。肌腱分为小腿部和跖部，小腿部止于足跟，可缺如，跖部演化为足底腱膜

图 1-114　小腿肌（后面观）（2）
Crus muscles (Posterior aspect) (2)

图 1-115　小腿肌（后面观）（3）
Crus muscles (Posterior aspect) (3)

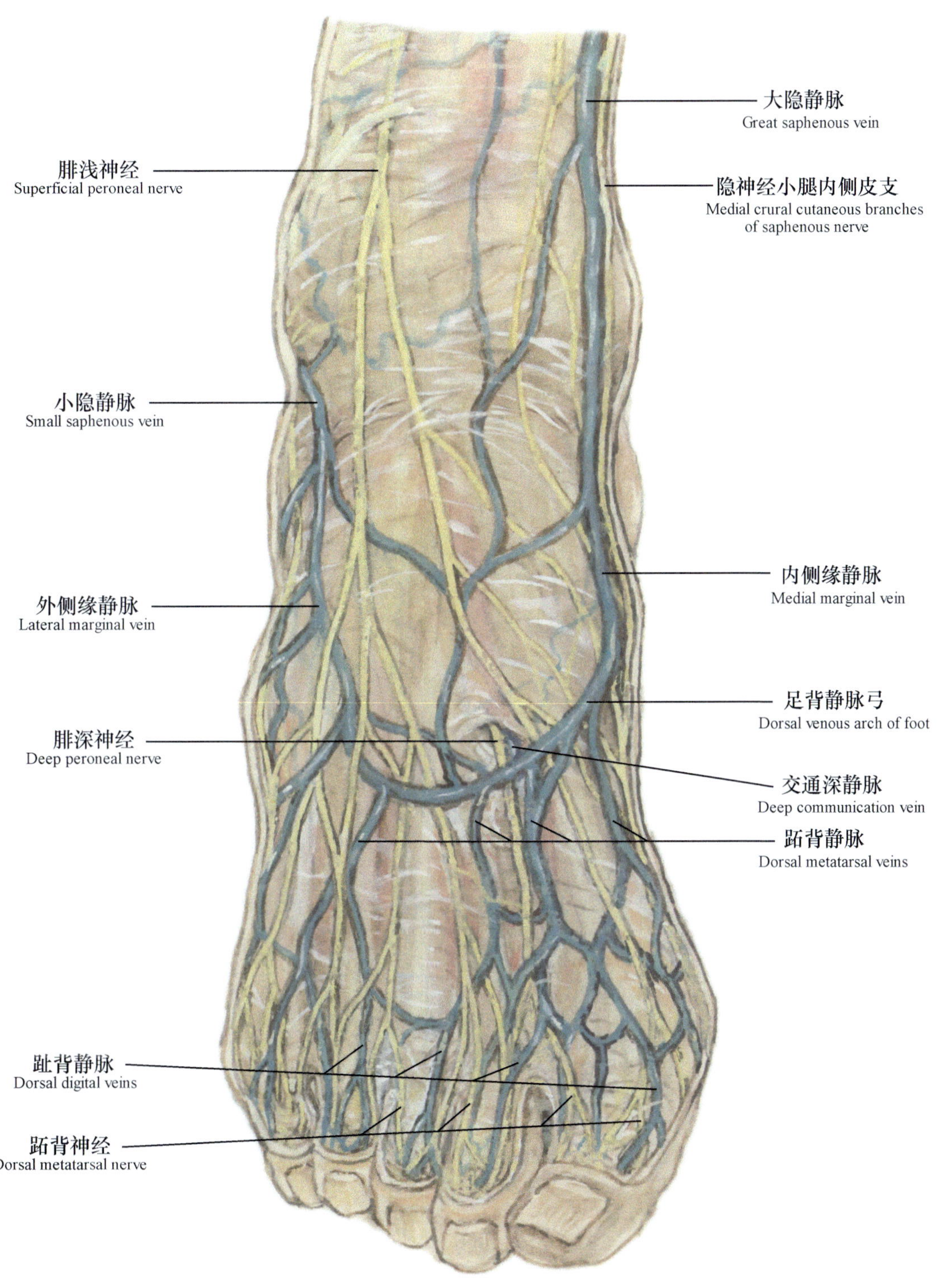

图 1-116 右侧足背（1）
The dorsum of the right foot (1)

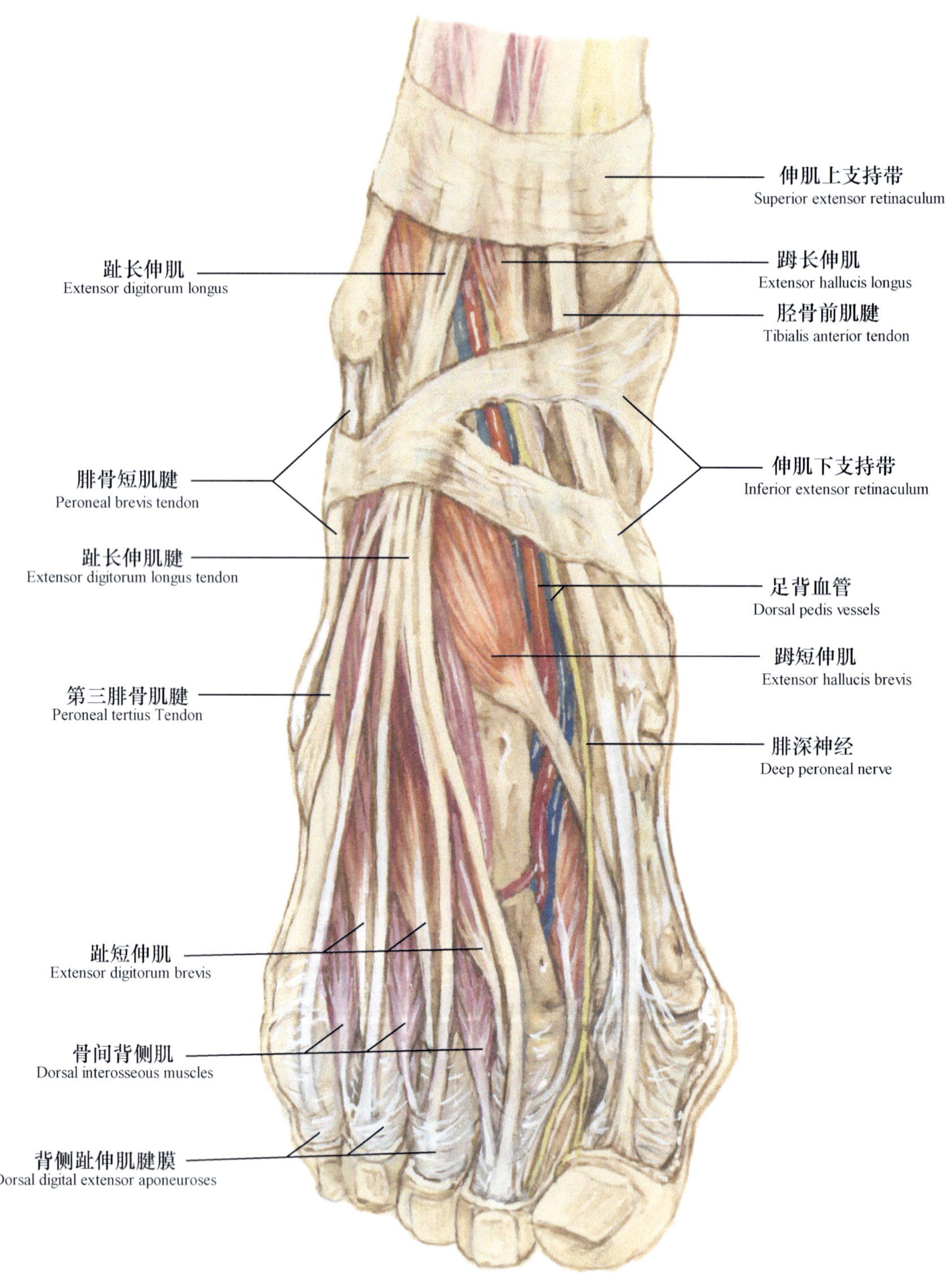

图 1-117 右侧足背（2）
The dorsum of the right foot (2)

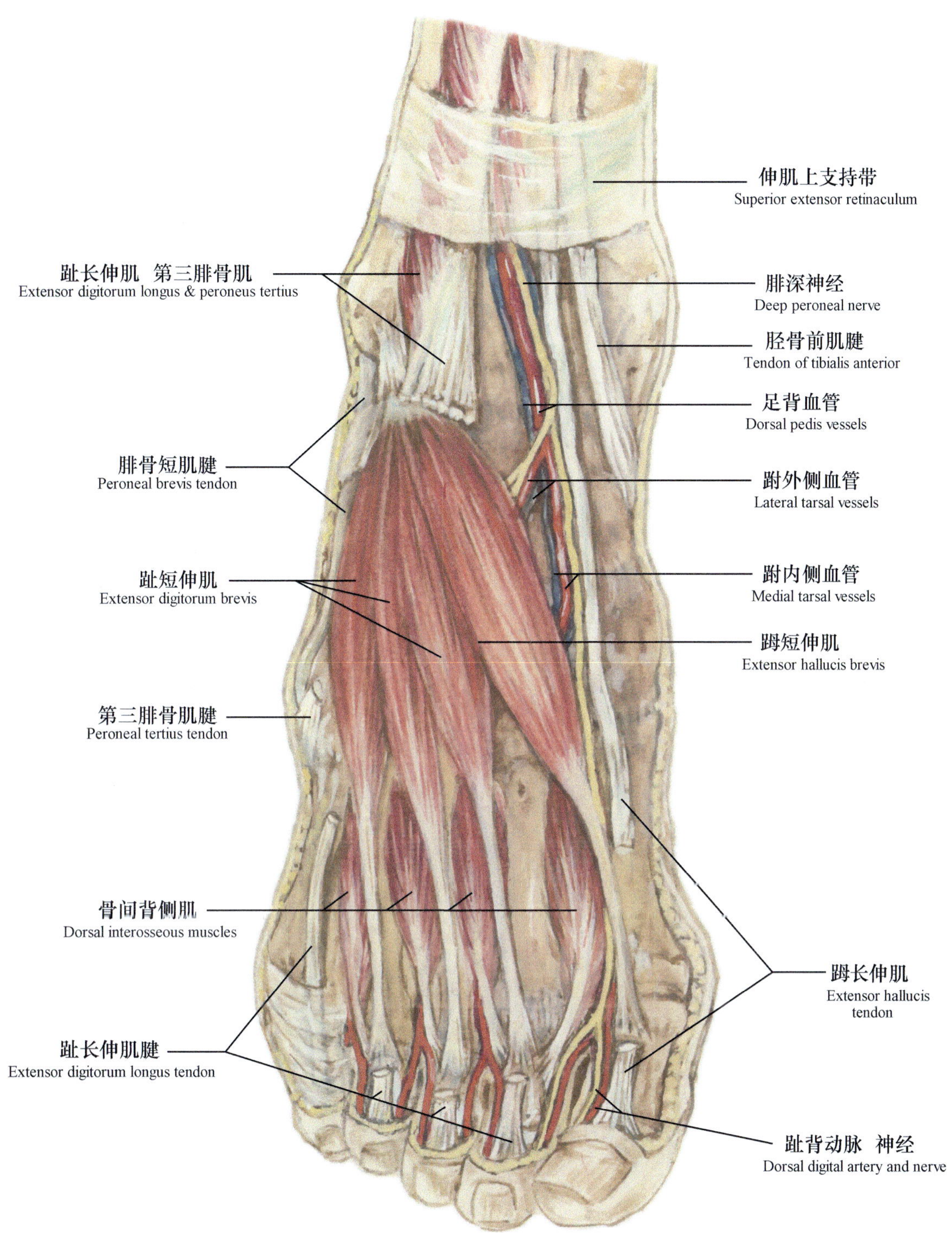

图 1-118 右侧足背（3）
The dorsum of the right foot (3)

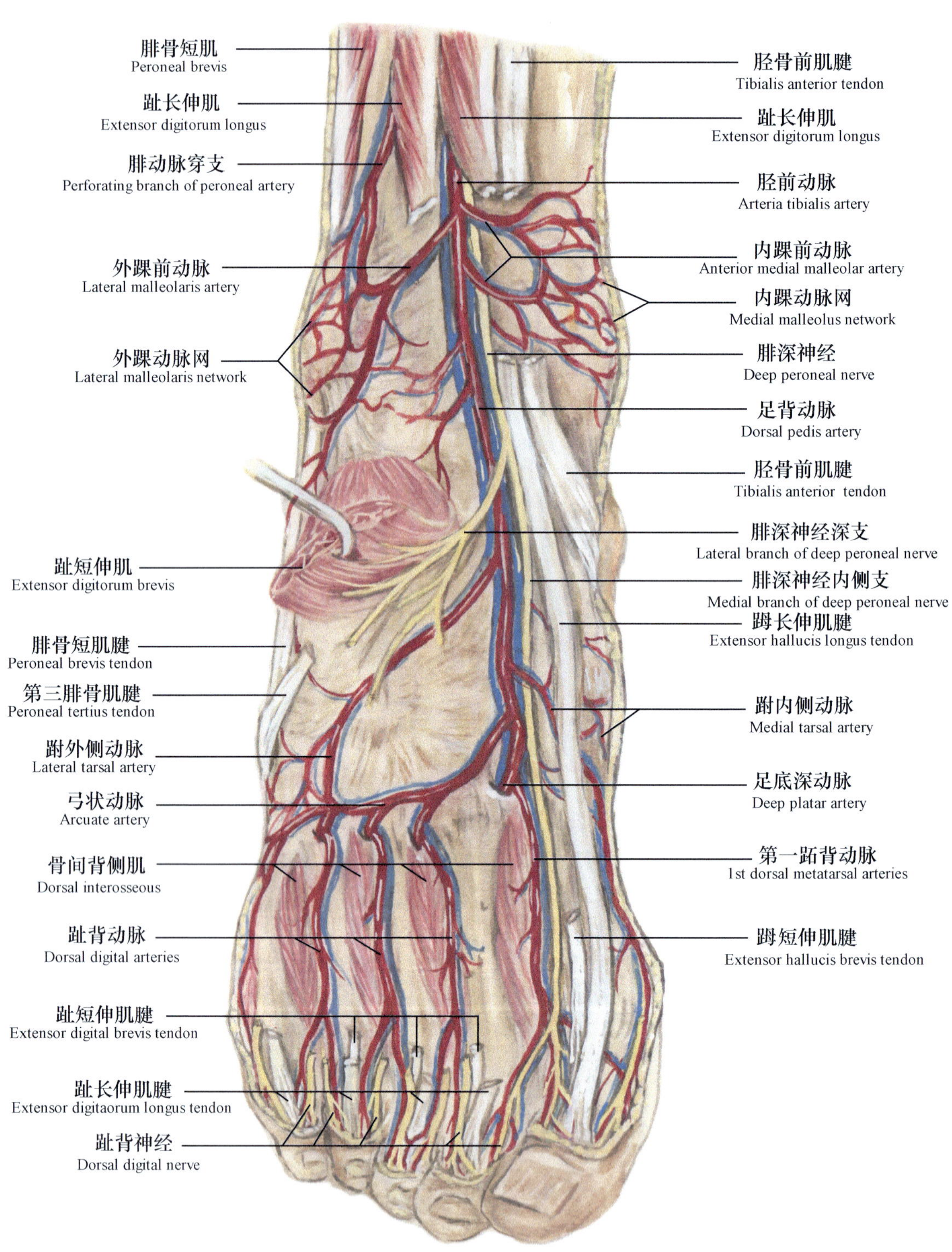

图 1-119 右侧足背（4）
The dorsum of the right foot (4)

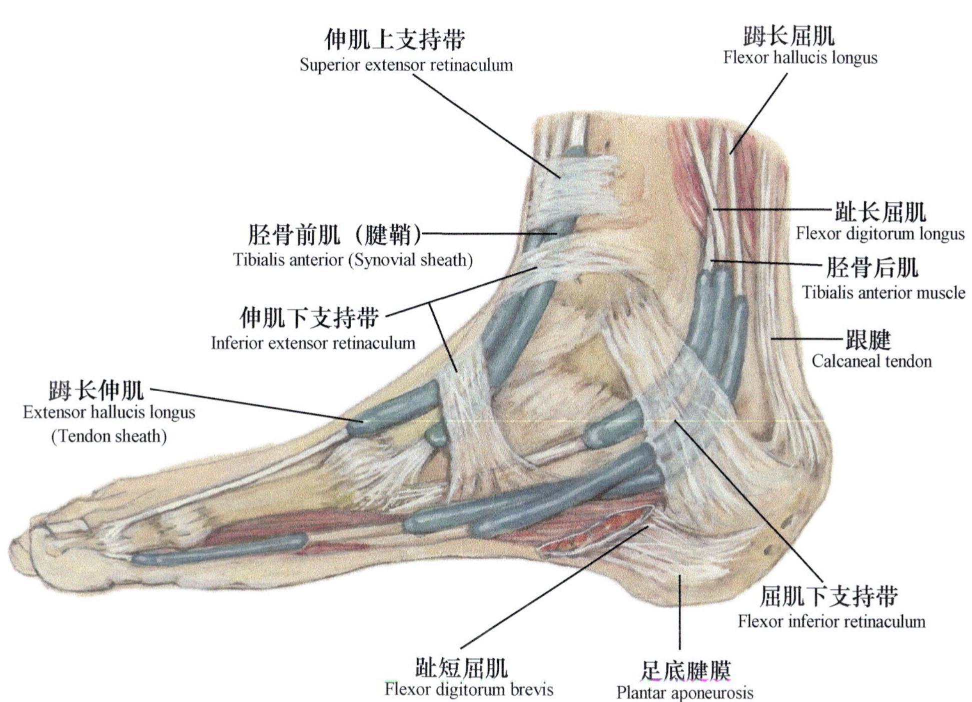

图 1-120　右侧足腱鞘（内侧面观）
Tendon sheathes of the right foot (Midial aspect)

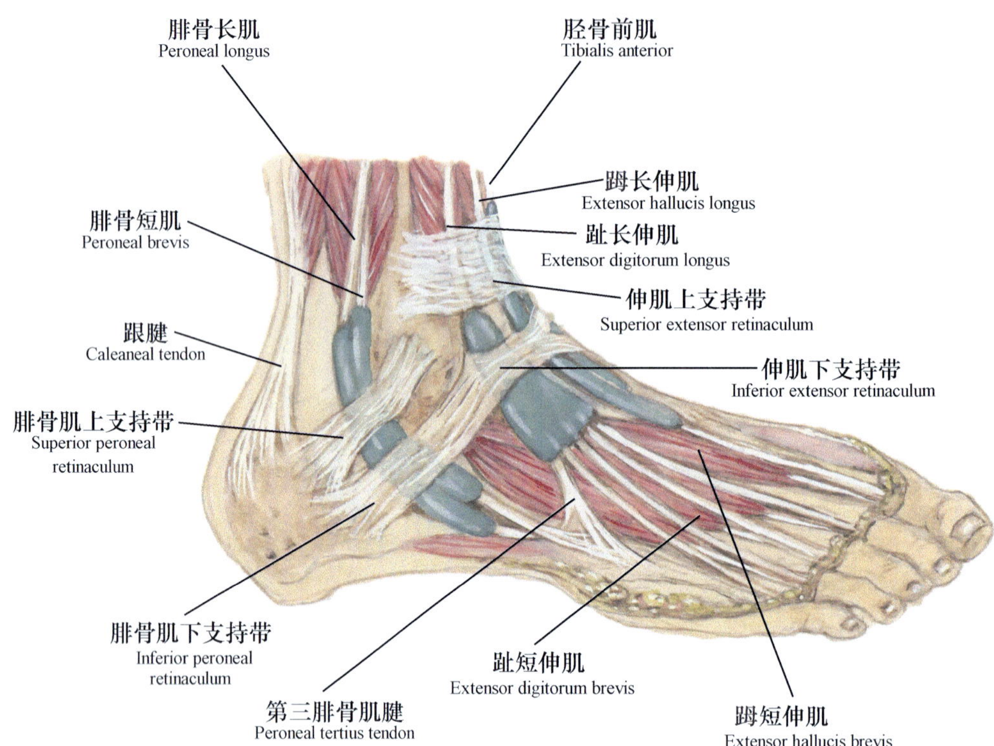

图 1-121　右侧足腱鞘（外侧面观）
Tendon sheathes of the right foot (Lateral aspect)

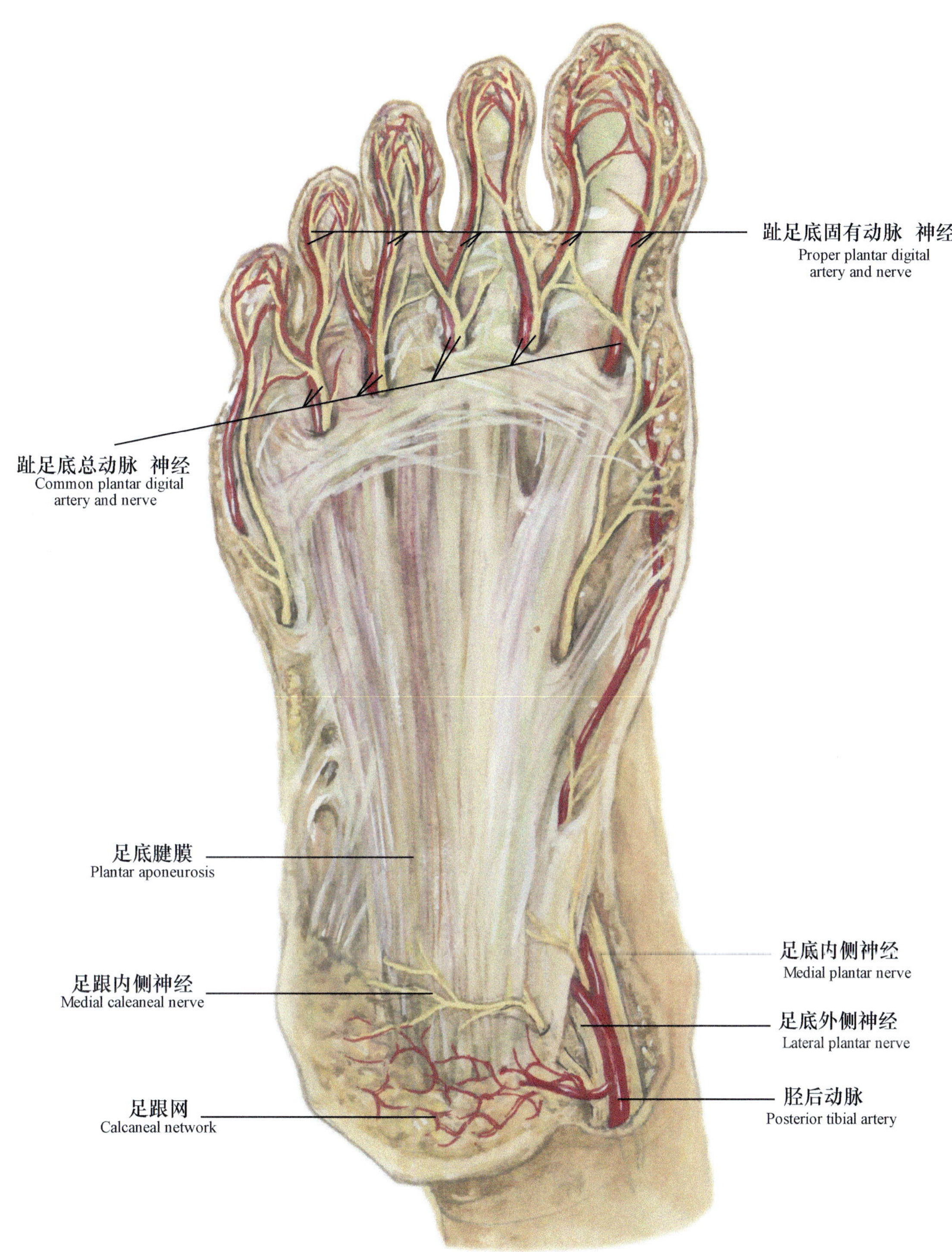

图 1-122 右侧足底（1）
The sole of the right foot (1)

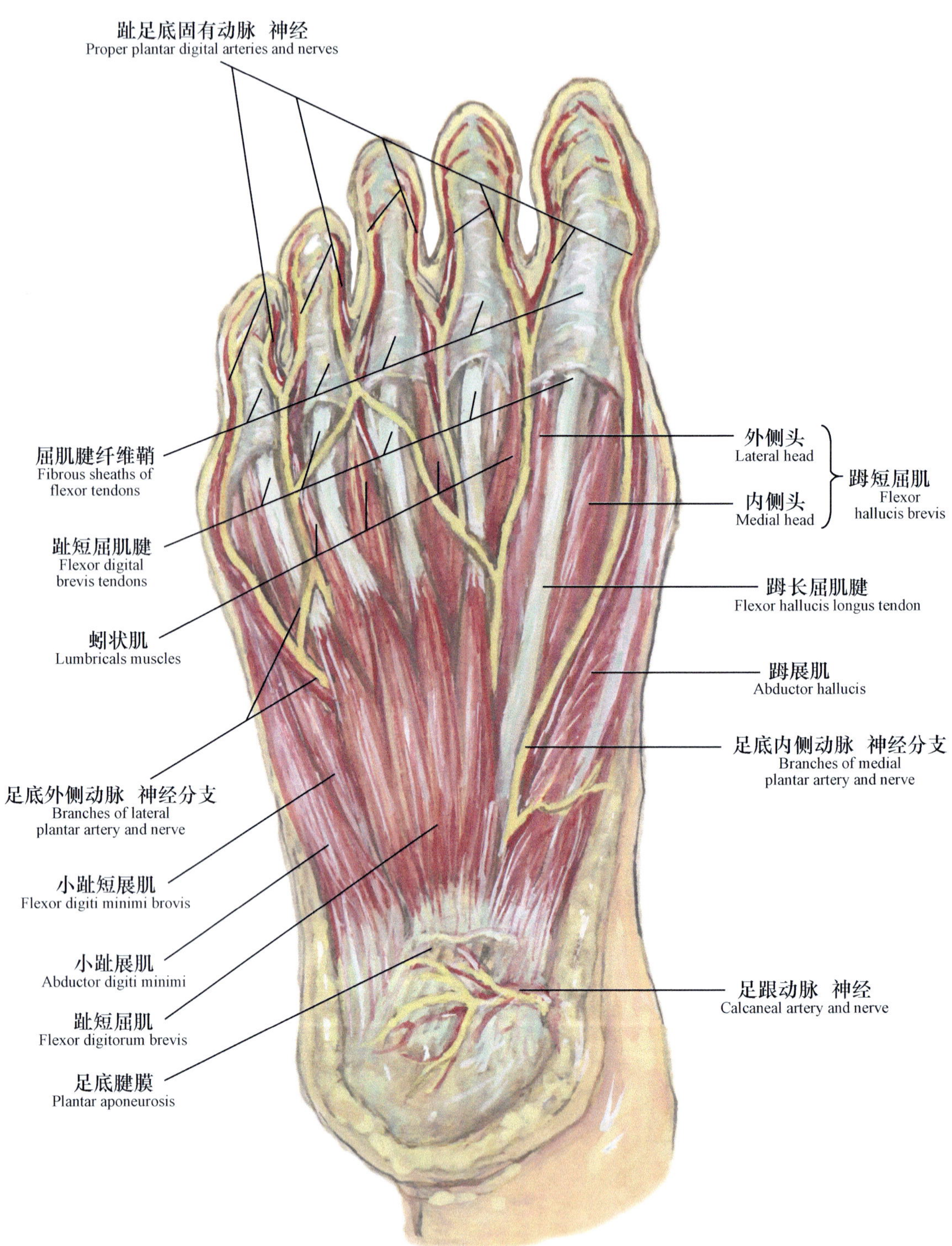

图 1-123 右侧足底（2）
The sole of the right foot (2)

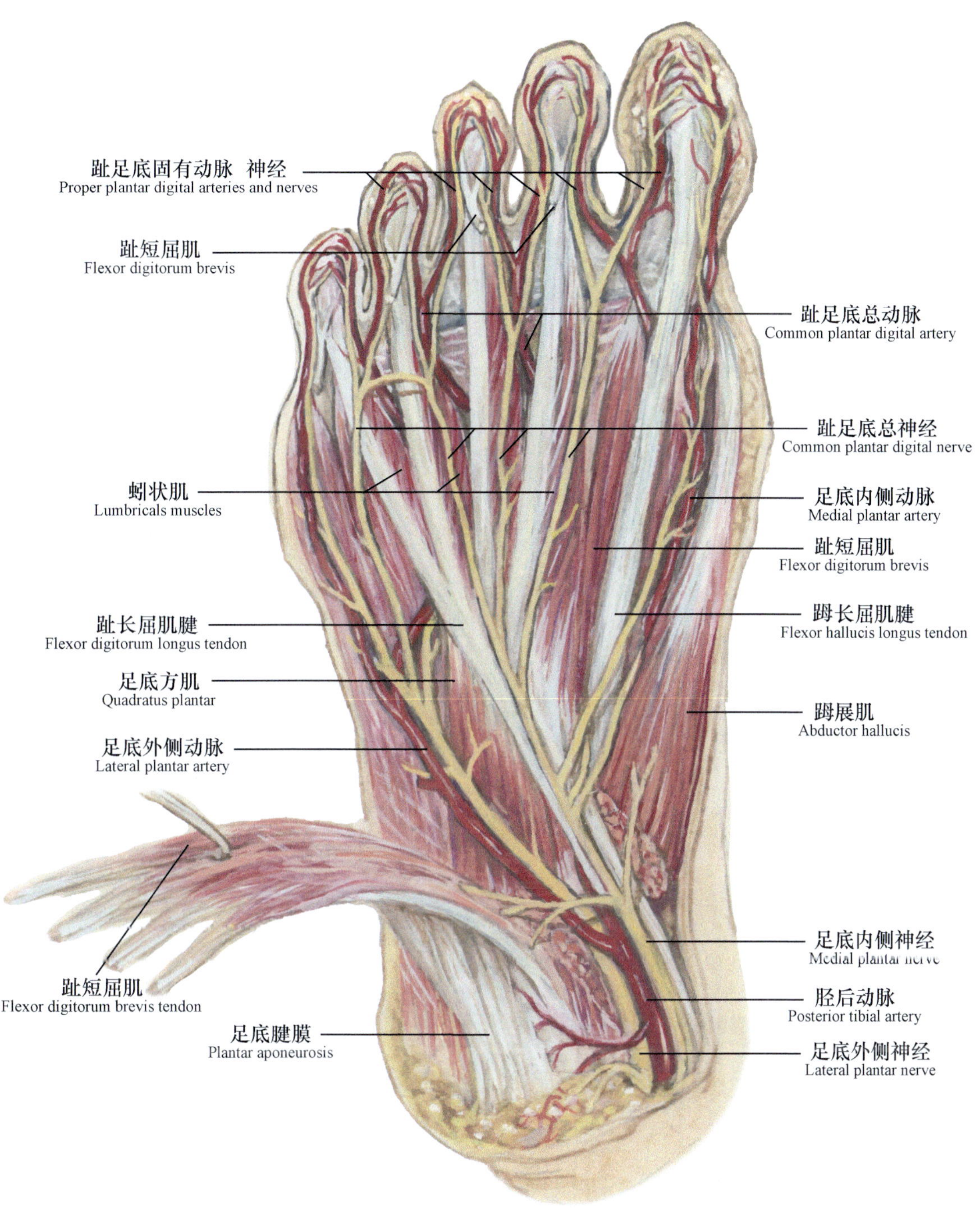

图 1-124　右侧足底（3）
The sole of the right foot (3)

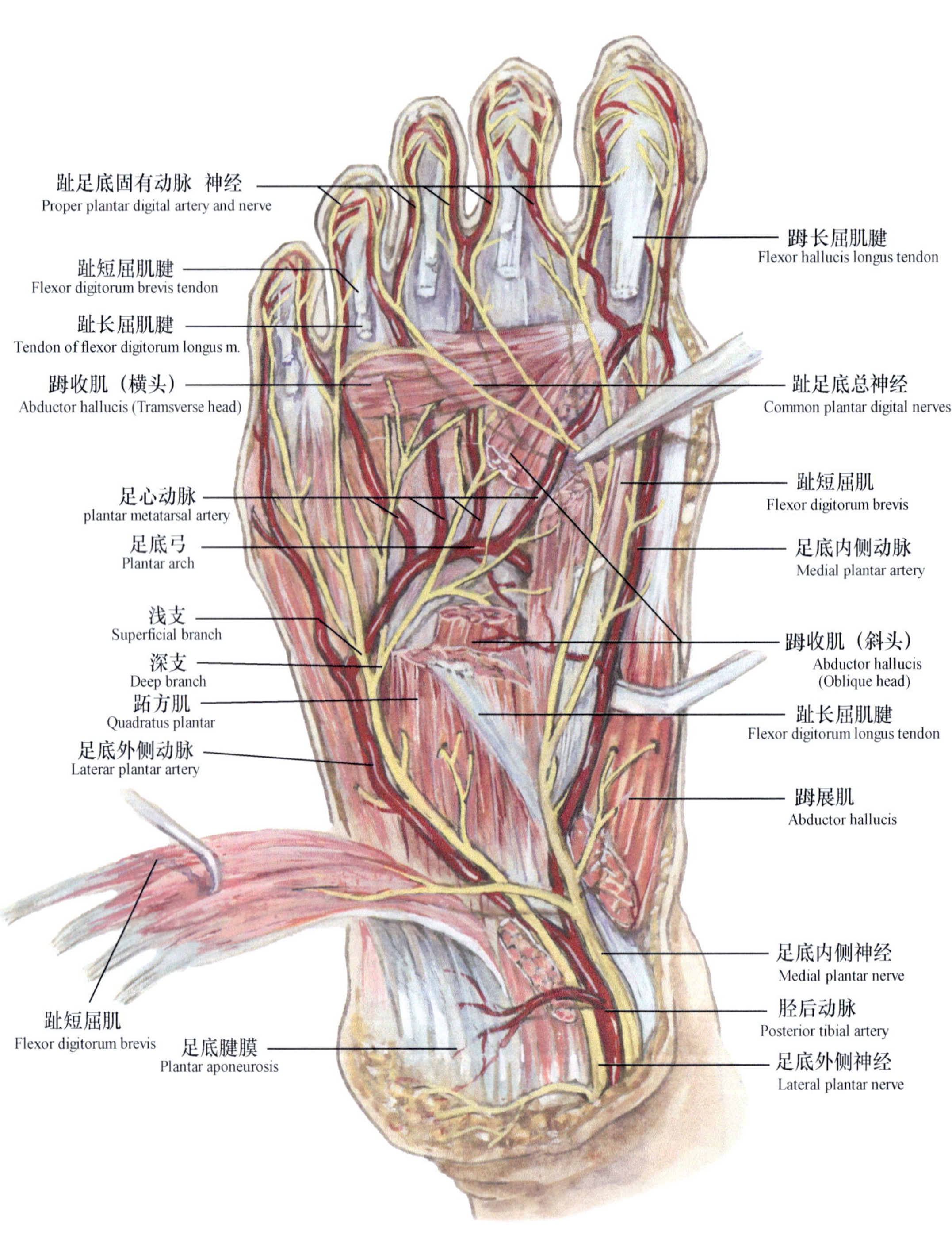

图 1-125 右侧足底（4）
The sole of the right foot (4)

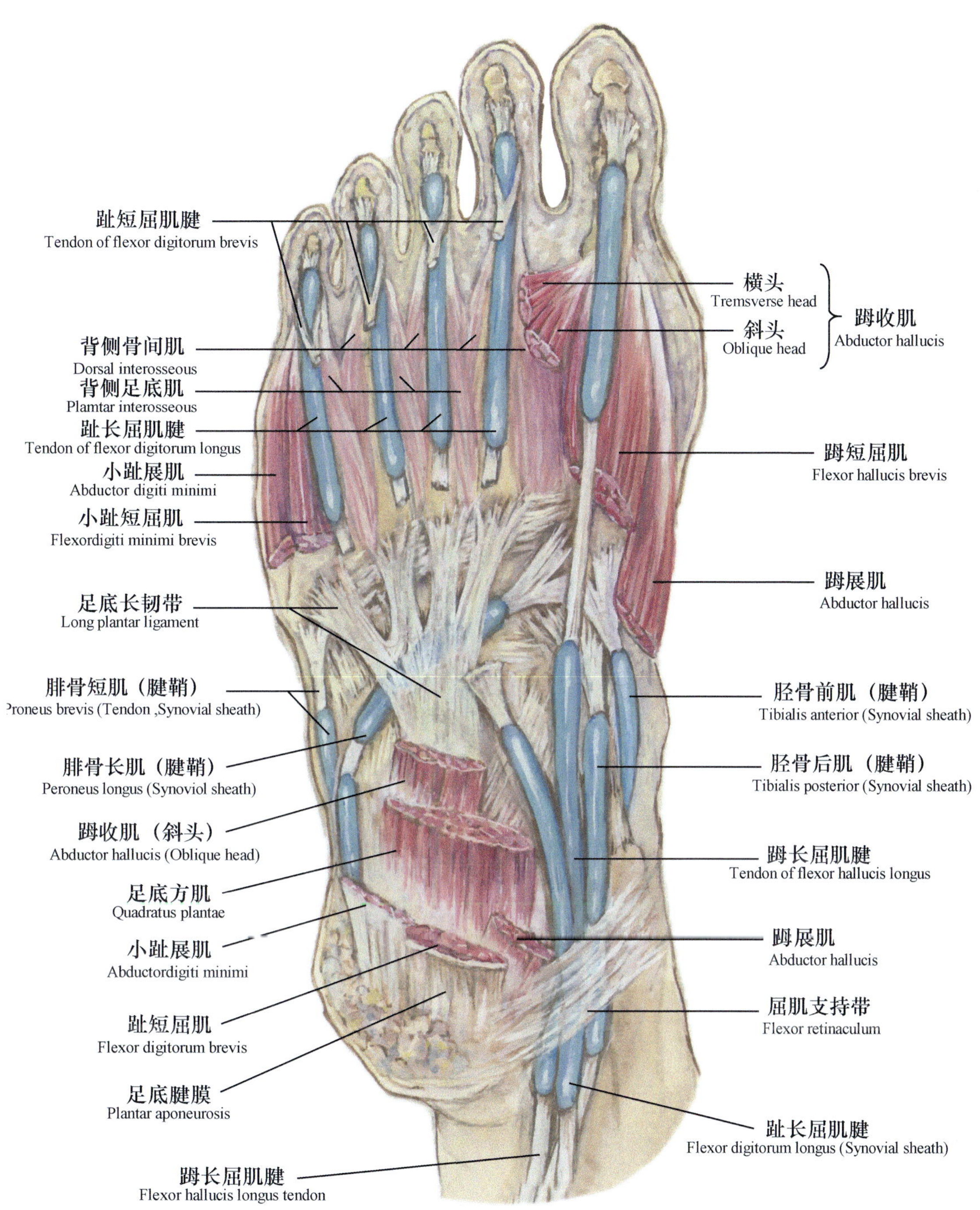

图 1-126　右侧足底腱鞘
Tendon sheath of the right foot

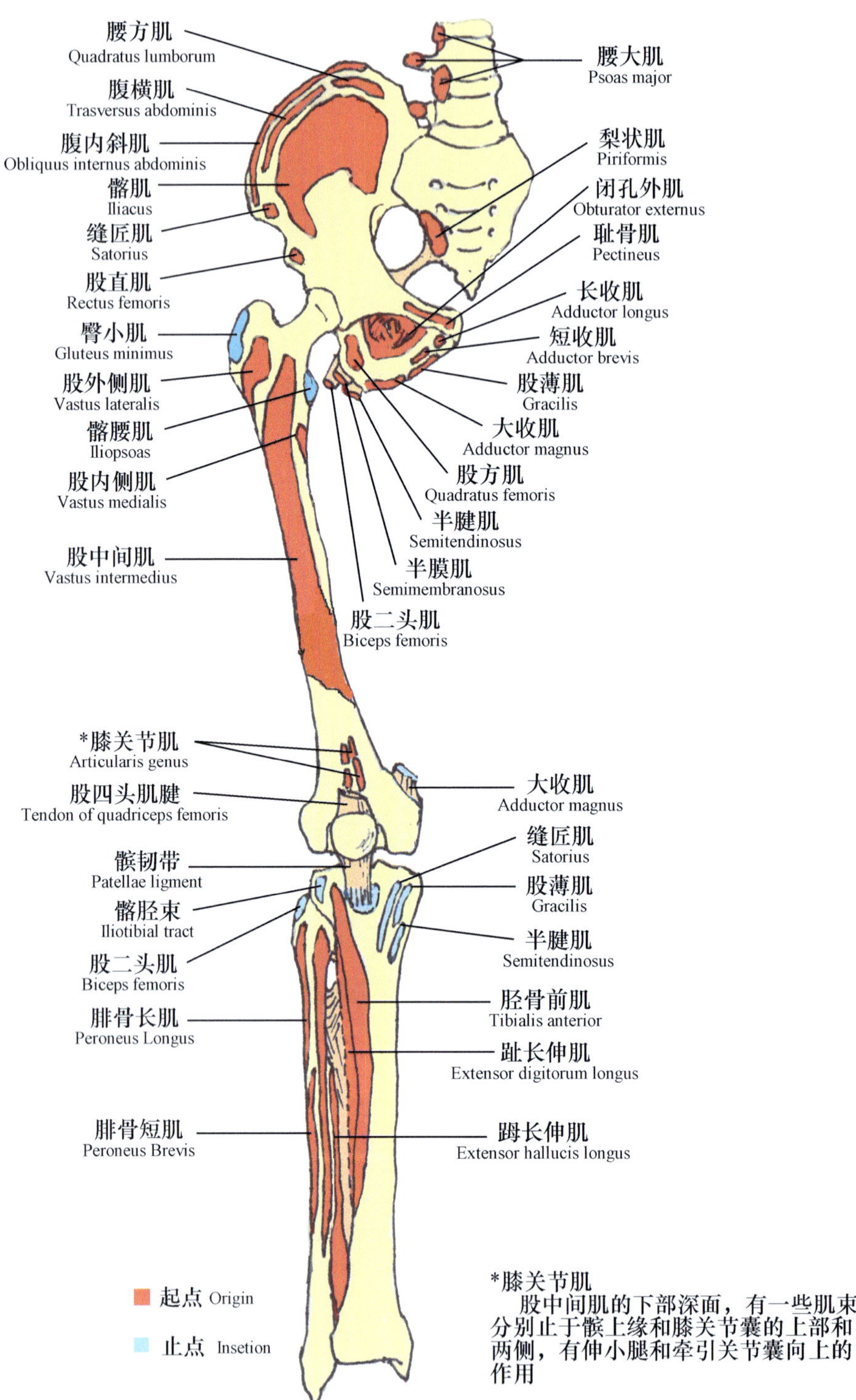

*膝关节肌

股中间肌的下部深面，有一些肌束分别止于髌上缘和膝关节囊的上部和两侧，有伸小腿和牵引关节囊向上的作用

图 1-127　右侧下肢肌前面的起止点示意图

Schematic diagram of the start and stop points of the front of the right lower limb muscle

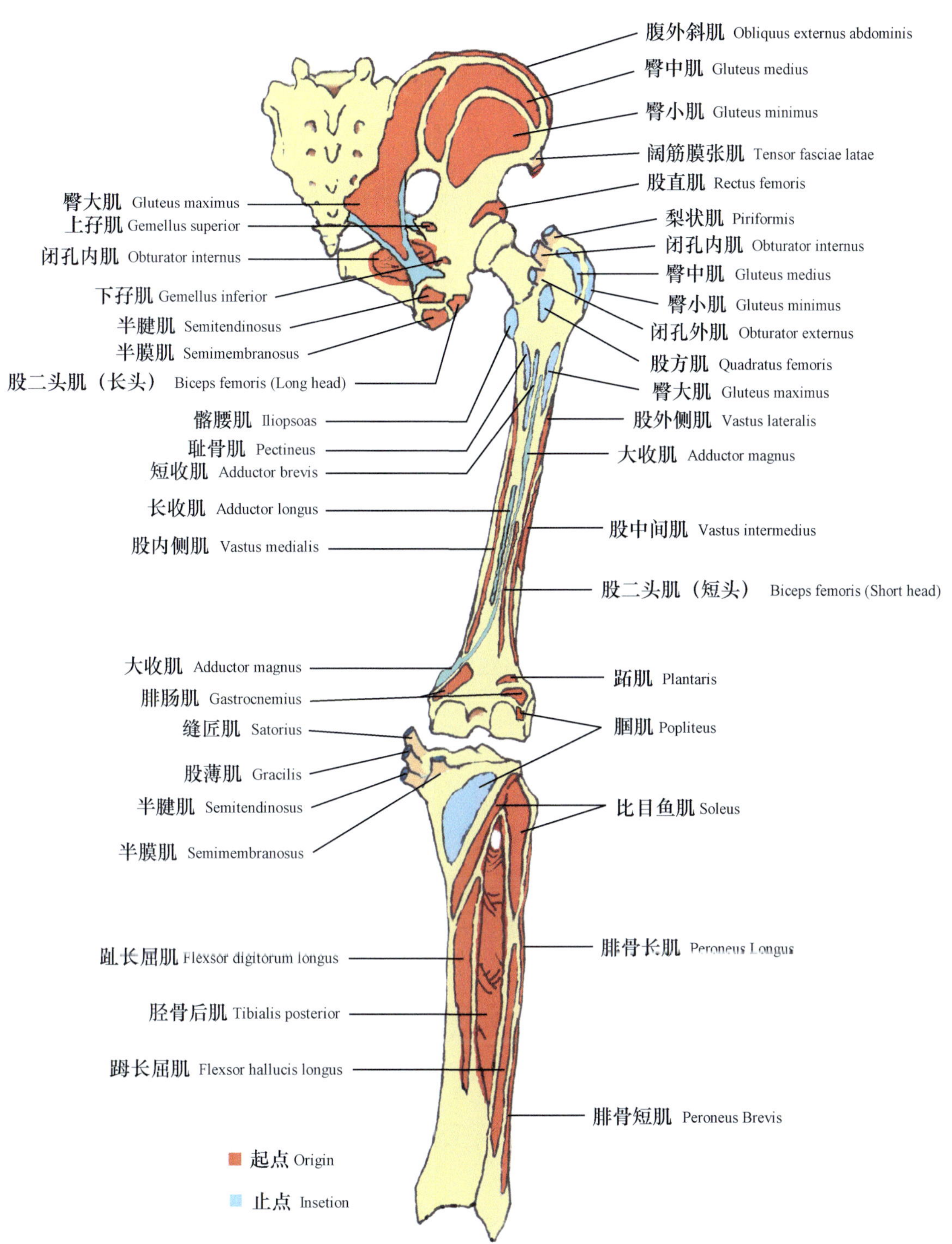

图 1-128 右侧下肢肌后面的起止点

The start and stop points of the back of the right lower limb muscle

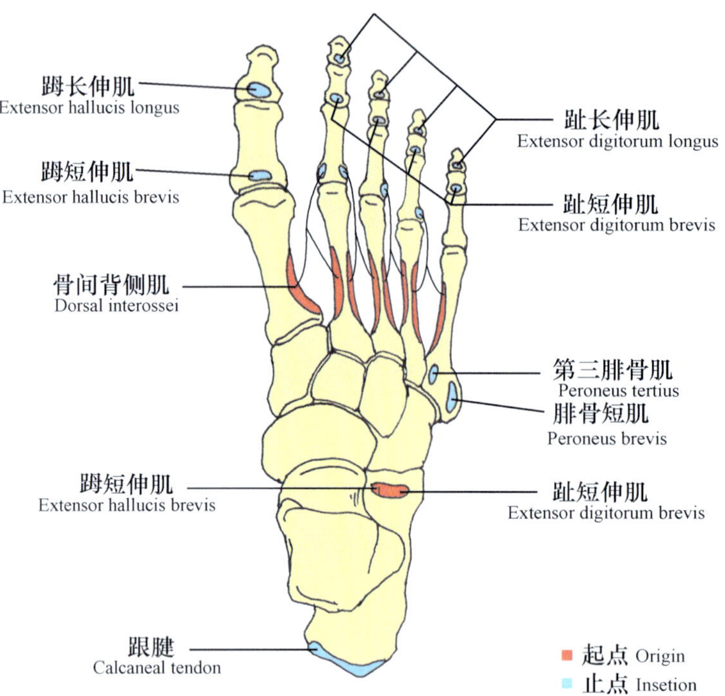

图 1-129 右侧足背肌起止点
The attachments of muscles of the right foot

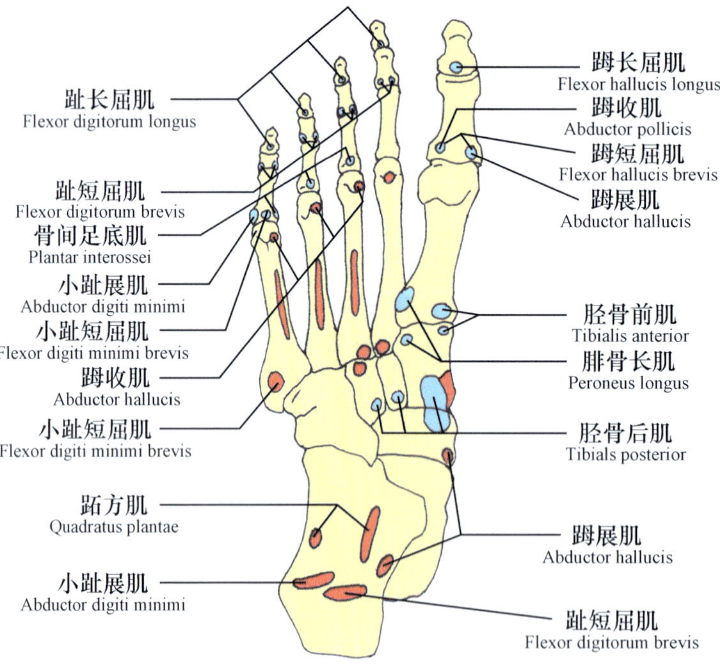

图 1-130 右侧足底肌起止点
The attachments of muscles of the right foot plantar aspect

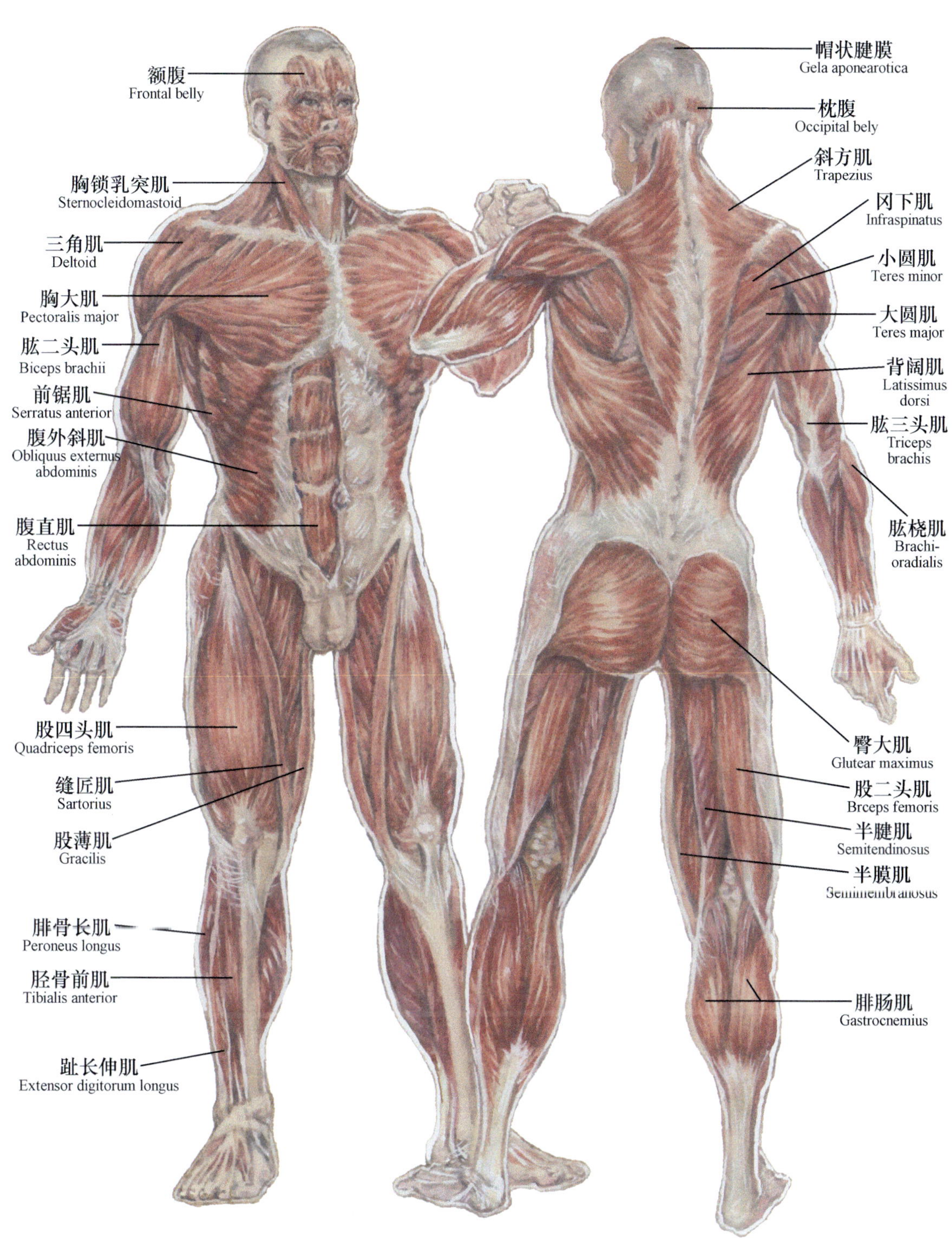

图 1-131　全身肌概观
A general view of muscles of the body

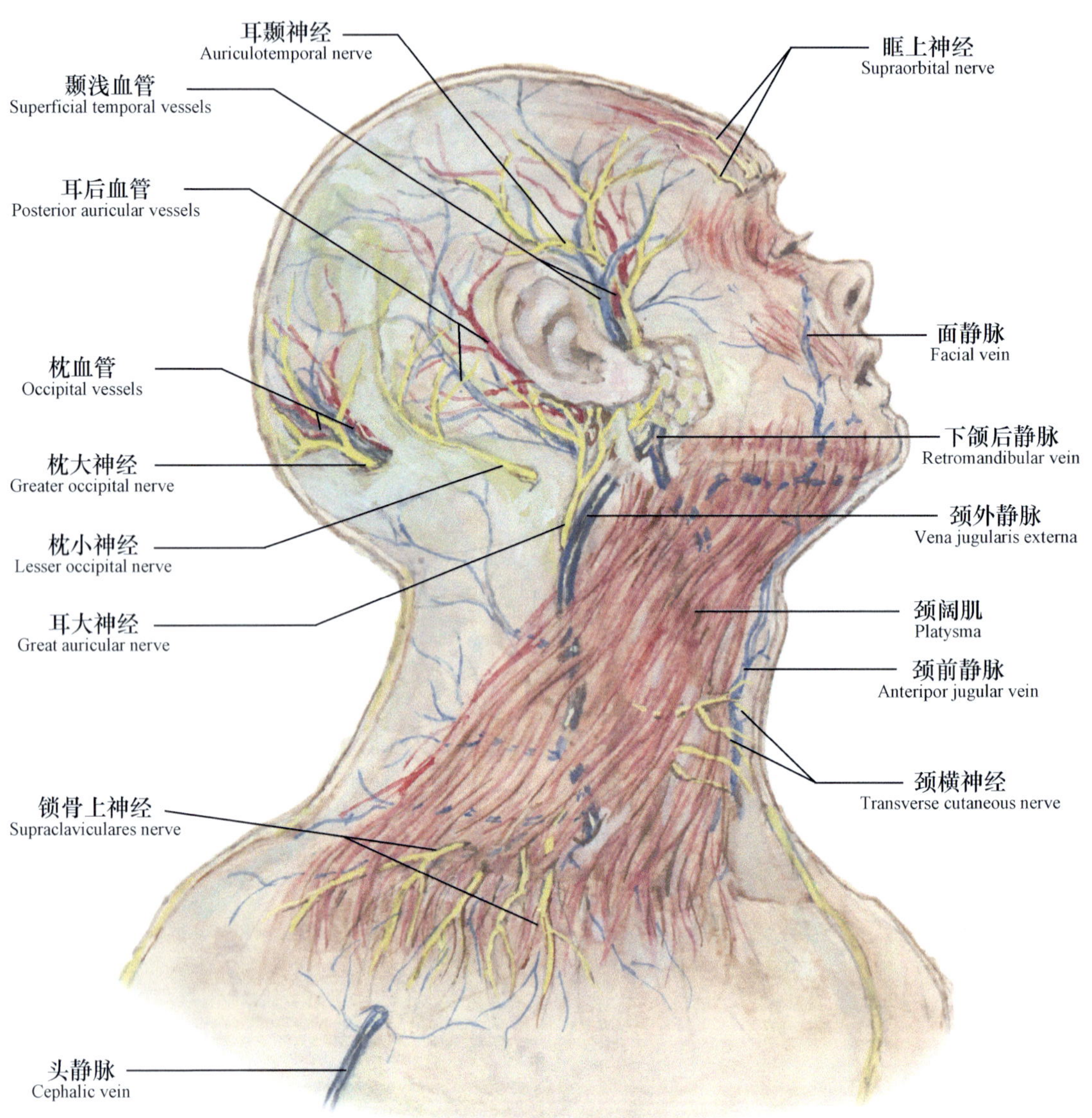

图 1-132 头颈（1）
The head and neck (1)

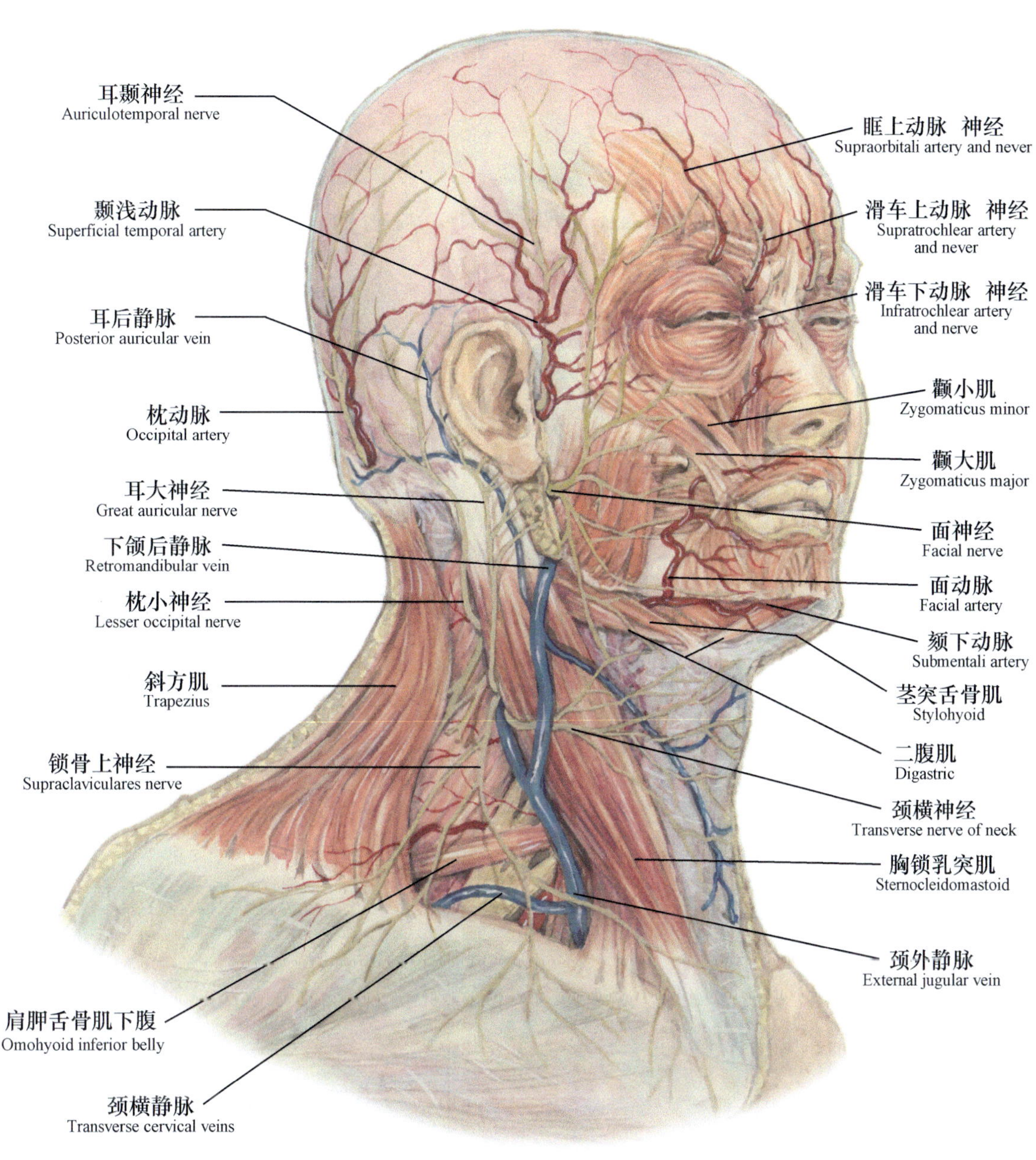

图 1-133 头颈（2）
The head and neck (2)

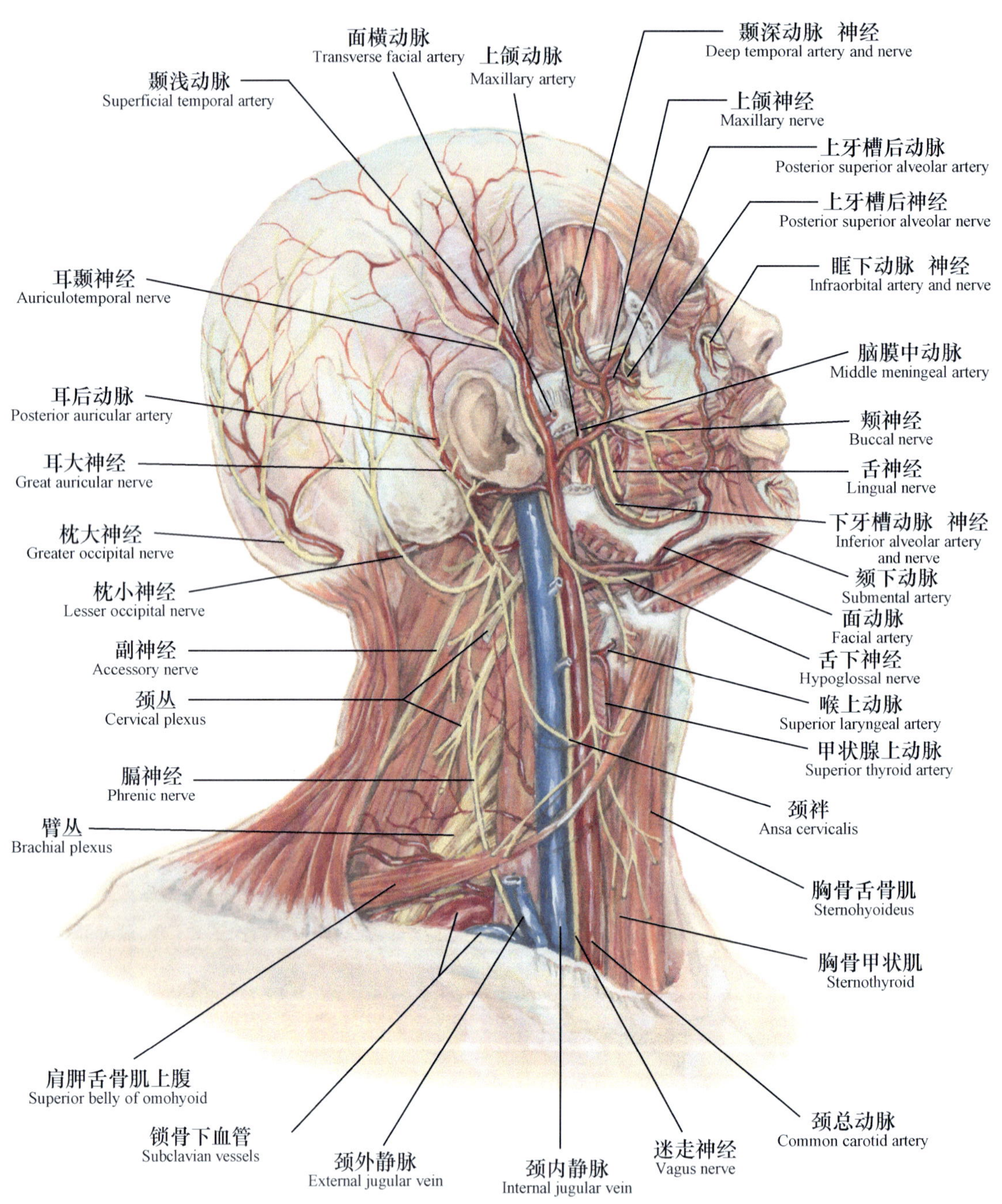

图 1-134 头颈（3）
The head and neck (3)

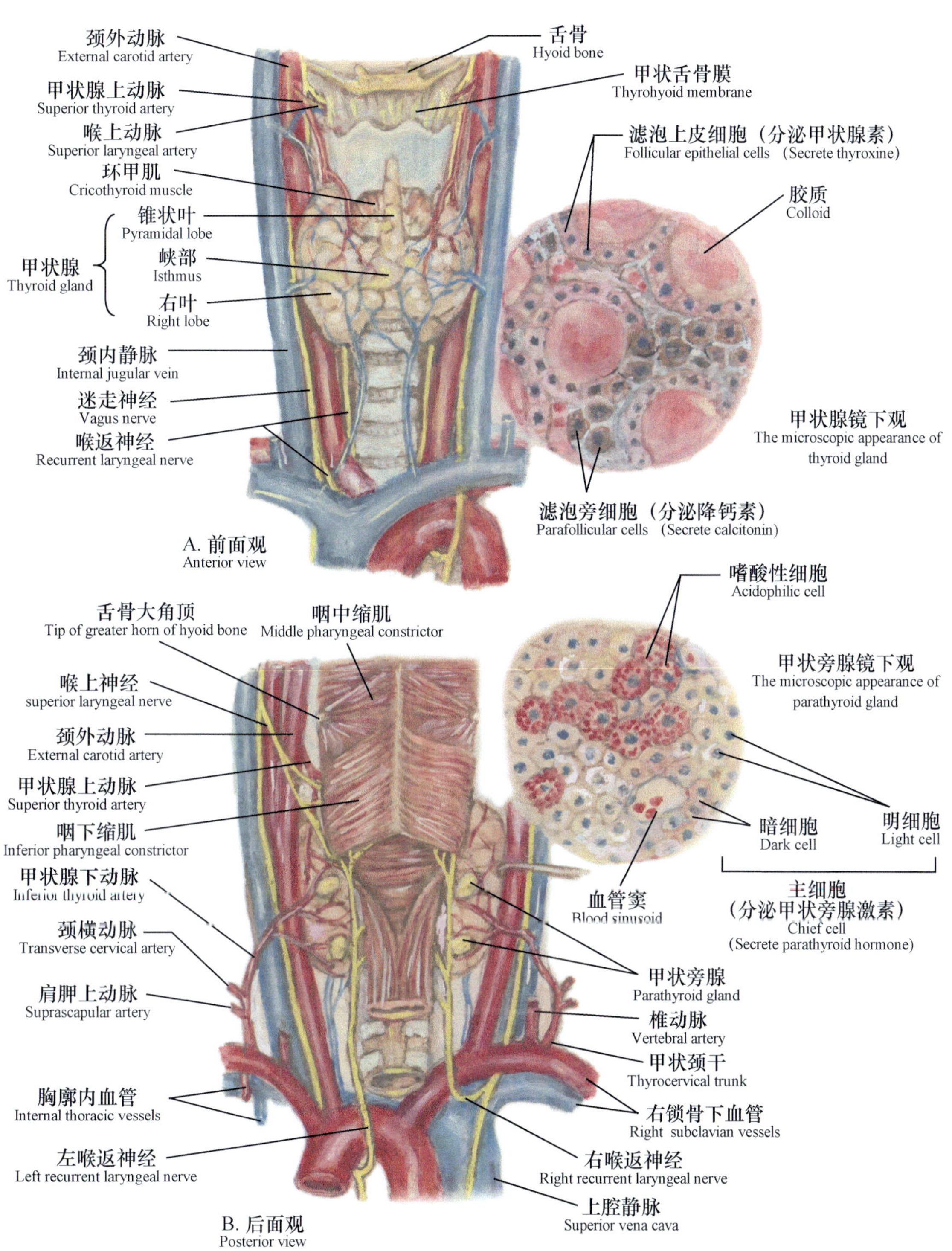

图 1-135 甲状腺与甲状旁腺
Thyroid gland and parathyroid gland

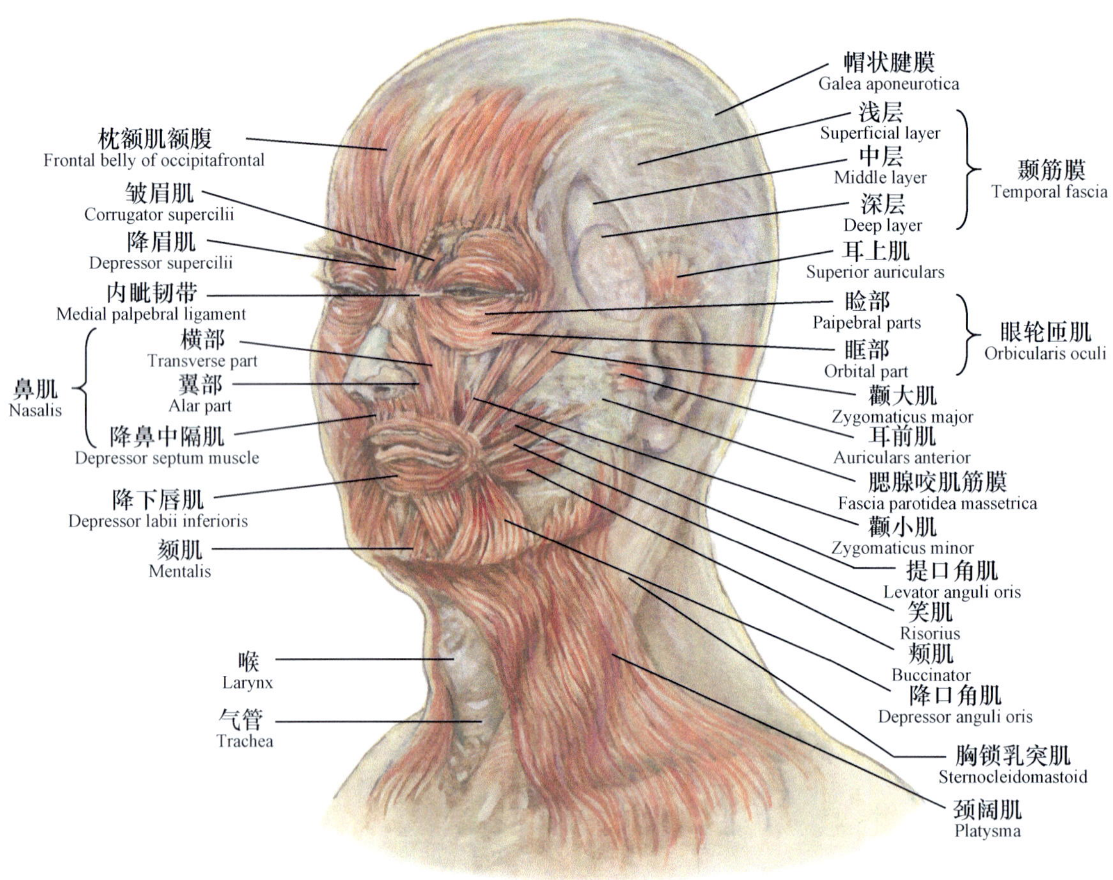

图 1-136 头颈肌（1）
Muscles of head and neck (1)

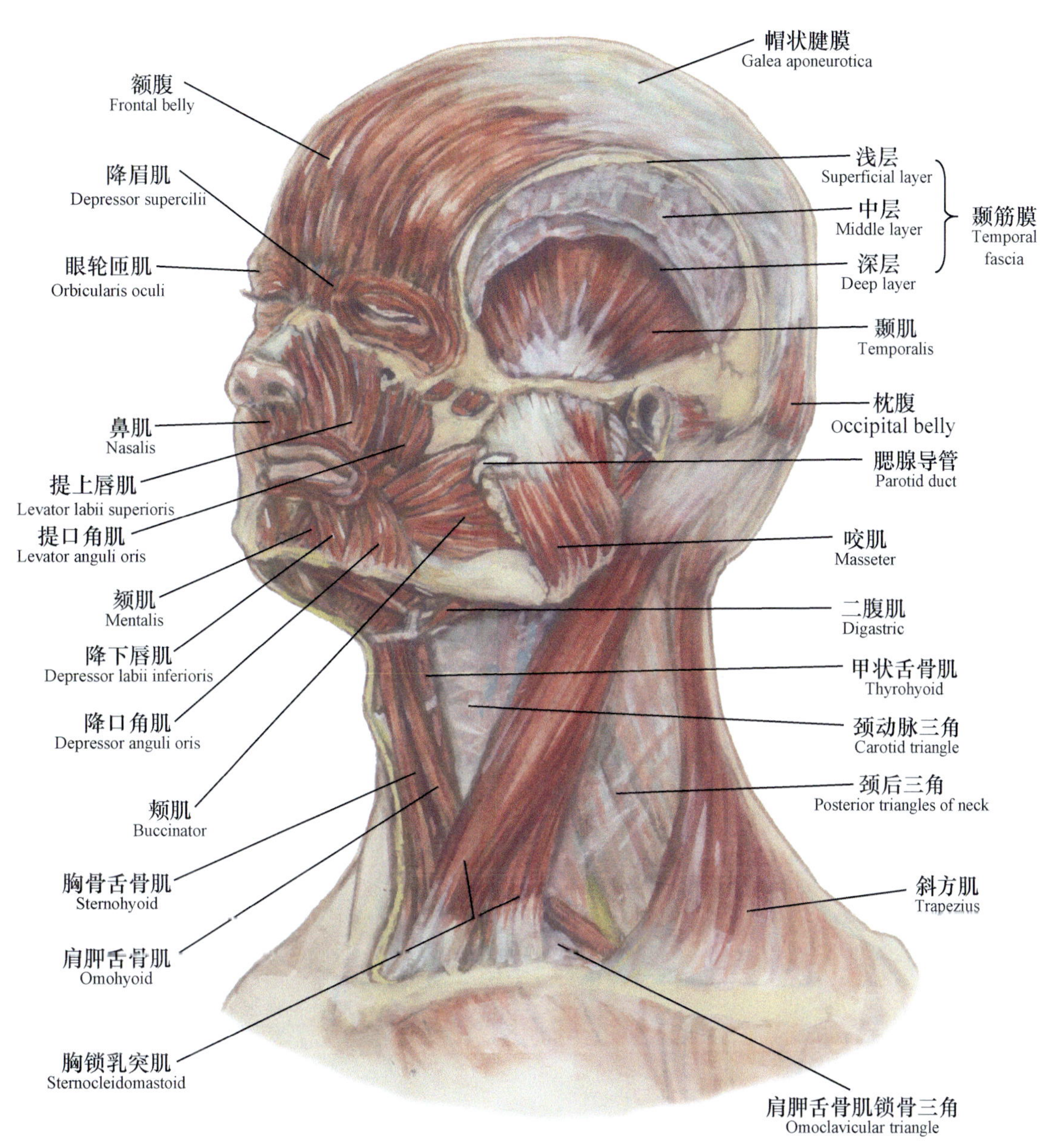

图 1-137 头颈肌（2）
Muscles of head and neck (2)

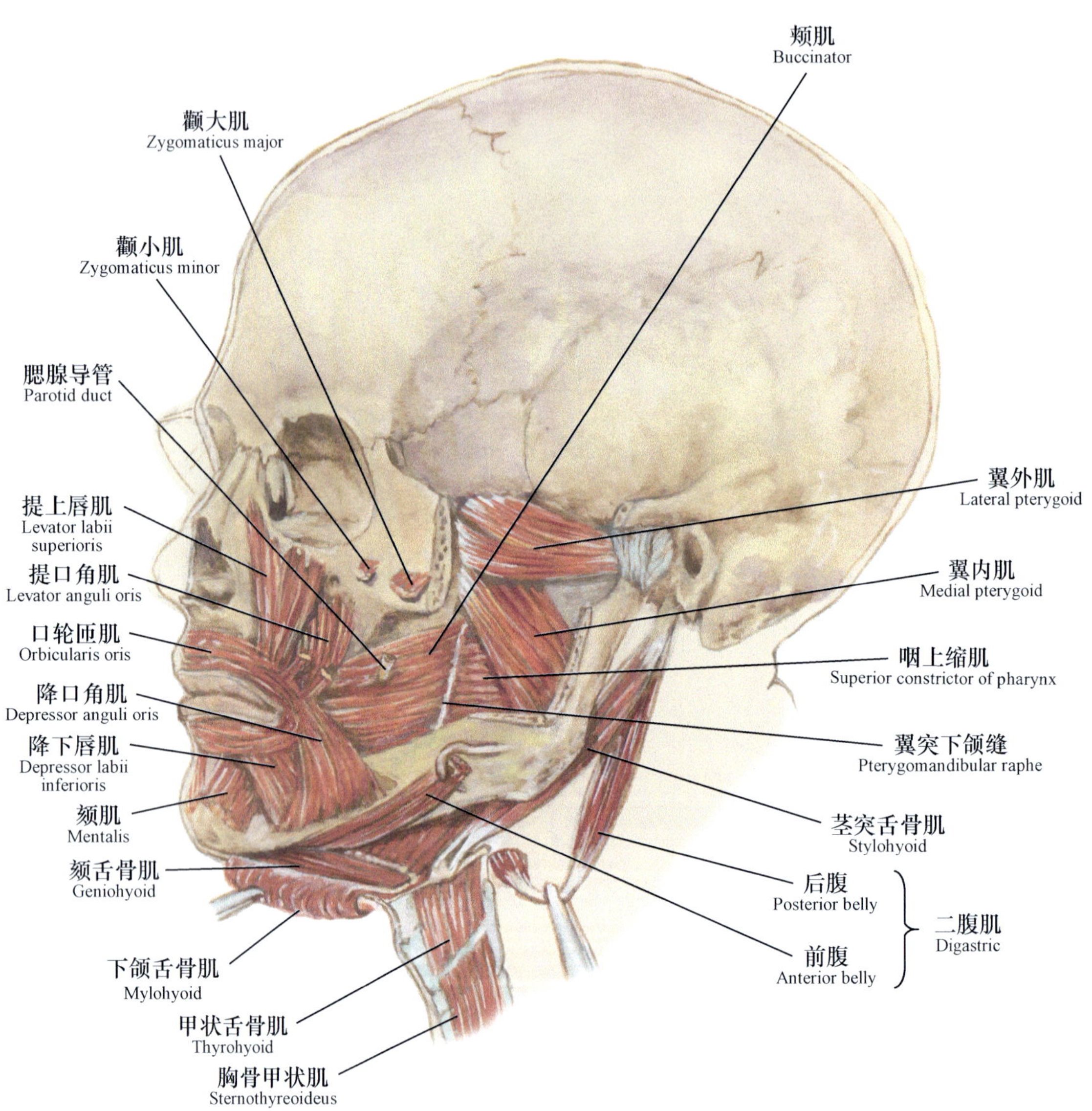

图 1-138 头颈肌（3）
Muscles of head and neck (3)

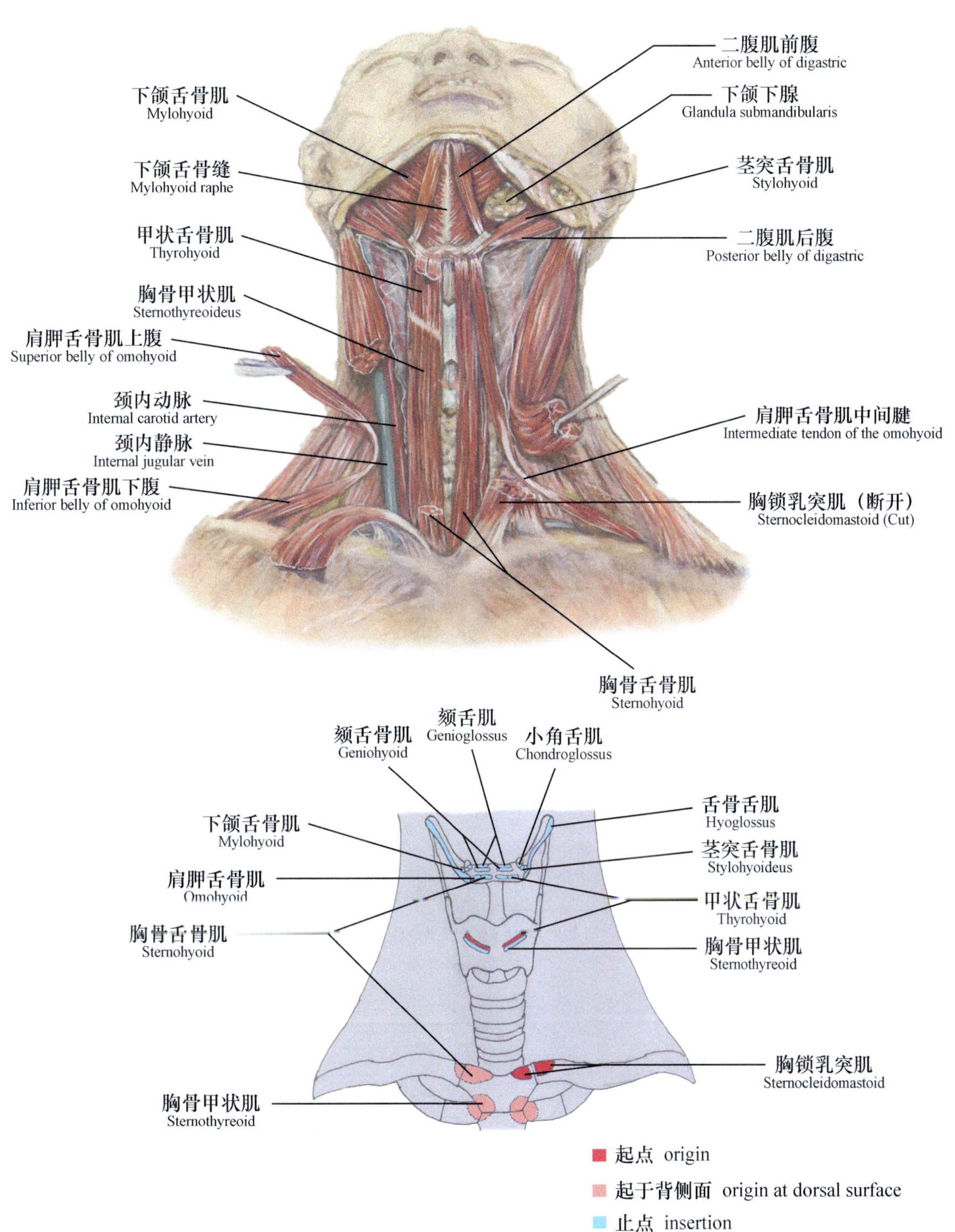

图 1-139　头颈肌（4）
Muscles of head and neck (4)

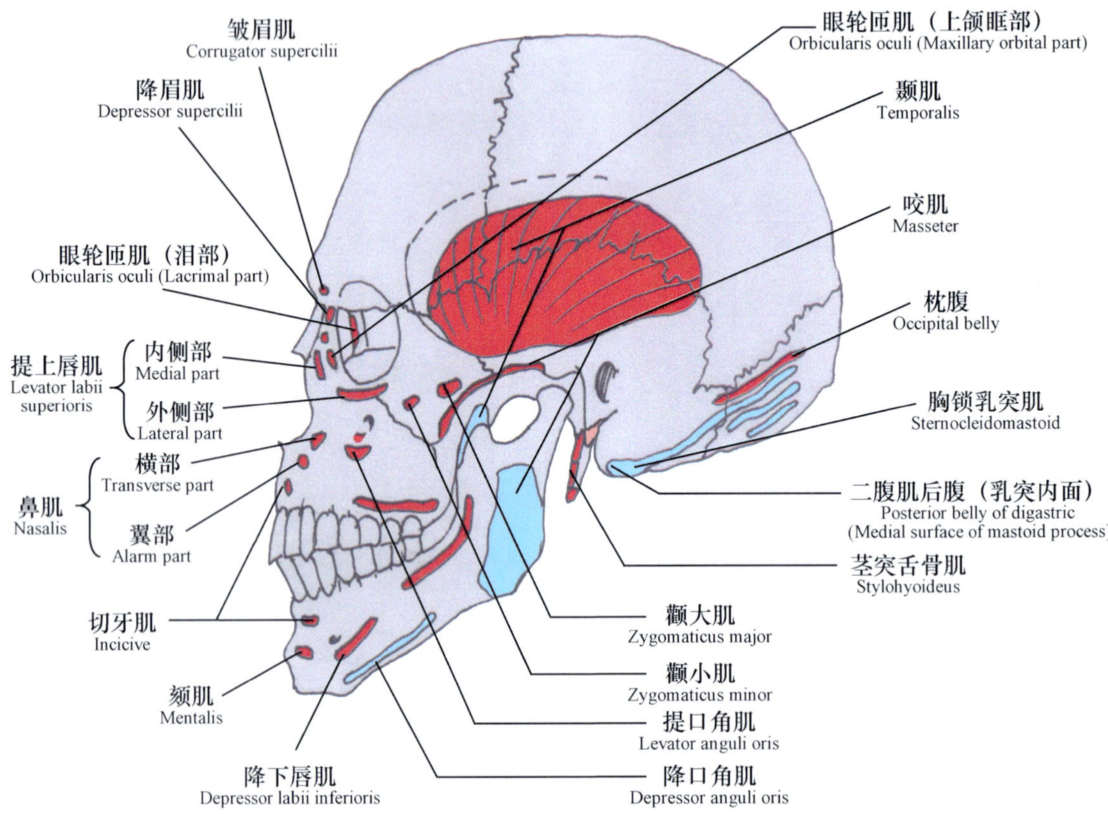

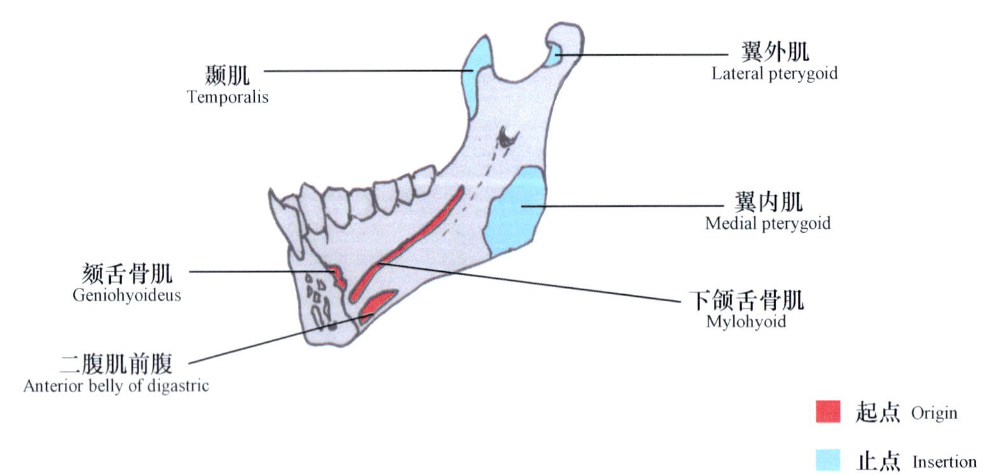

图 1-140 头肌起止示意图

A diagram showing attachment of muscles of the head

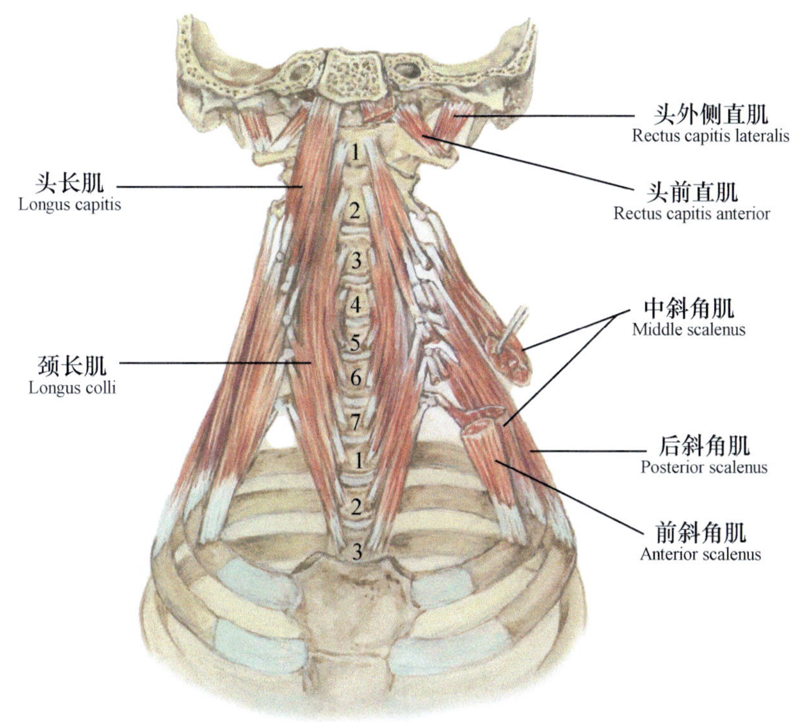

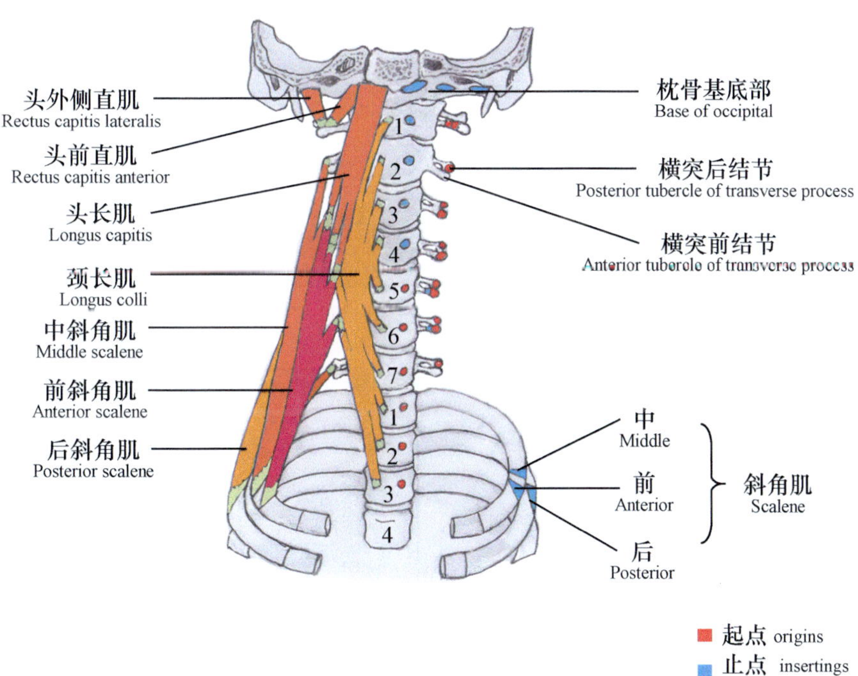

图 1-141 头颈肌和椎前肌

Muscles of the head and neck, the anterior vertebral muscles

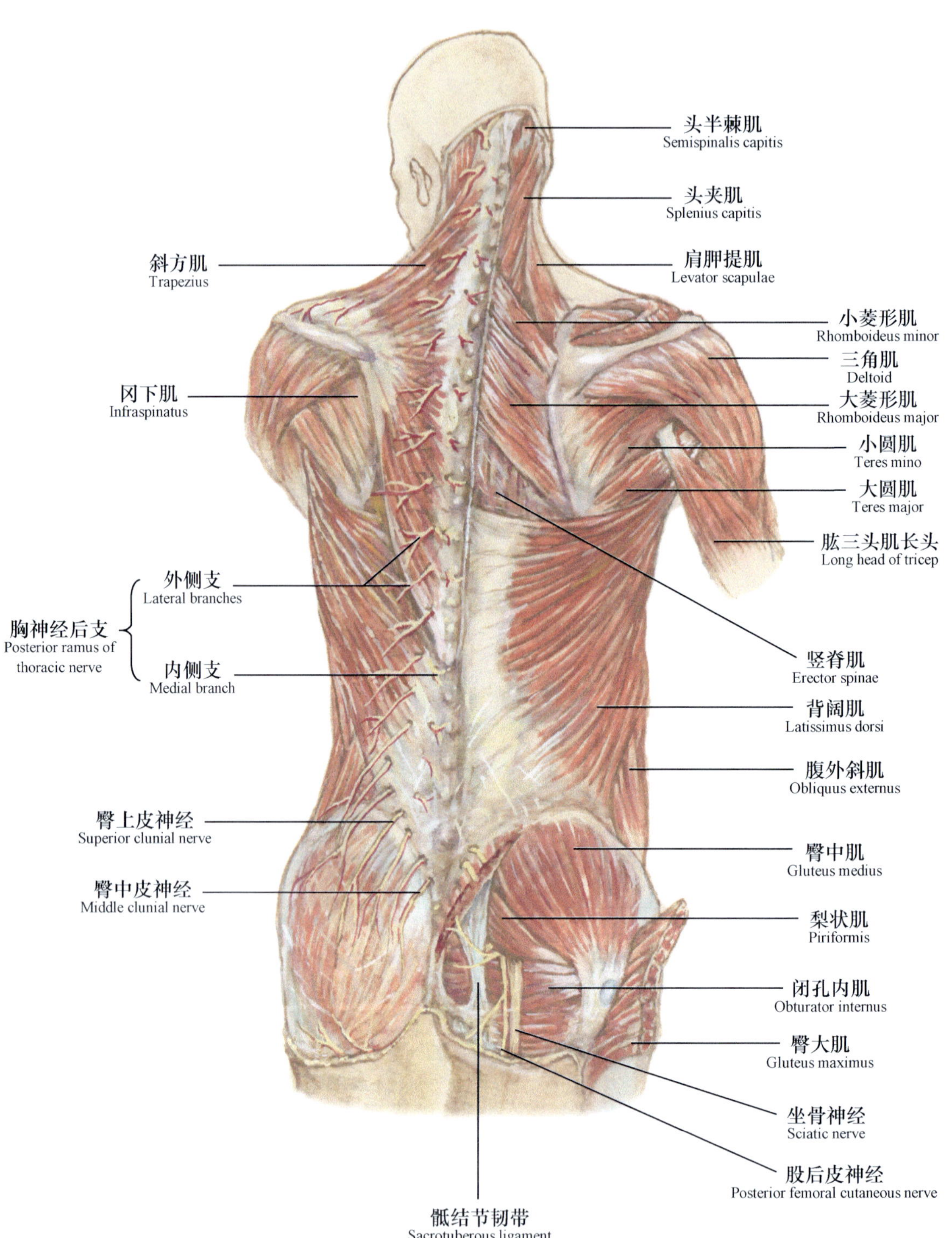

图 1-142 背肌（1）
Muscles of the back (1)

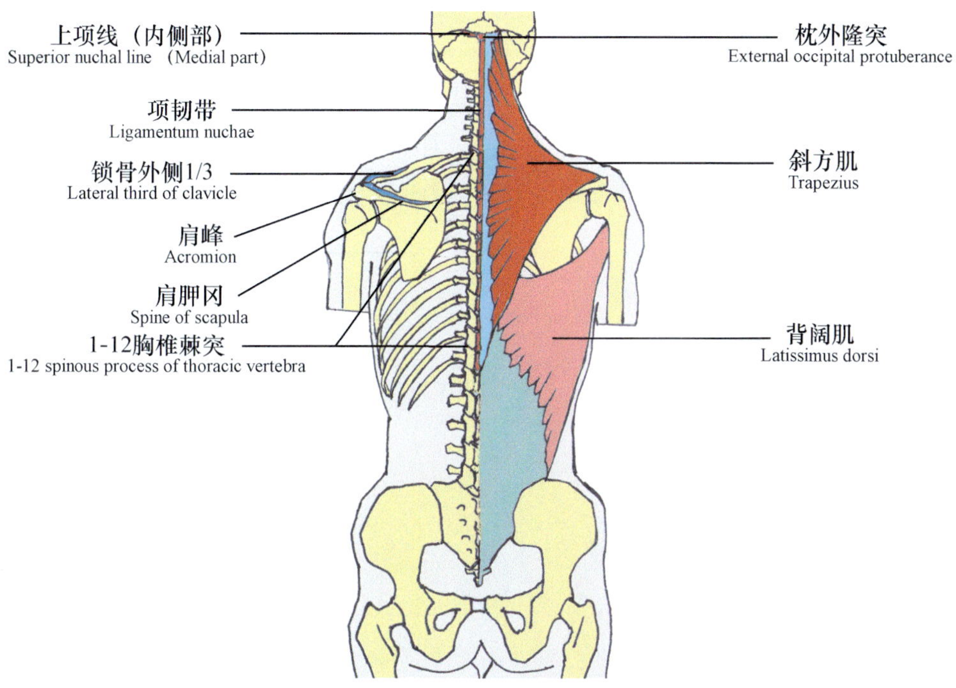

图 1-143 斜方肌的起止
Trapezius and its origins and insertions

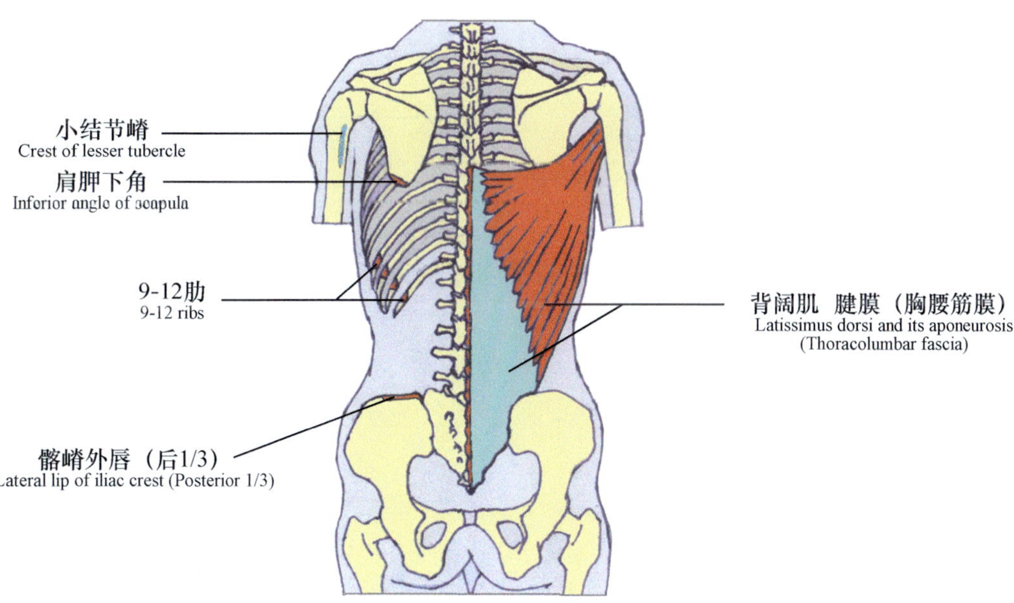

图 1-144 背阔肌的起止
Latissimus dorsi and its origins and insertions

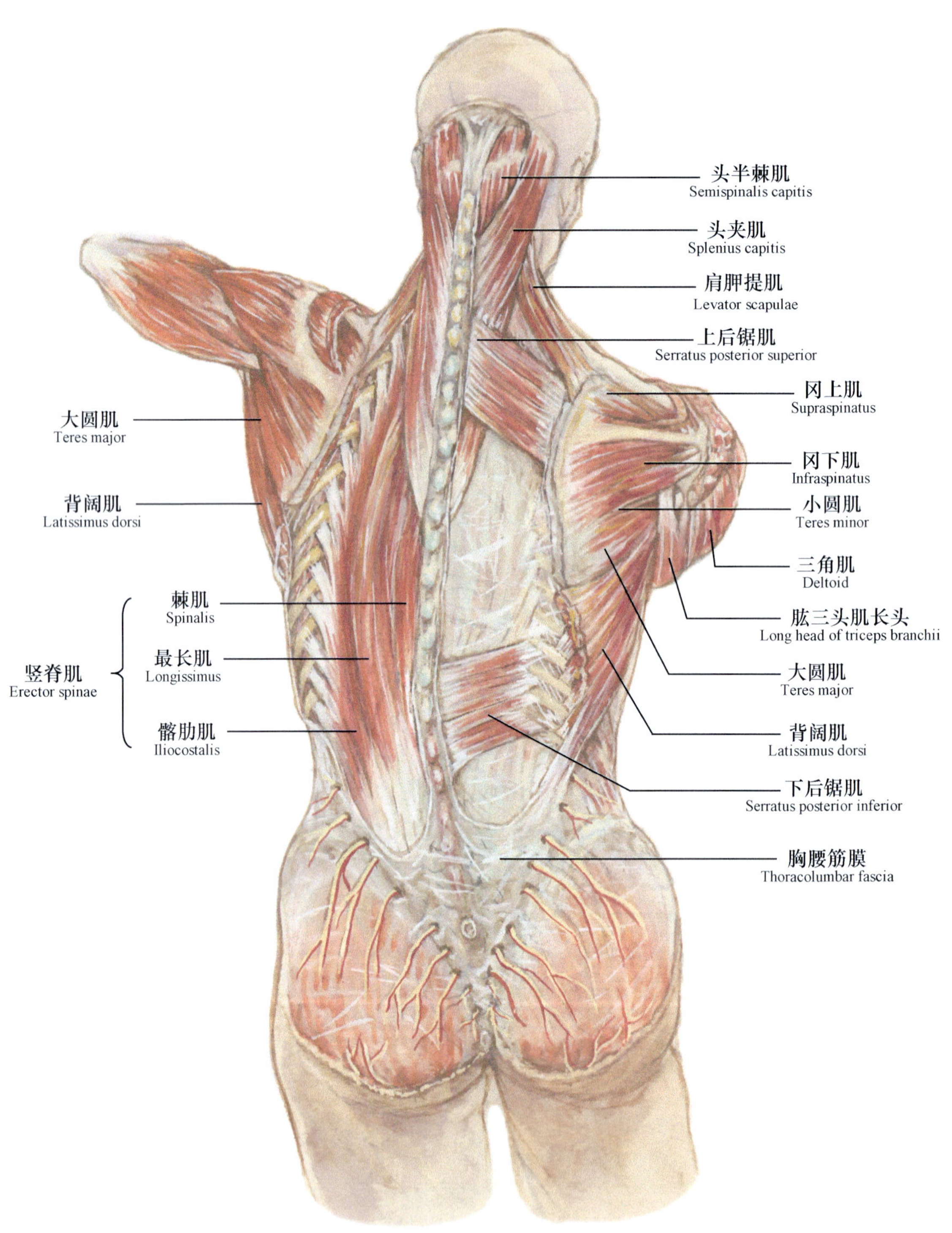

图 1-145　背肌（2）
Muscles of back (2)

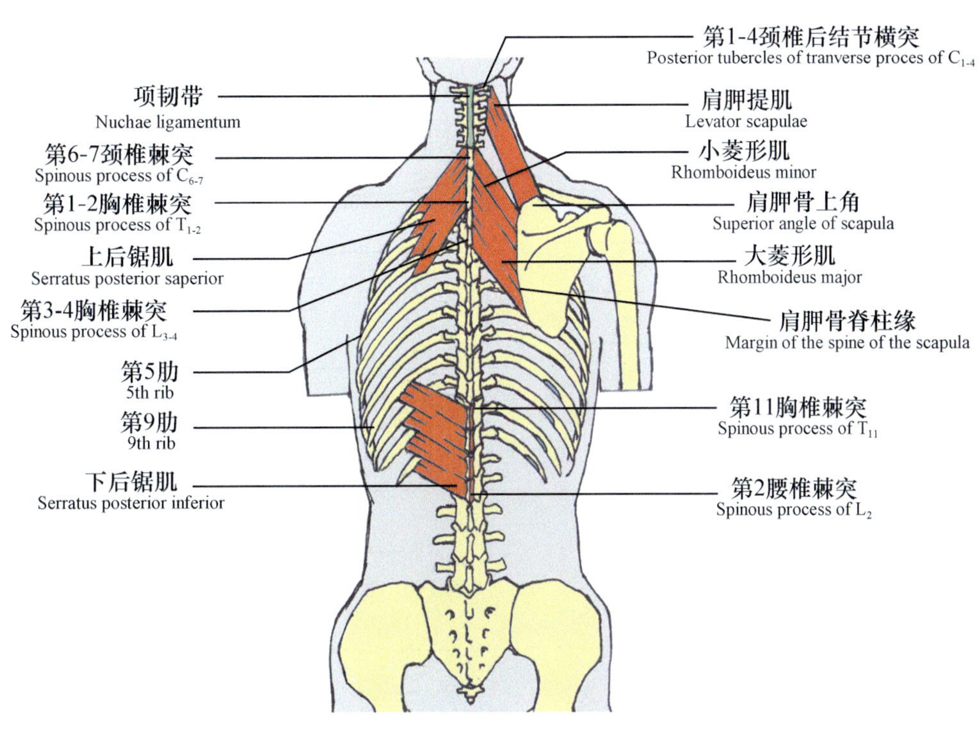

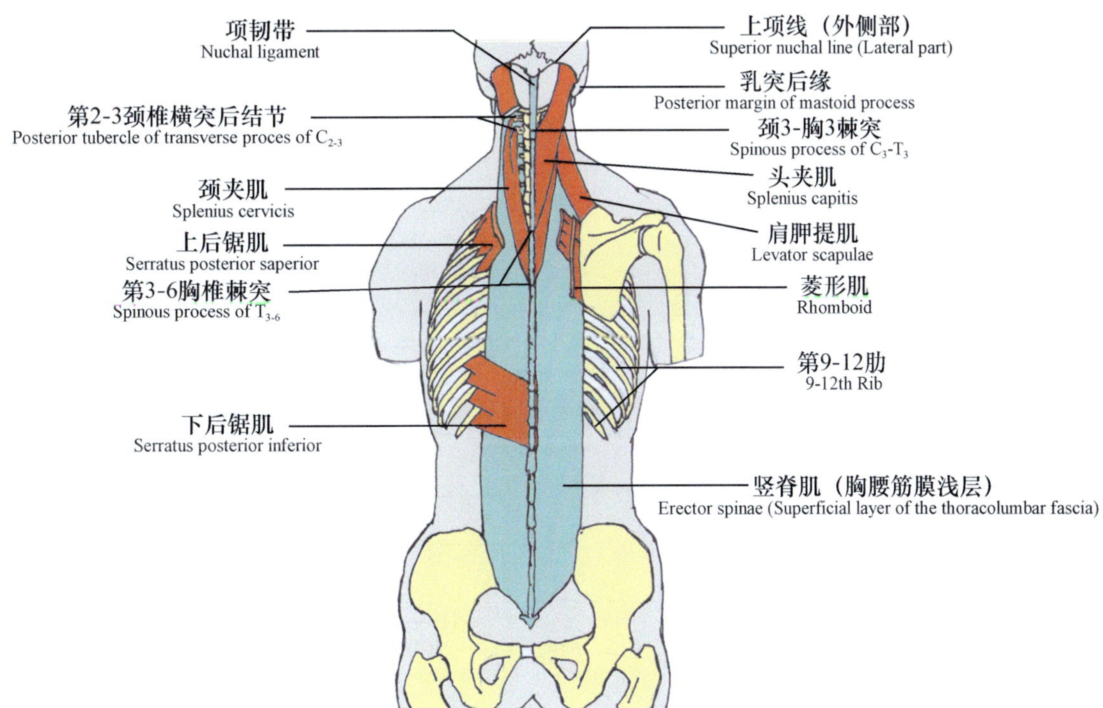

图 1-146 背部深肌简图

A brief diagram of the deep muscle of the back

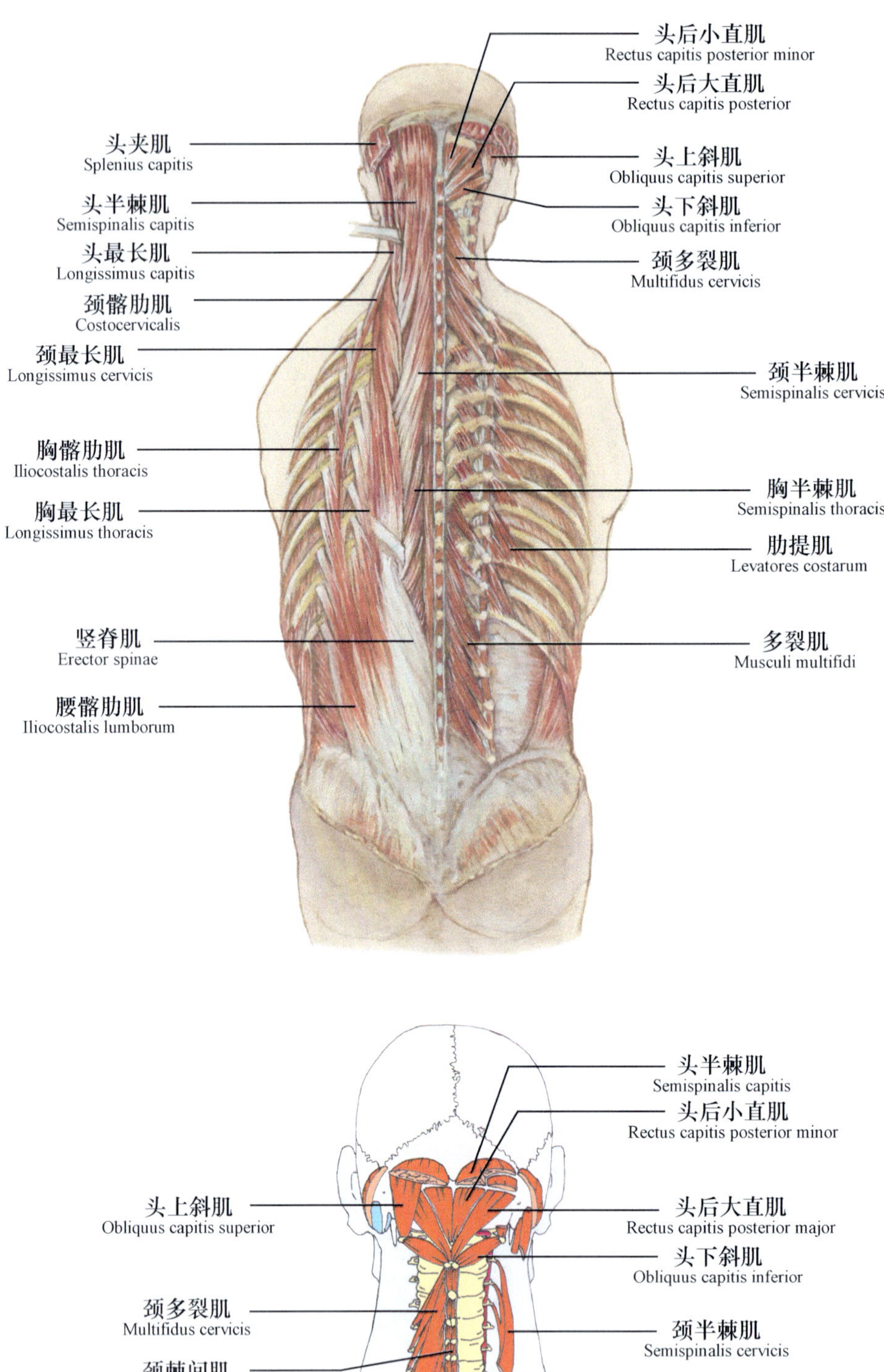

图 1-147 背肌（3）
Muscles of back (3)

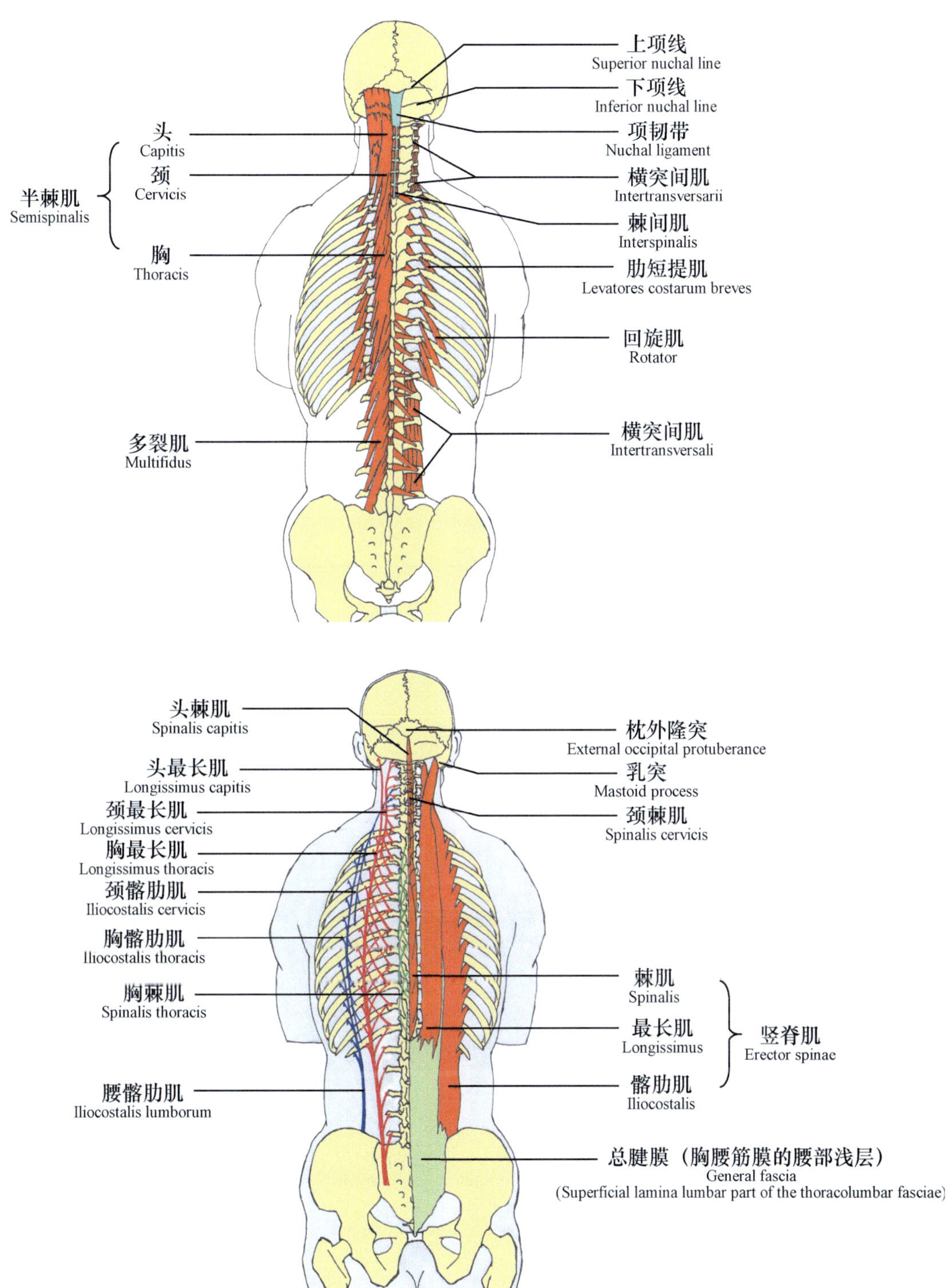

图 1-148 背部深层肌群

Scheme of deep muscles of the back

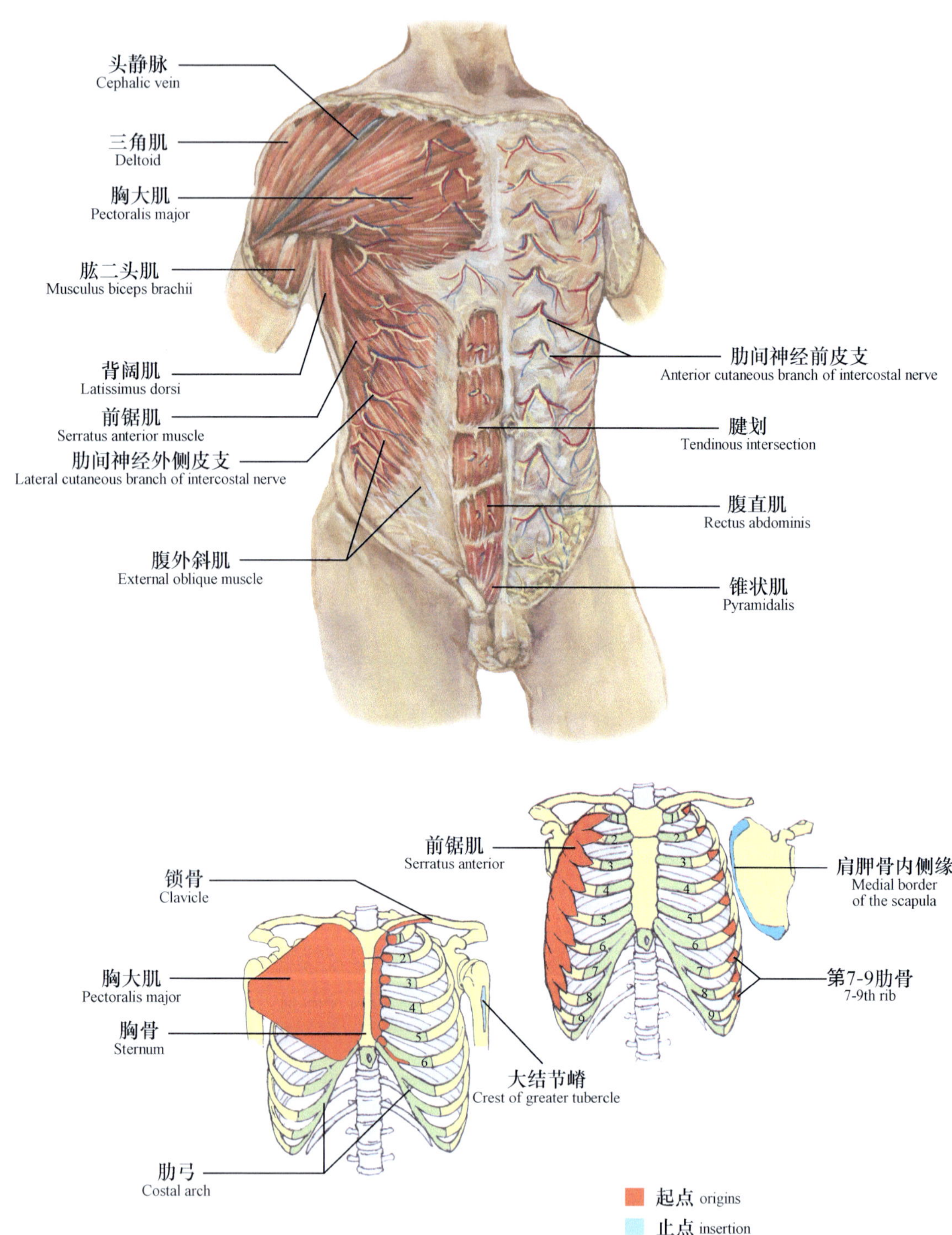

图 1-149 胸腹前壁（1）
Anterior thoracicoabdominal wall (1)

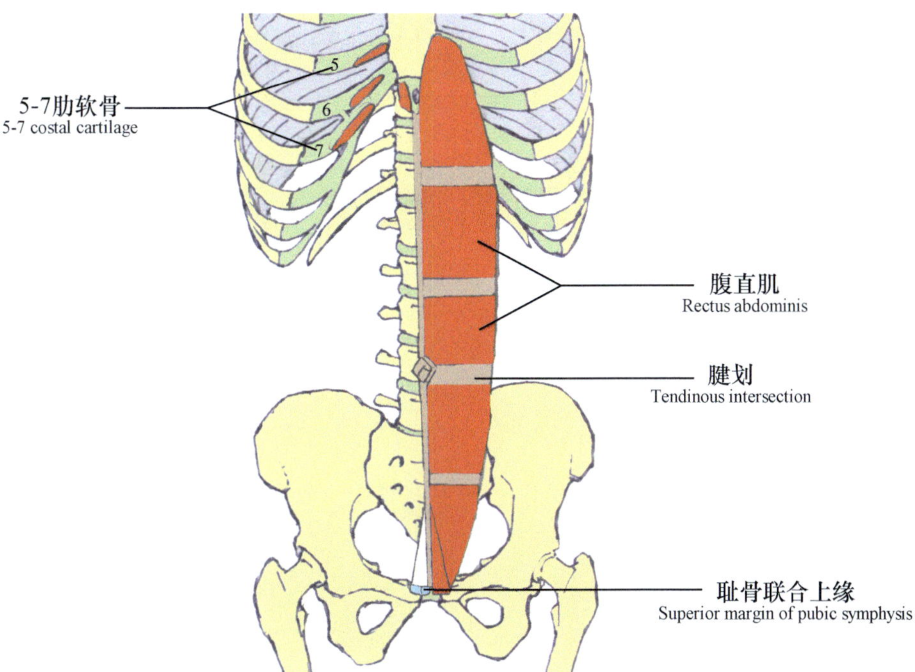

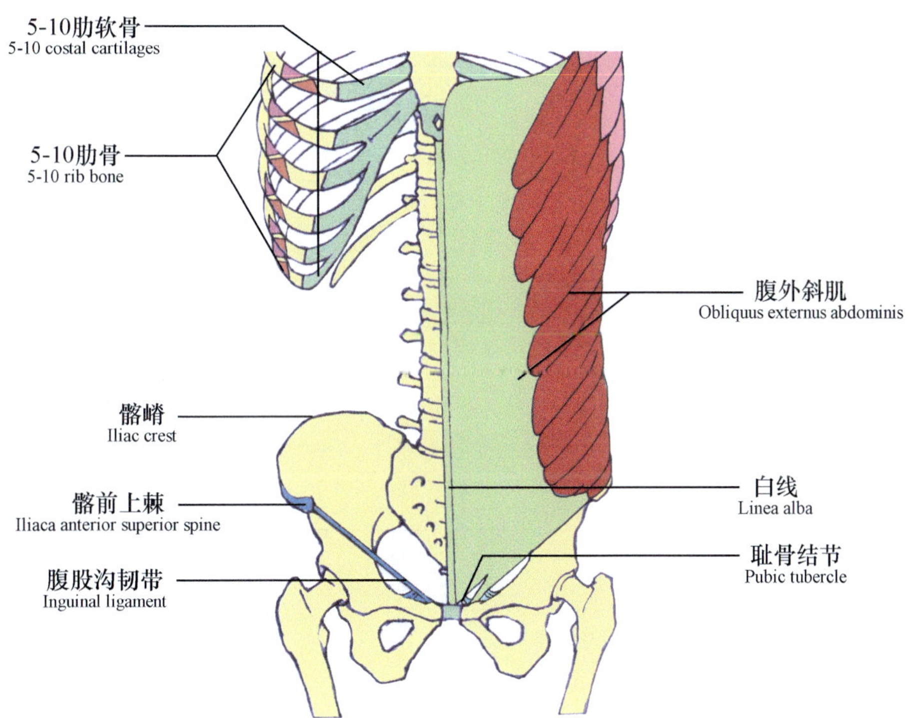

图 1-150 腹前壁
Anterior thoracicoabdominal wall

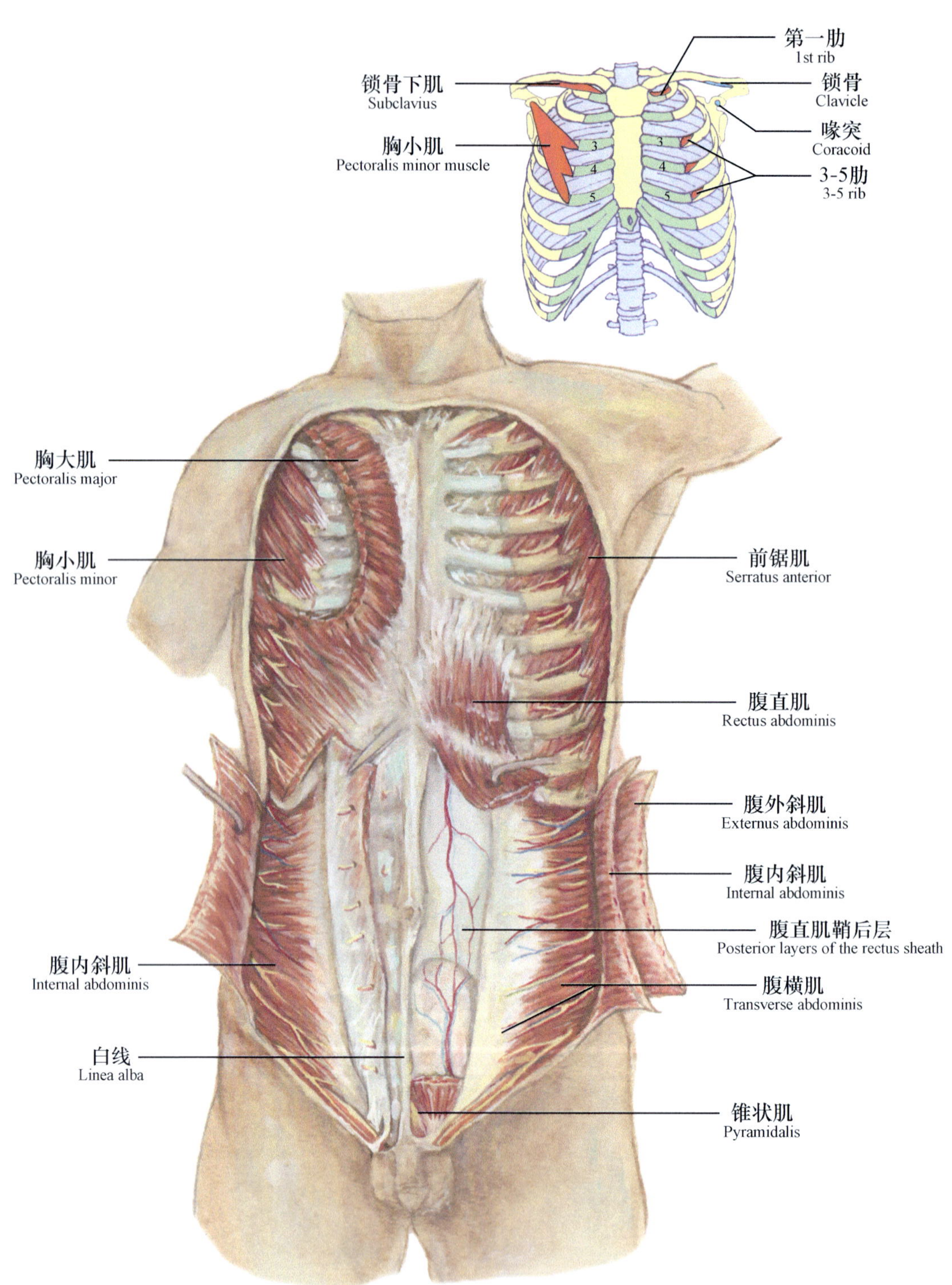

图 1-151　胸腹前壁（2）
Anterior thoracicoabdominal wall (2)

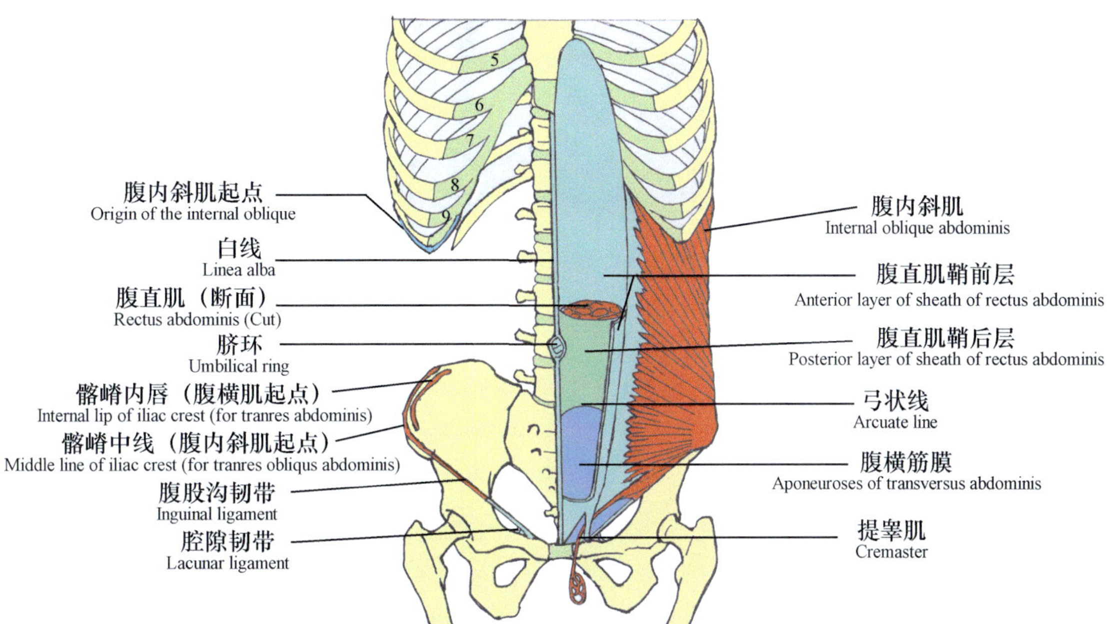

图 1-152 腹内斜肌示意图
Scheme of obliquus intermus abdominis

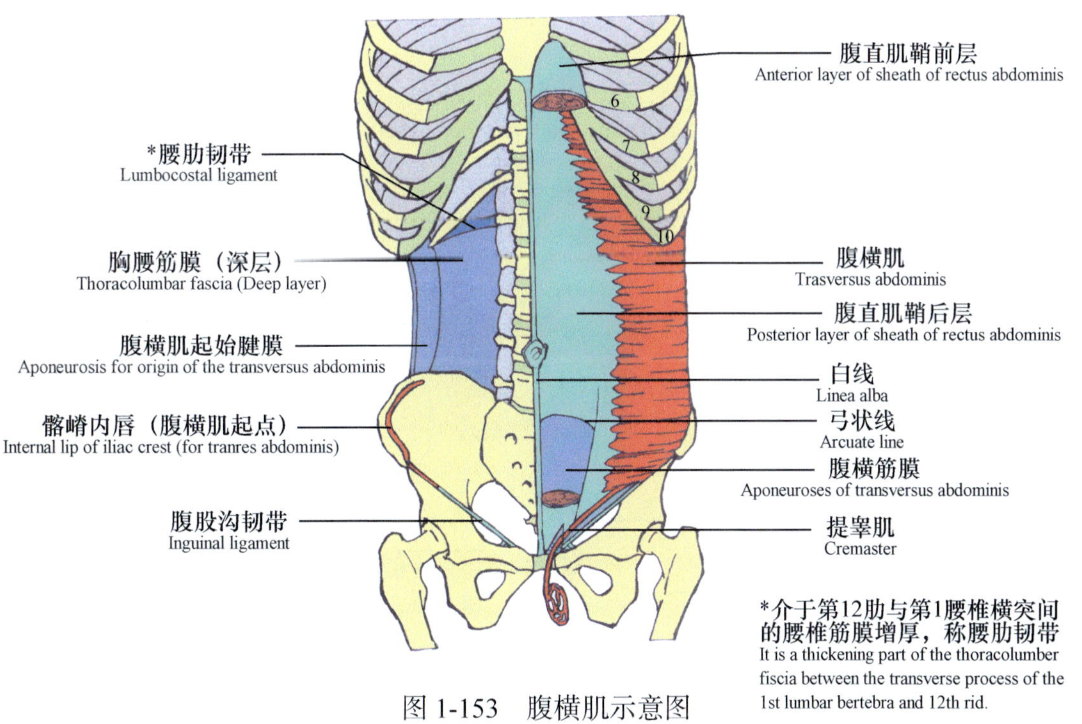

*介于第12肋与第1腰椎横突间的腰椎筋膜增厚，称腰肋韧带
It is a thickening part of the thoracolumber fiscia between the transverse process of the 1st lumbar bertebra and 12th rid.

图 1-153 腹横肌示意图
Scheme of transversus abdominis

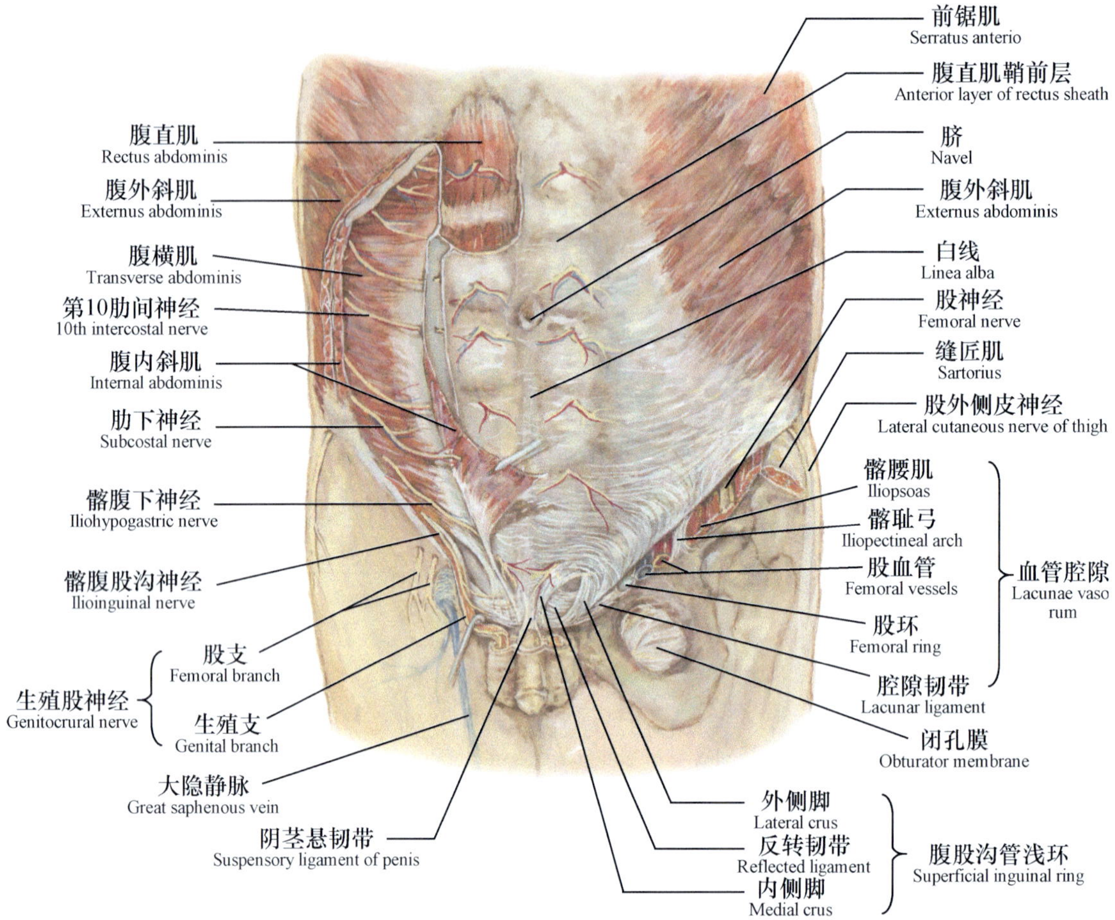

前锯肌
Serratus anterio
腹直肌鞘前层
Anterior layer of rectus sheath
腹直肌
Rectus abdominis
脐
Navel
腹外斜肌
Externus abdominis
腹外斜肌
Externus abdominis
腹横肌
Transverse abdominis
白线
Linea alba
第10肋间神经
10th intercostal nerve
股神经
Femoral nerve
腹内斜肌
Internal abdominis
缝匠肌
Sartorius
肋下神经
Subcostal nerve
股外侧皮神经
Lateral cutaneous nerve of thigh
髂腰肌
Iliopsoas
髂腹下神经
Iliohypogastric nerve
髂耻弓
Iliopectineal arch
髂腹股沟神经
Ilioinguinal nerve
股血管
Femoral vessels
血管腔隙
Lacunae vaso rum
股环
Femoral ring
股支
Femoral branch
生殖股神经
Genitocrural nerve
腔隙韧带
Lacunar ligament
生殖支
Genital branch
闭孔膜
Obturator membrane
大隐静脉
Great saphenous vein
外侧脚
Lateral crus
阴茎悬韧带
Suspensory ligament of penis
反转韧带
Reflected ligament
腹股沟管浅环
Superficial inguinal ring
内侧脚
Medial crus

图 1-154 腹壁（前面观）
The abdominal wall (Anterior aspect)

肋间后动脉
Posterior intercostal arteries
竖脊肌
Erector spinae
后支
Posterior branch
胸神经
Thoracic nerve
肋间外肌
External intercostals
前支
Anterior branch
肋间内肌
Internal intercostals
肋间神经外侧皮支
Lateral cutaneous branch of intercostal nerve
肋间最内肌
Intermost intercostals
半奇静脉
Hemizaygos vein
上腔静脉 ← 奇静脉
Superior vena cava Azygos vein
胸横肌
Transversus thoracis
胸廓内动静脉
Internal thoracic artery and vein
肋间神经前皮支
Anterior cutaneous branch of intercostal nerve

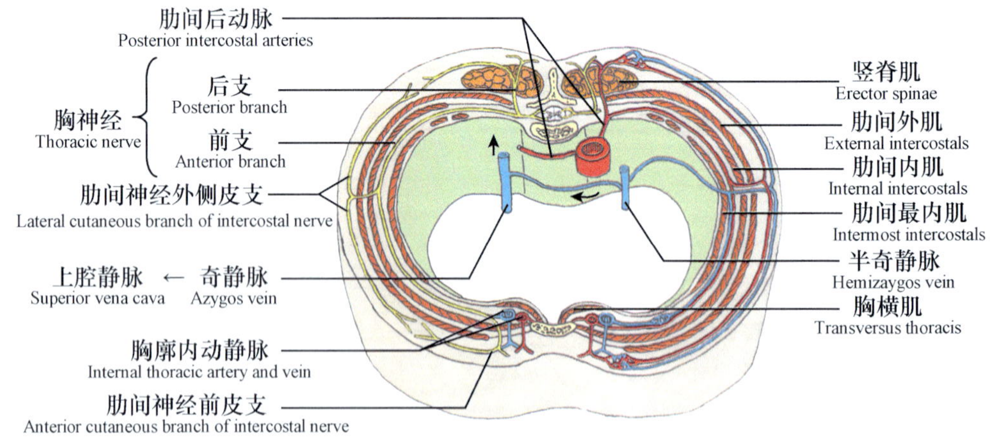

图 1-155 肋间神经、血管示意图
A diagram of intercostal nerves and blood vessel

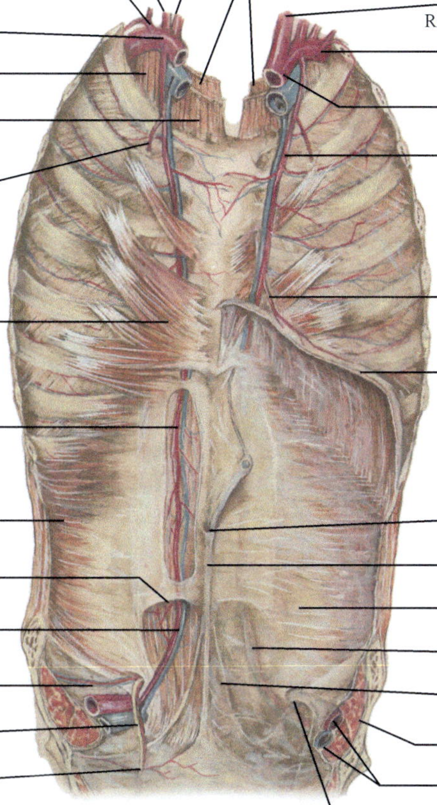

椎动脉
Vertebral artery
甲状颈干
Thyrocervical trunk
胸骨舌骨肌
Sternohyoid
肋颈干
Costocervical trunk
右颈总动脉
Right common carotid artery
左锁骨下血管
Left subclavian vessels
右锁骨下静脉
Right subclavian artery
前斜角肌
Scalenus anterior
头臂干
Truncus brachiocephalicus
胸骨甲状肌
Sternothyroid
胸廓内动脉
Internal thoracic artery
心包膈动脉
Pericardiacophrenic artery
肌膈动脉
Musculophrenic artery
胸横肌
Transversus thoracis
膈
Diaphragm
腹壁上血管
Superior epigastric vessels
脐环
Umbilical ring
腹横肌
Trasversus abdominis
脐正中襞
Median umbilical fold
弓状线
Arcuate line
腹横筋膜
Fascia trans
腹壁下血管
Inferior epigastric vessels
脐外侧襞
Lateral umbilical folds
睾丸血管
Testiculus vessels
脐内侧襞
Medial umbilical fold
输精管
Ductus deferens
髂肌
Iliacus
膀胱上动脉
Superior vesical artery
髂外血管
External iliac vessels
腹股沟管深环
Deep inguinal ring

胸横肌
Transversus thoracis
止点
Ending points
起点
Arising points
肋间内肌
Intercostales interni
肋间最内肌
Intercostals intimi
胸横肌
Transverse thoracic
膈肌起点
Arising point of diaphragm
肋骨部
Part of rids
胸骨部
Part of stermum
膈
Diaphragm
腹横肌起点
Arising point of transversus abdominis

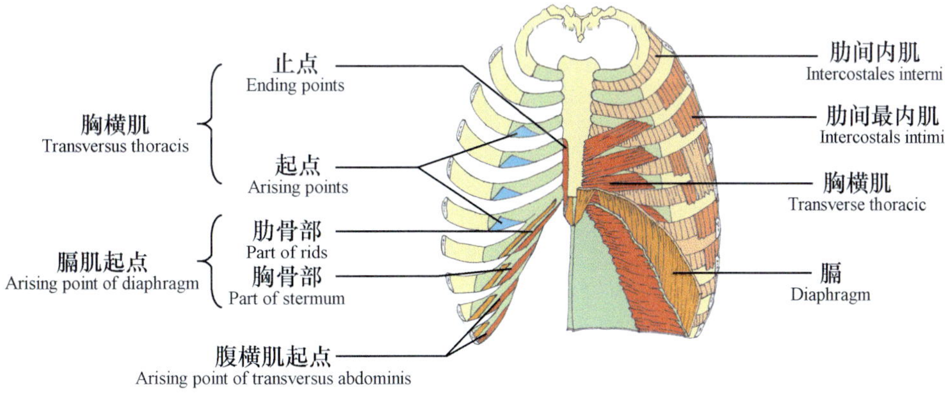

图 1-156 胸腹前壁（内面观）
The anterior thoracic and abdominal wall (Interial aspect)

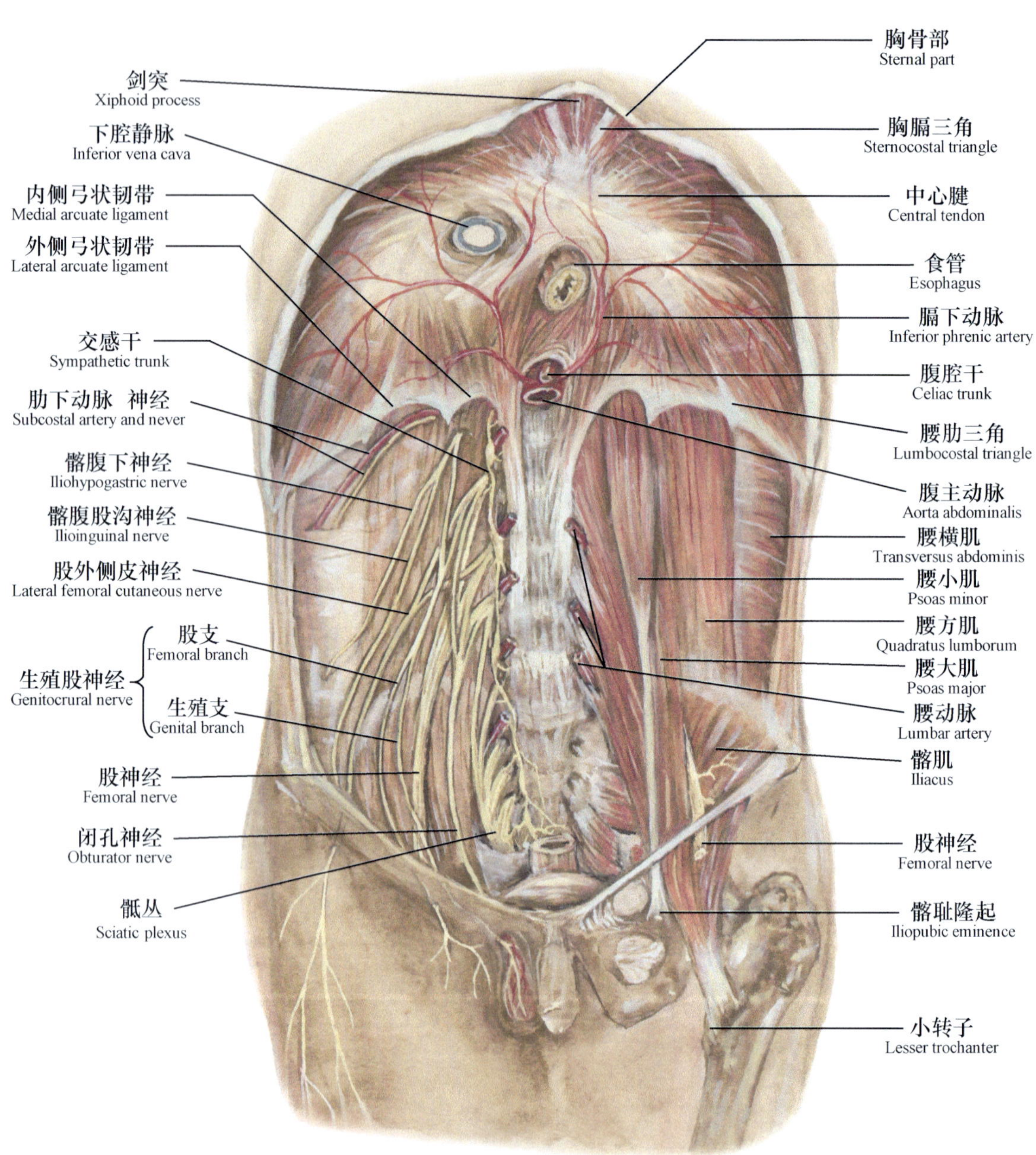

图 1-157 膈肌与腹后壁

The diaphragm and the posterior abdominal wall

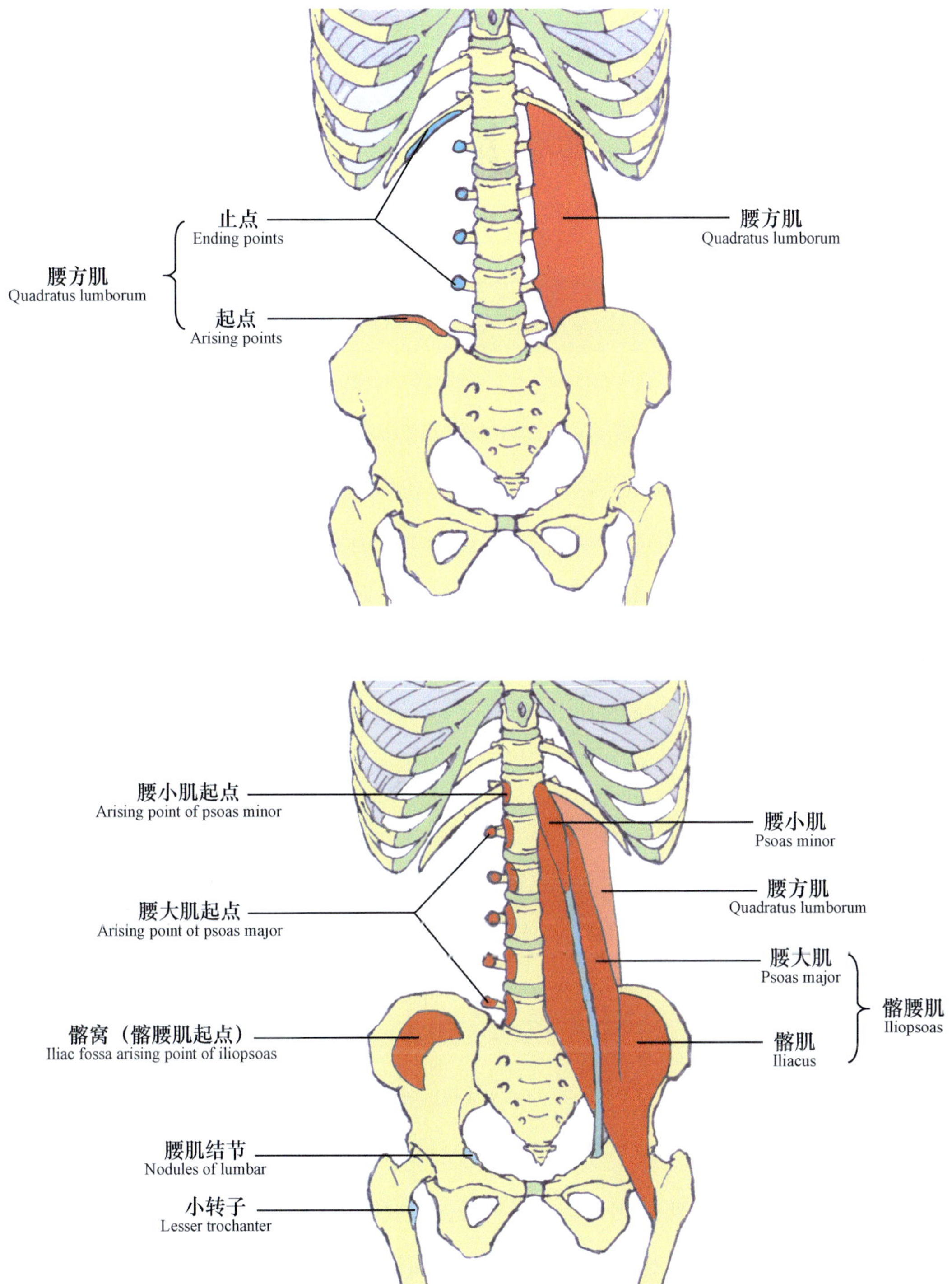

图 1-158 腹后壁肌群起止点示意图
Schematic diagram of starting point of posterior abdominal wall muscle group

第2章

内　脏　学

SPLANCHNOLOGY

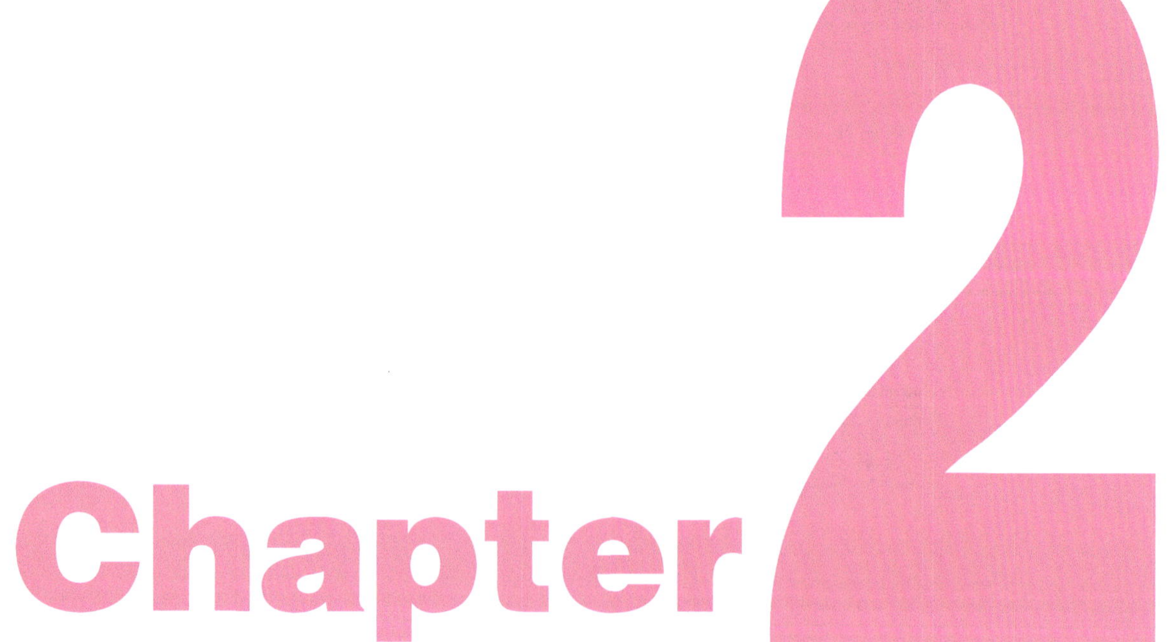

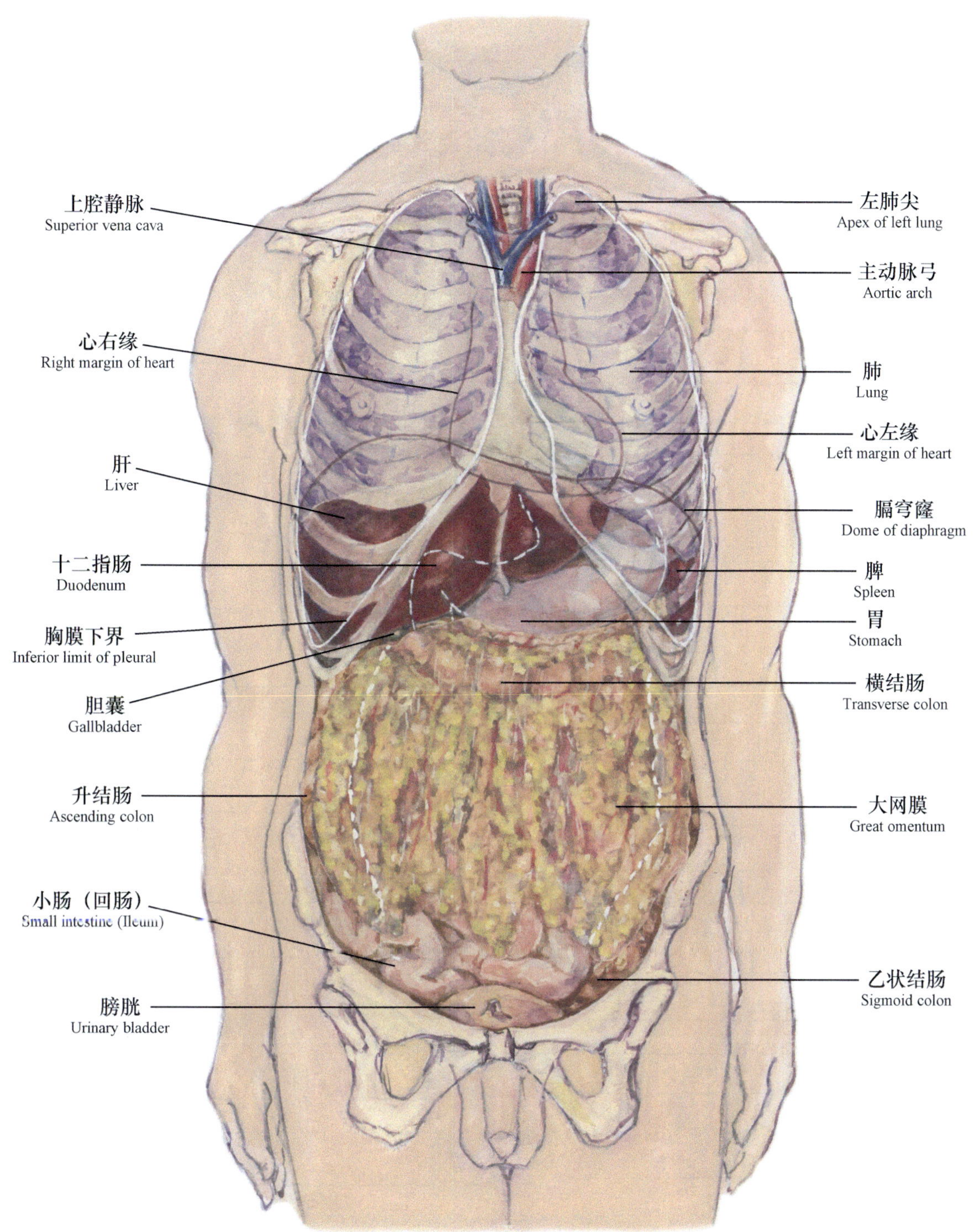

图 2-1　胸膜内脏投影（腹侧观）
Projection of thoracic and abdominal viscera (Frontal aspect)

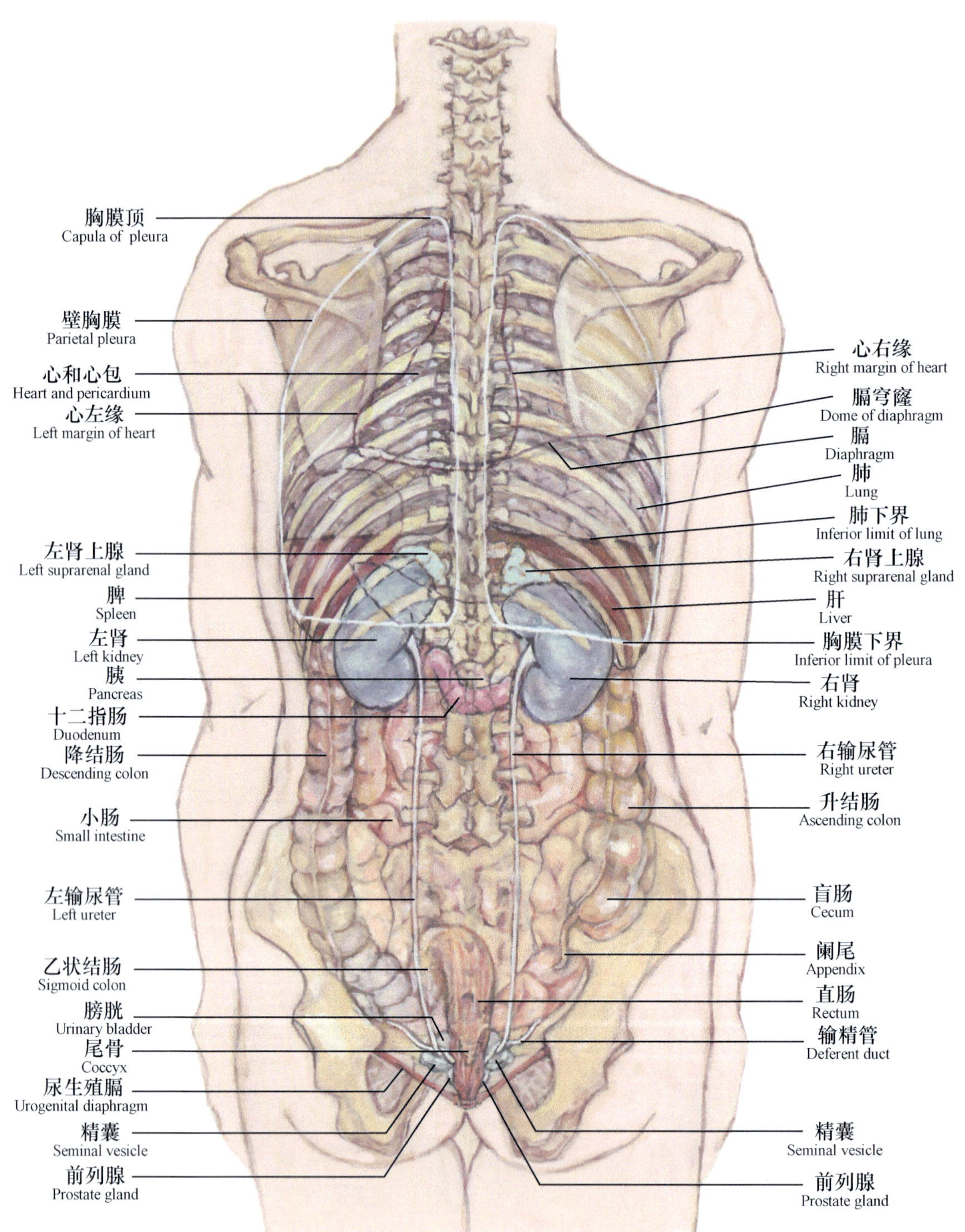

图 2-2 胸腹内脏投影（背侧观）
Projection of thoracic and abdominal viscerd (Dorsal aspect)

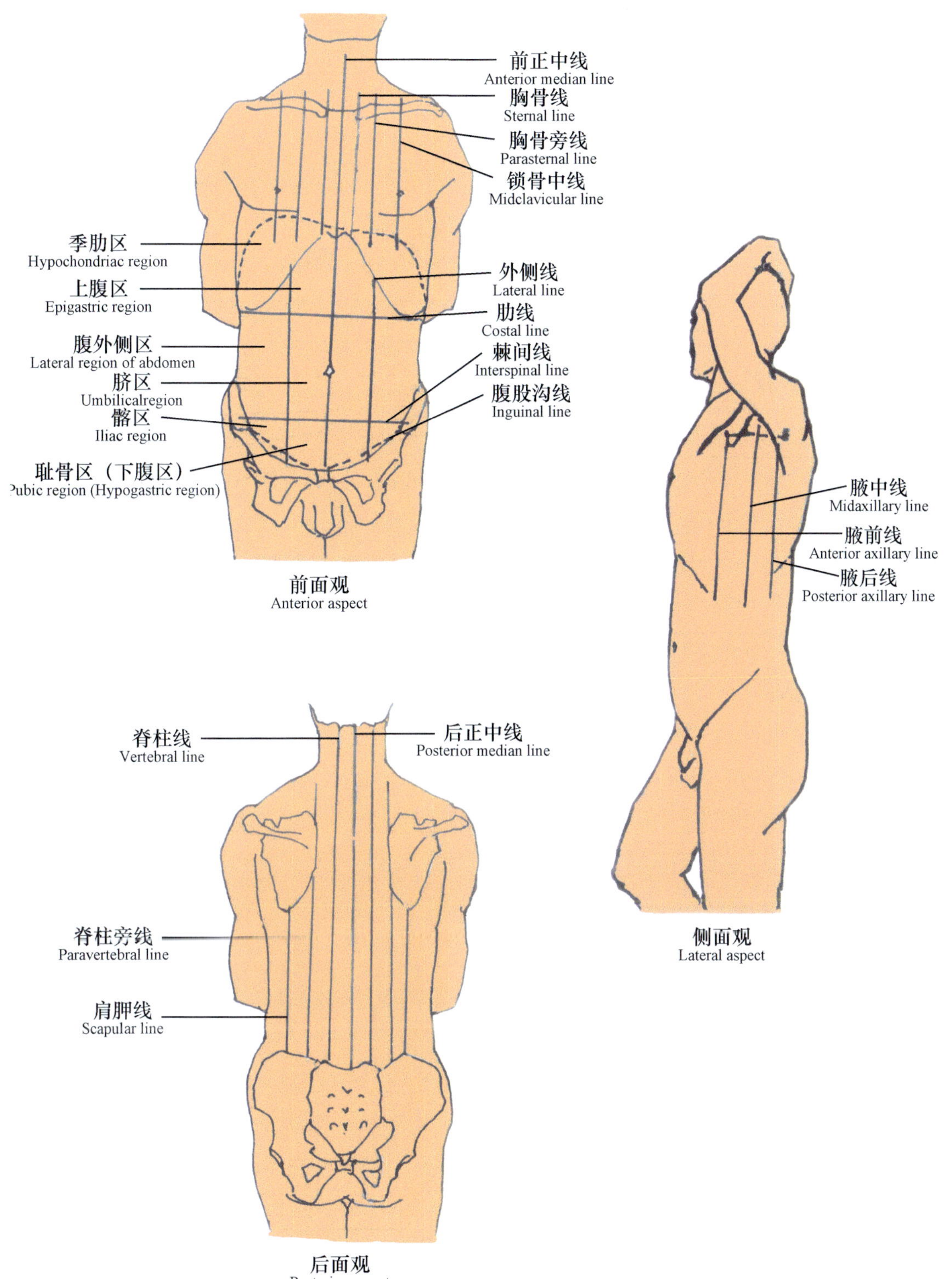

图 2-3 人体标志线和分区
Reference lines and regions of the body

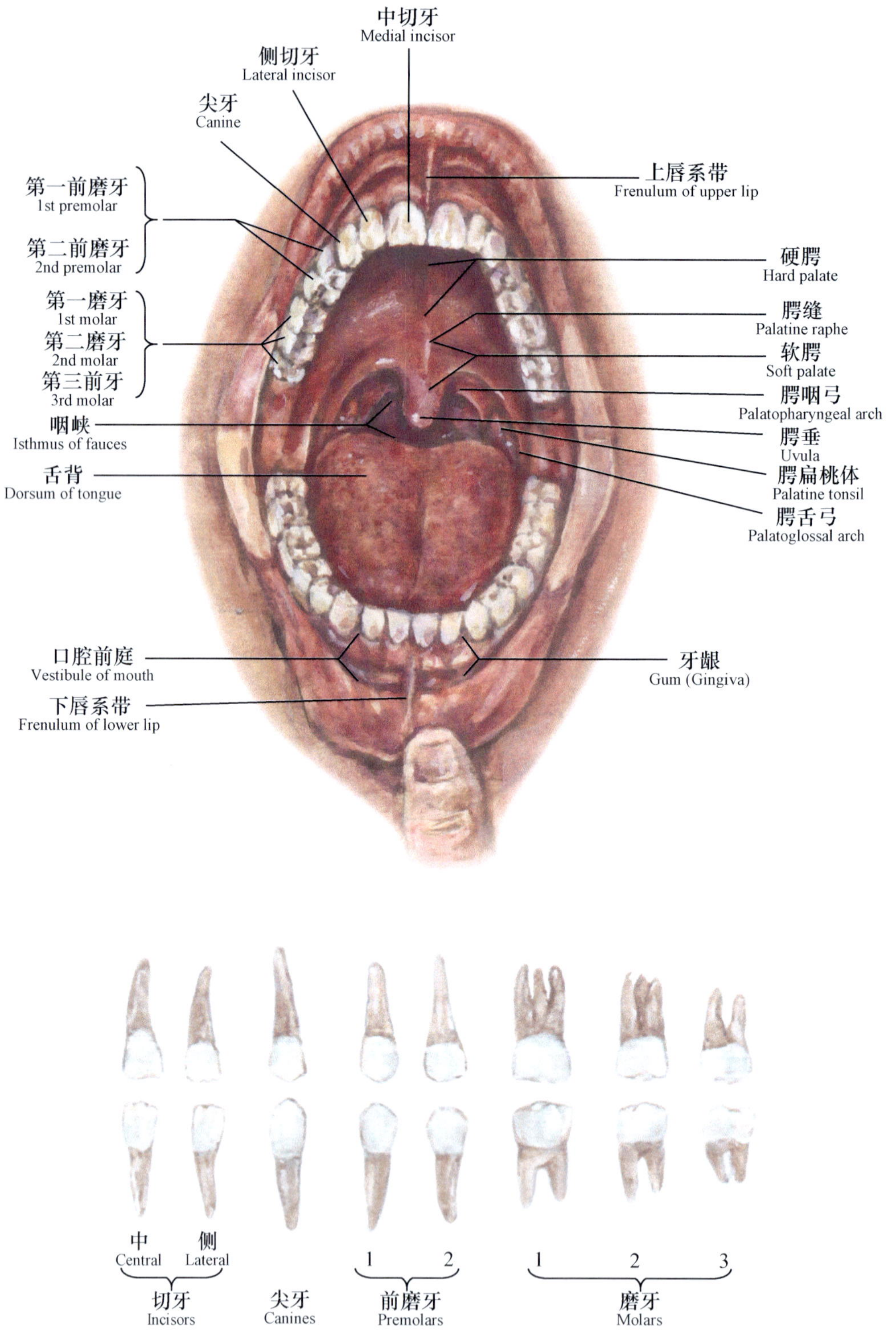

图 2-4 口腔
The mouth

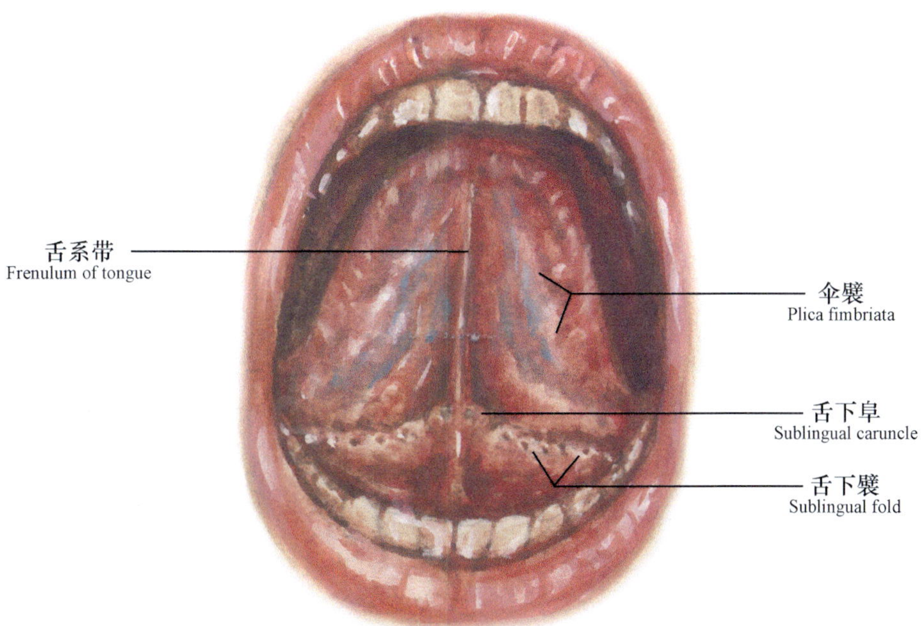

舌下面
Sublingual Region

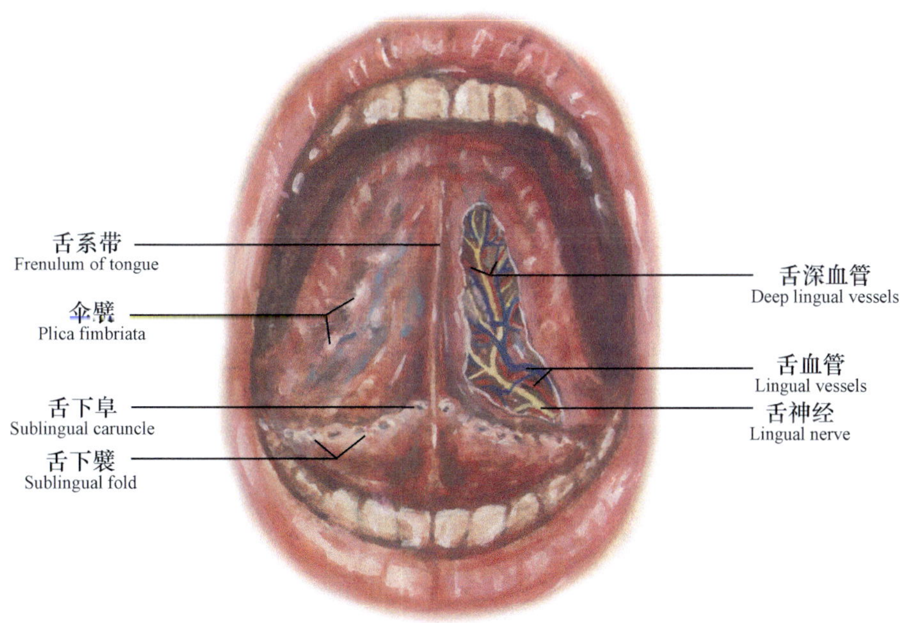

舌下面
Sublingual Region

图 2-5 舌下面
Sublingual Region

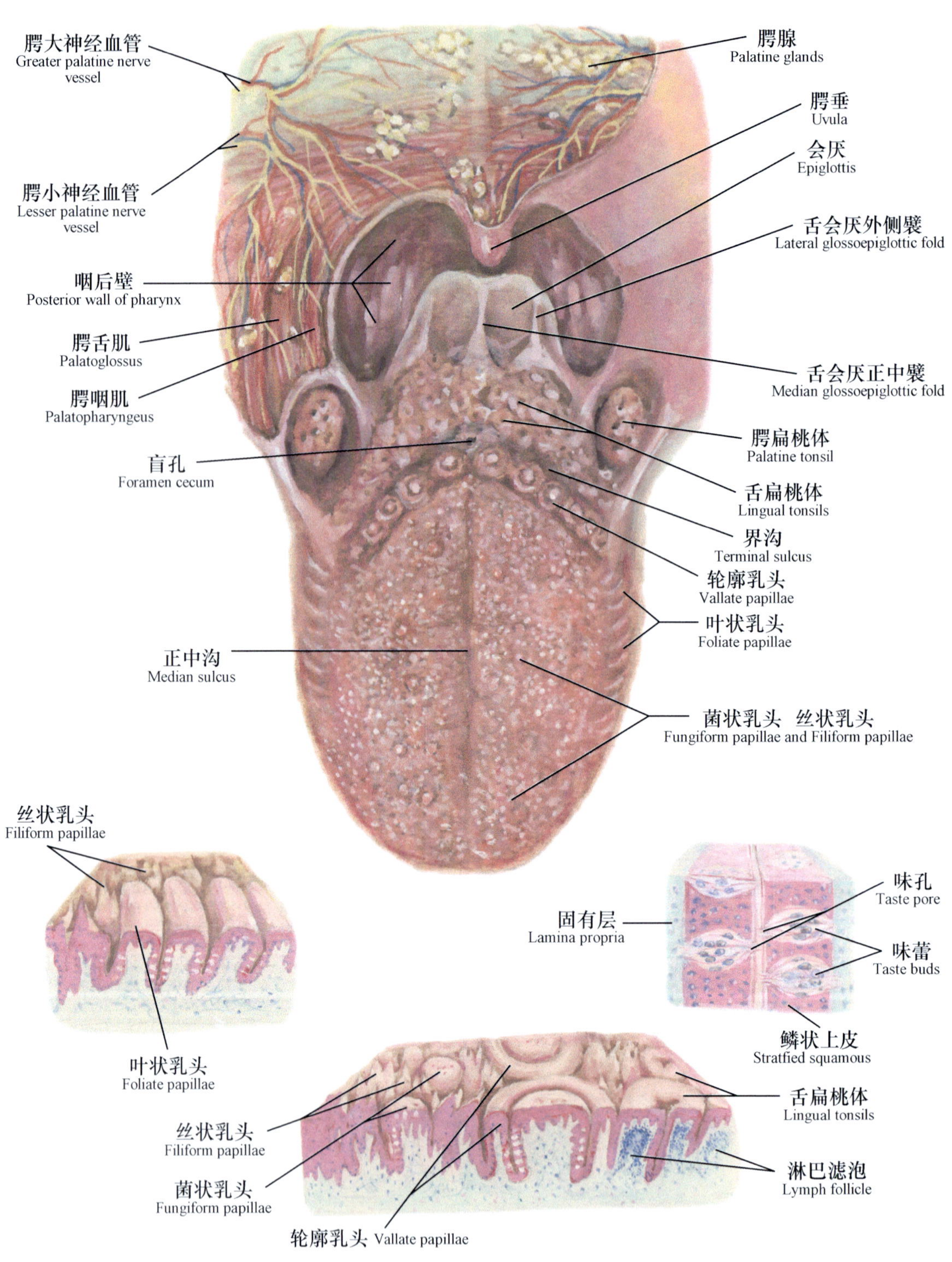

图 2-6 舌背
The dorsum of the tongue

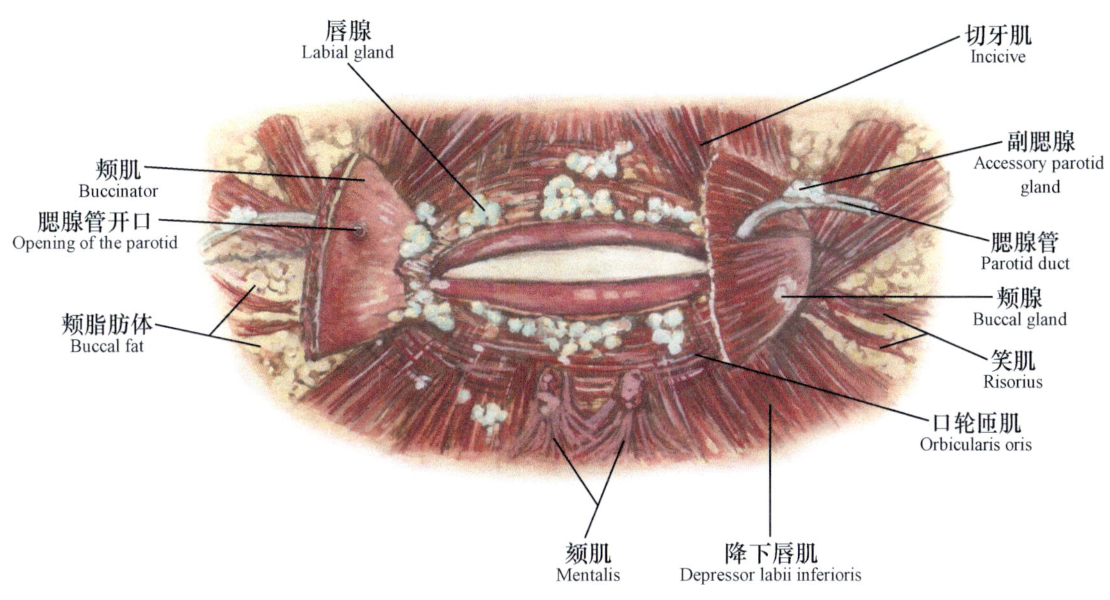

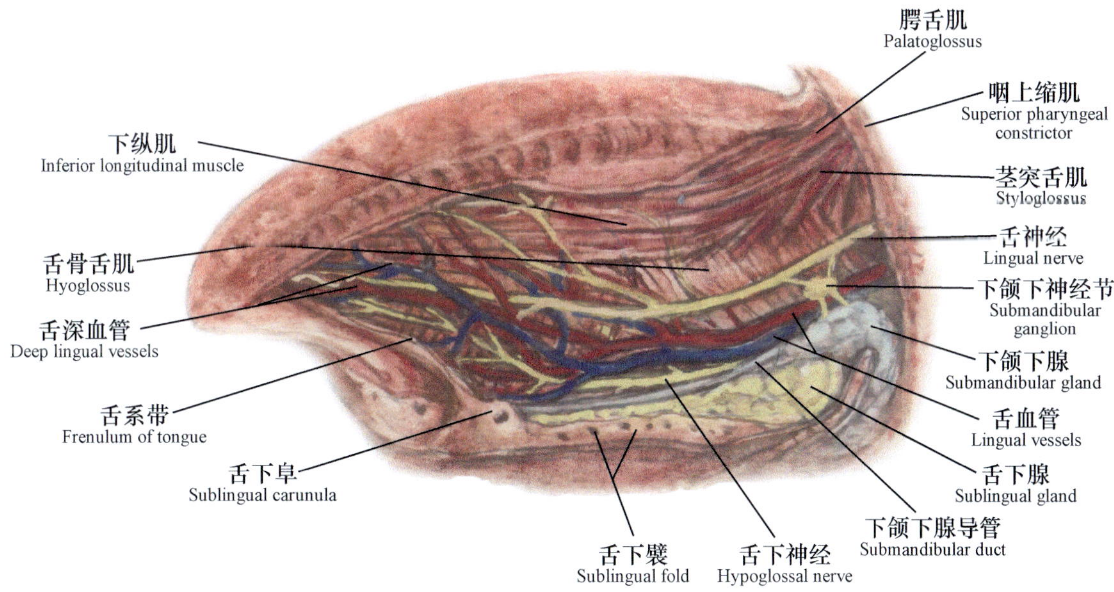

图 2-7 口唇周围腺（口腔内面观）
Glands around lips viewed from within the oral cavity

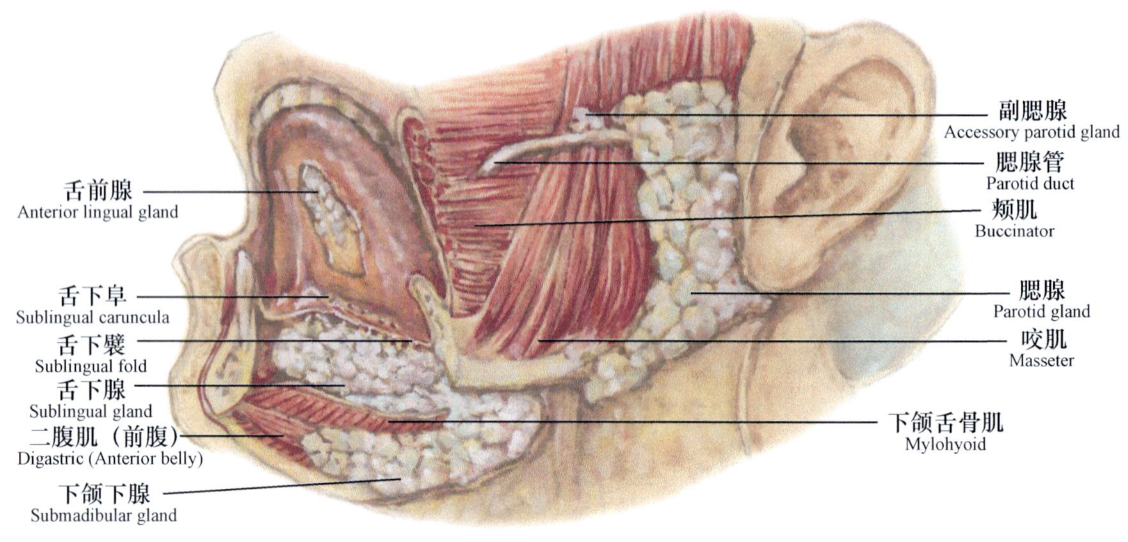

图 2-8　口腔和颜面的左侧部，自同侧观察
The left side of oral cavity and face, viewed form the same side

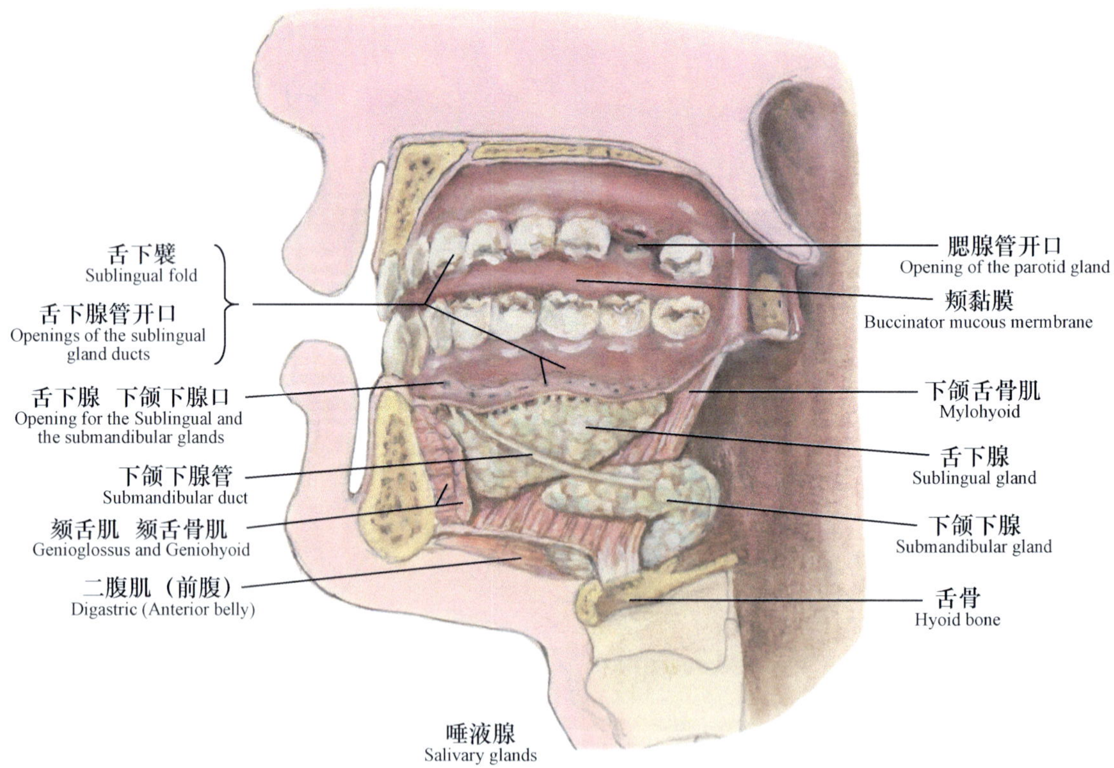

图 2-9　口腔的右半部，自左侧观察
The right half of the oral cavity (Viewed form the left)

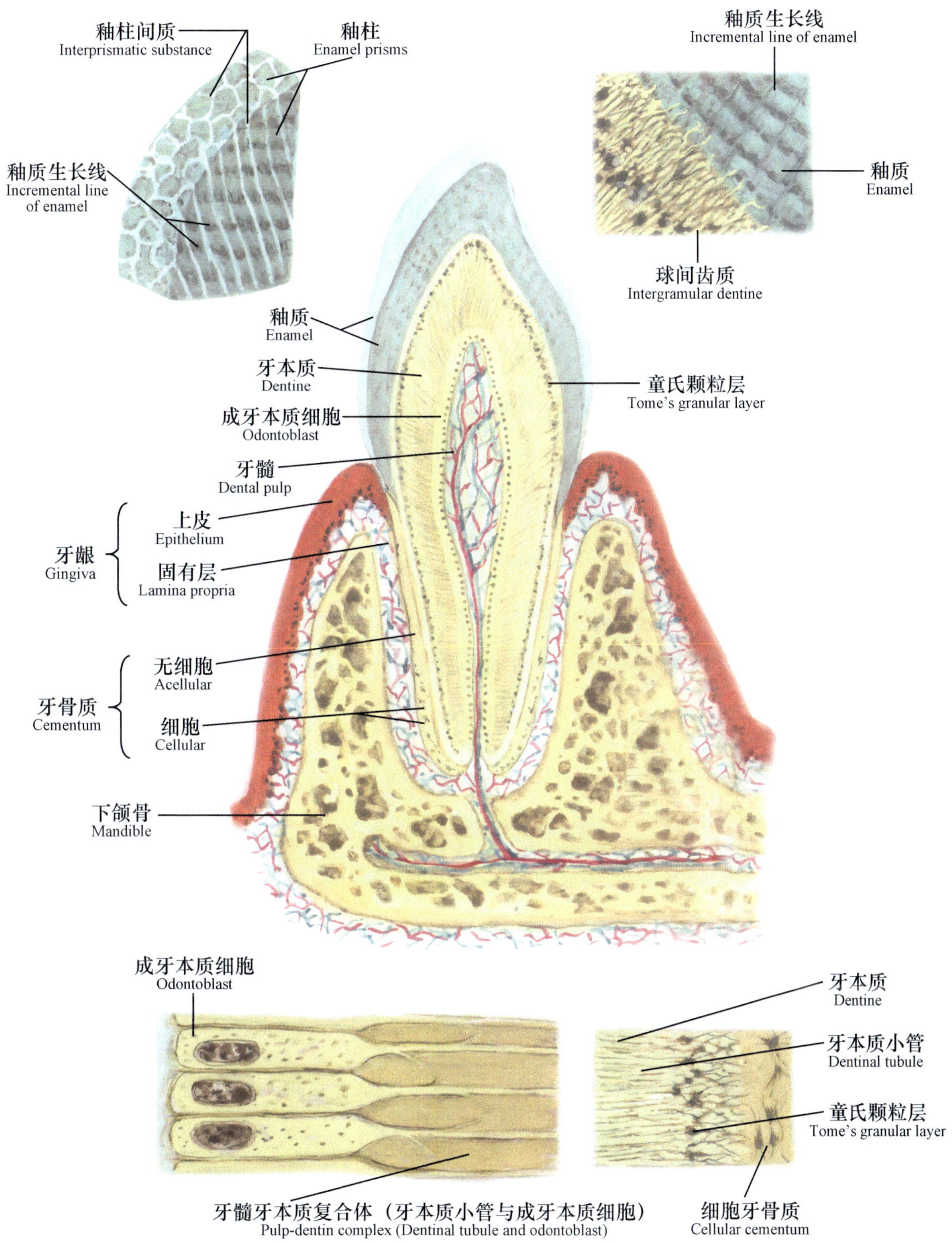

图 2-10　原位切牙纵剖面示意图
Diagram of longitudinal section of incisor in situ

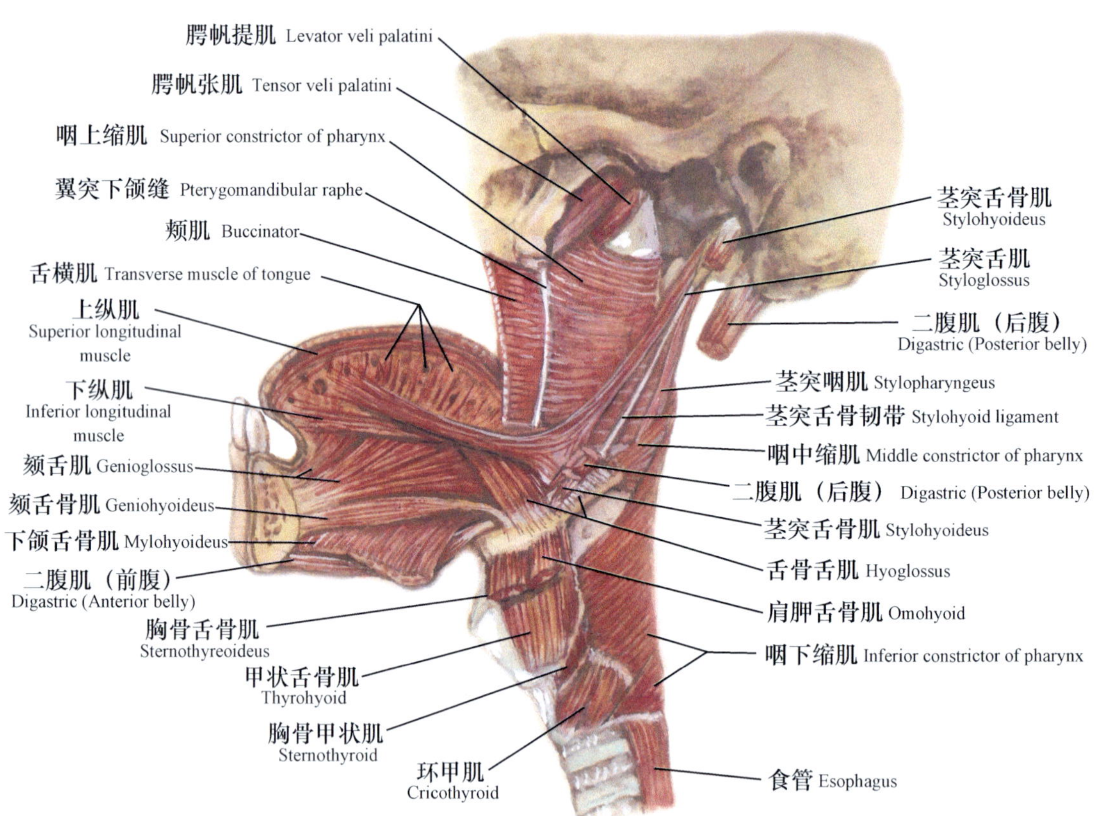

图 2-11 舌肌与咽缩肌
The lingual musculature and the pharyngeal constrictors

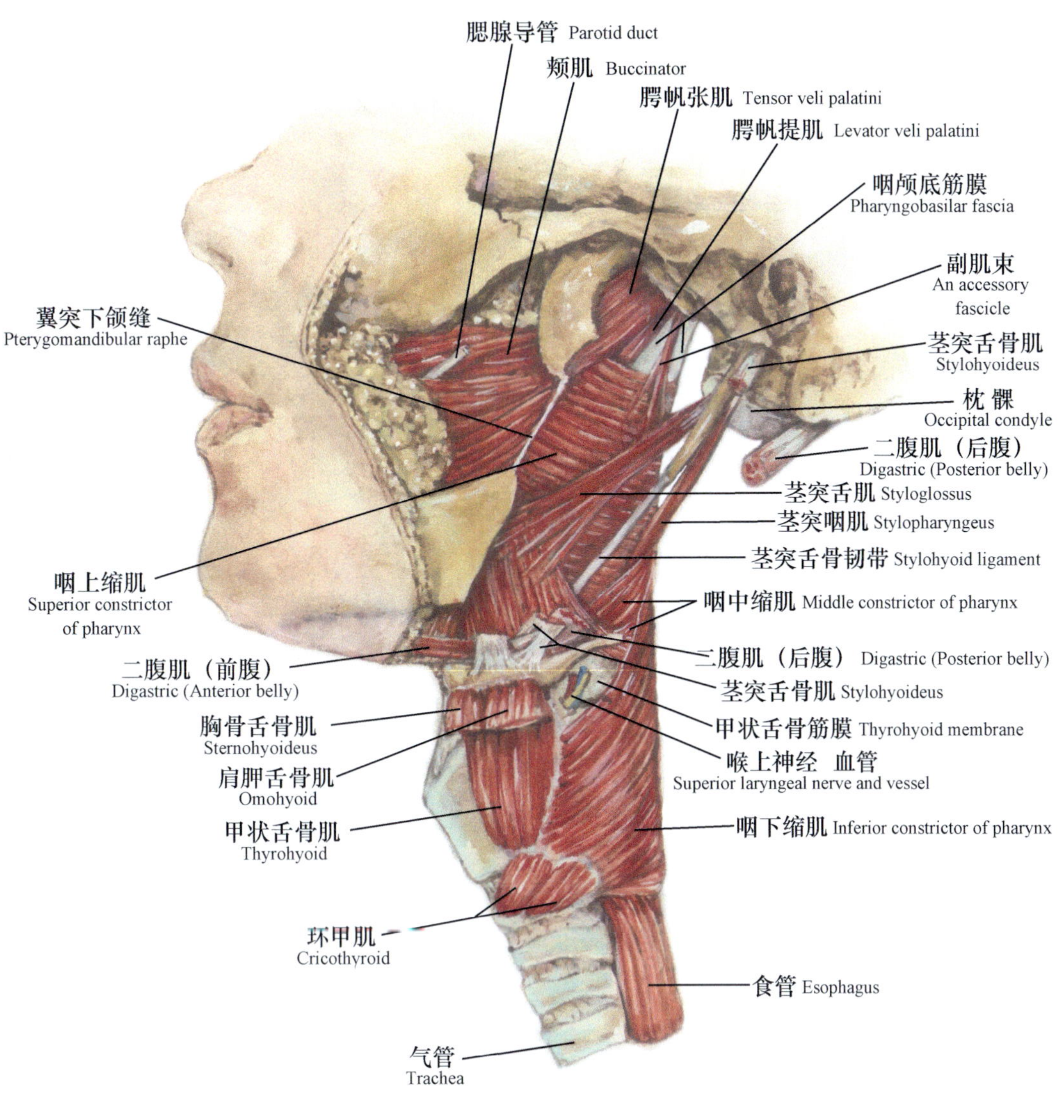

图 2-12 咽肌（侧面观）
The pharyngeal muscles (Laeral aspect)

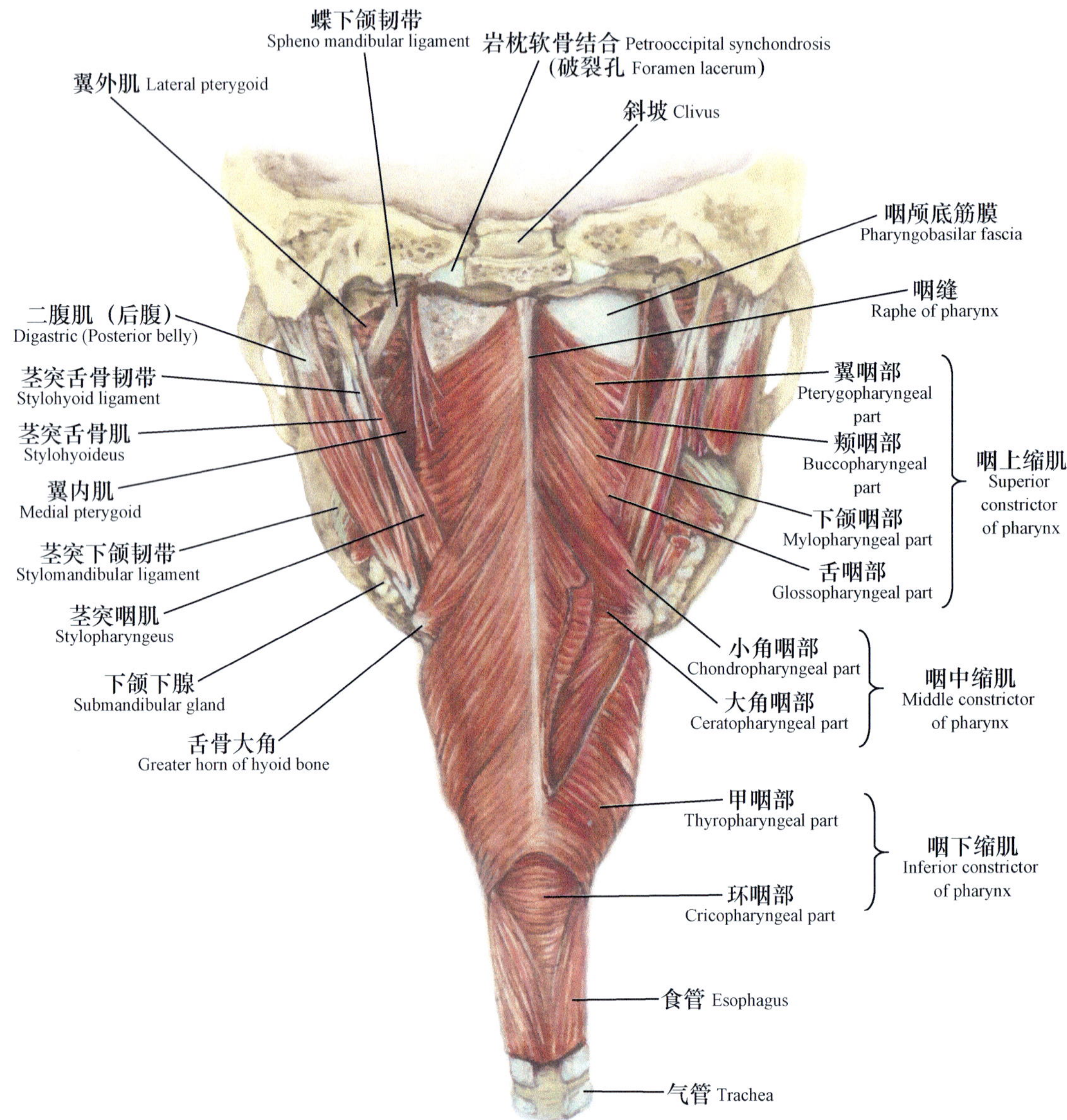

图 2-13 咽肌（背侧观）
The pharyngeal muscles (Dorsal aspect)

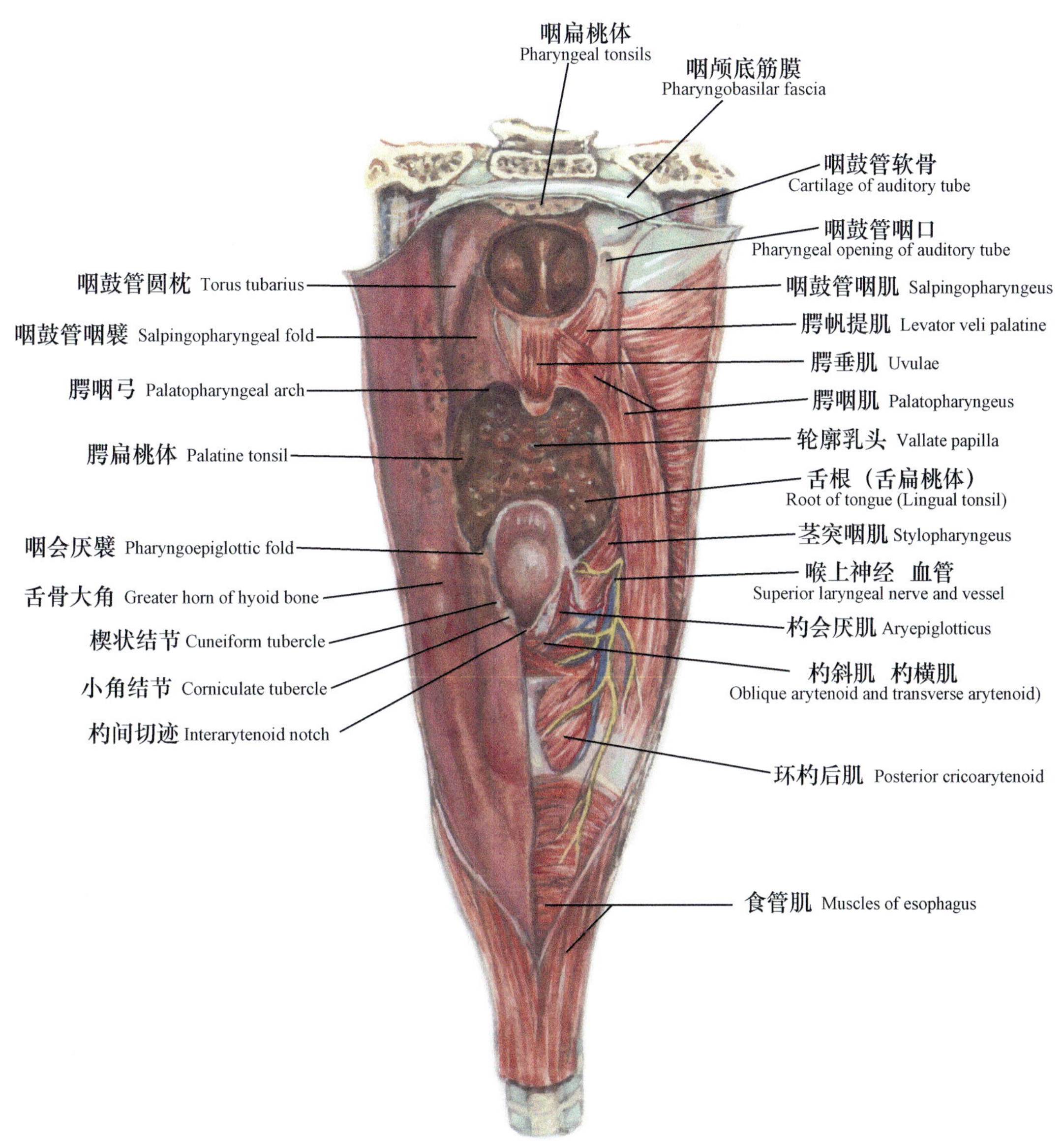

图 2-14 咽腔（切开咽后壁）
Pharyngeal cavity (Open the posterior pharyngeal wall)

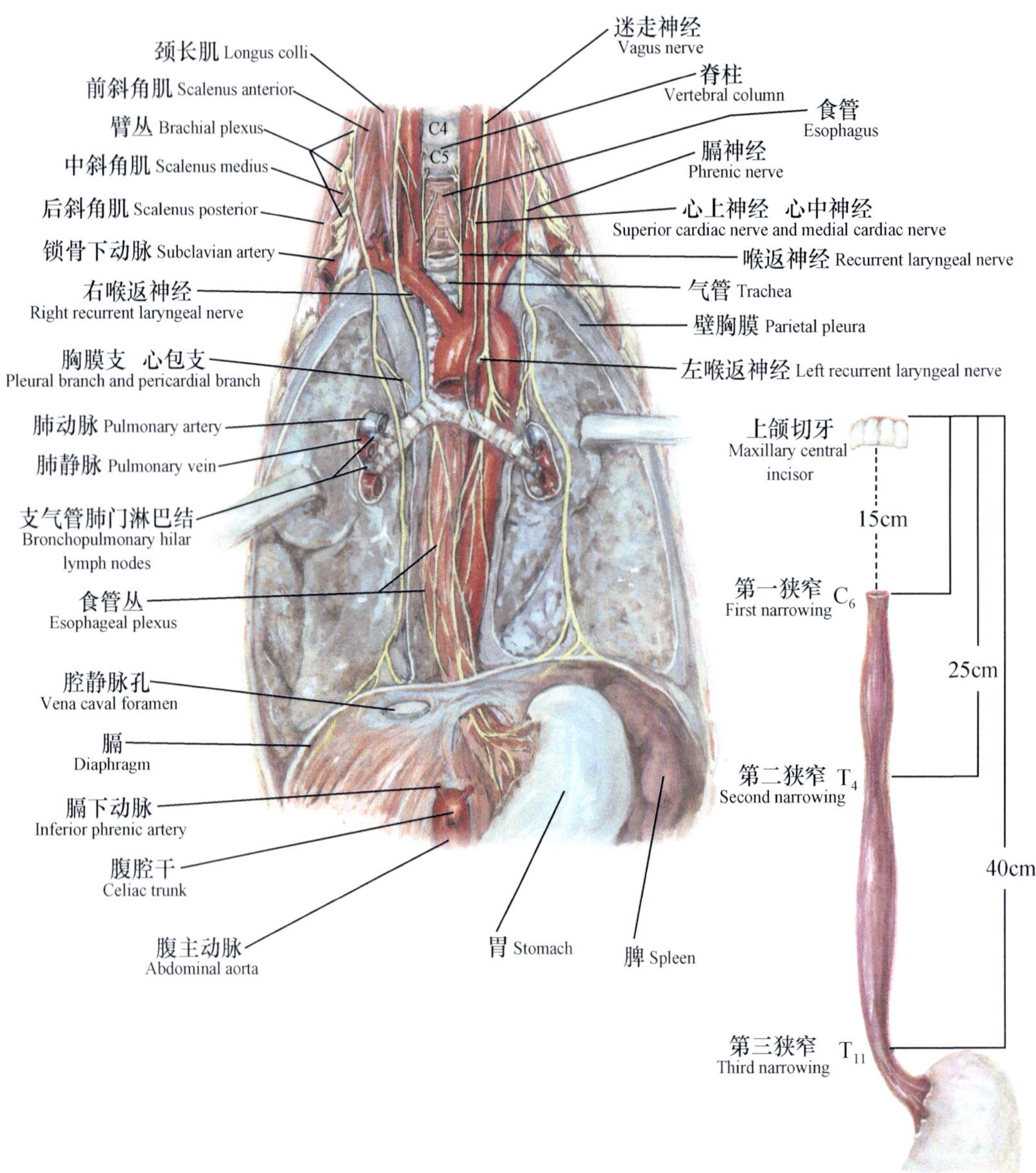

图 2-15 纵隔
The mediastinum

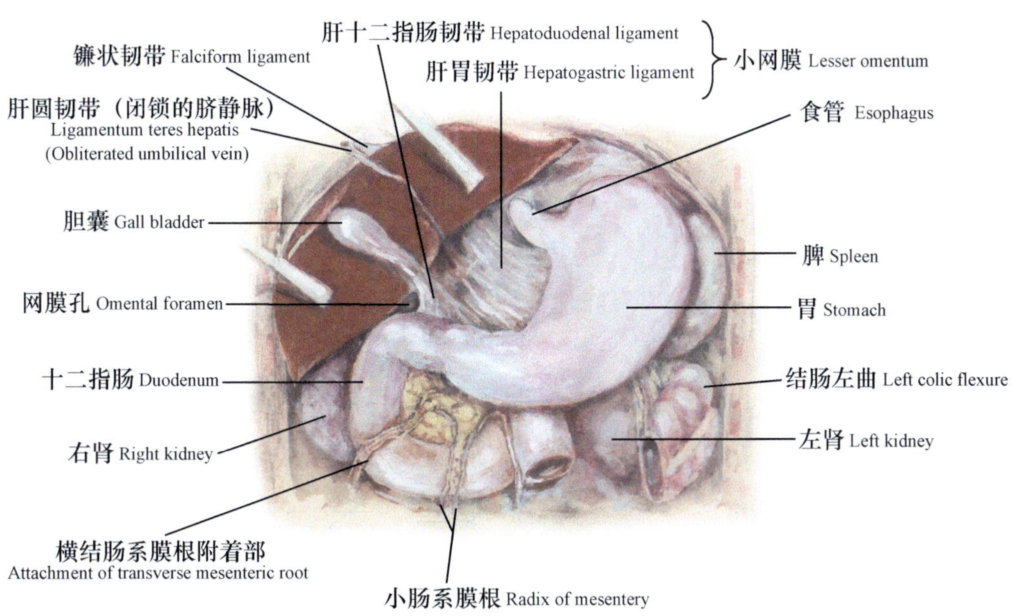

图 2-16 胃
Stomach

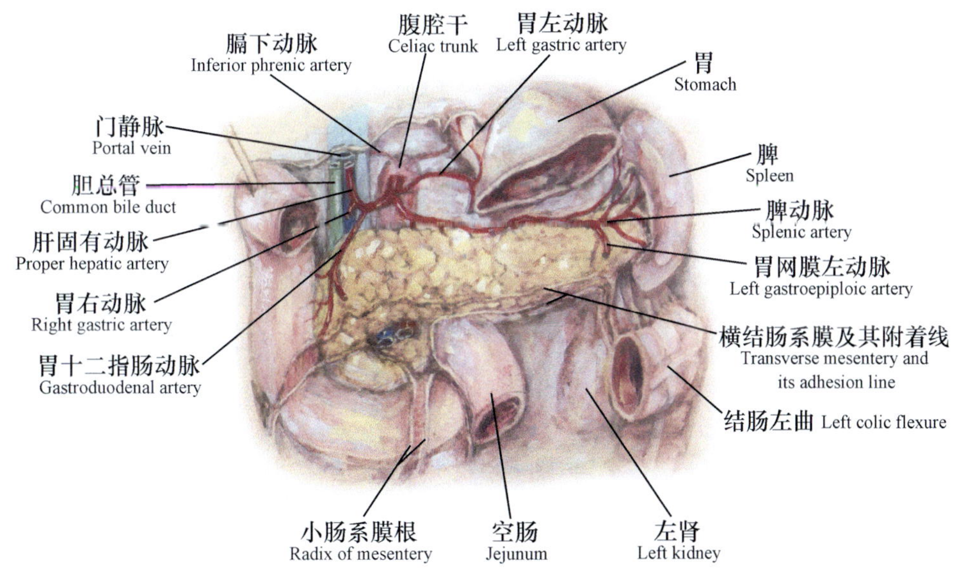

图 2-17 胰
Pancreas

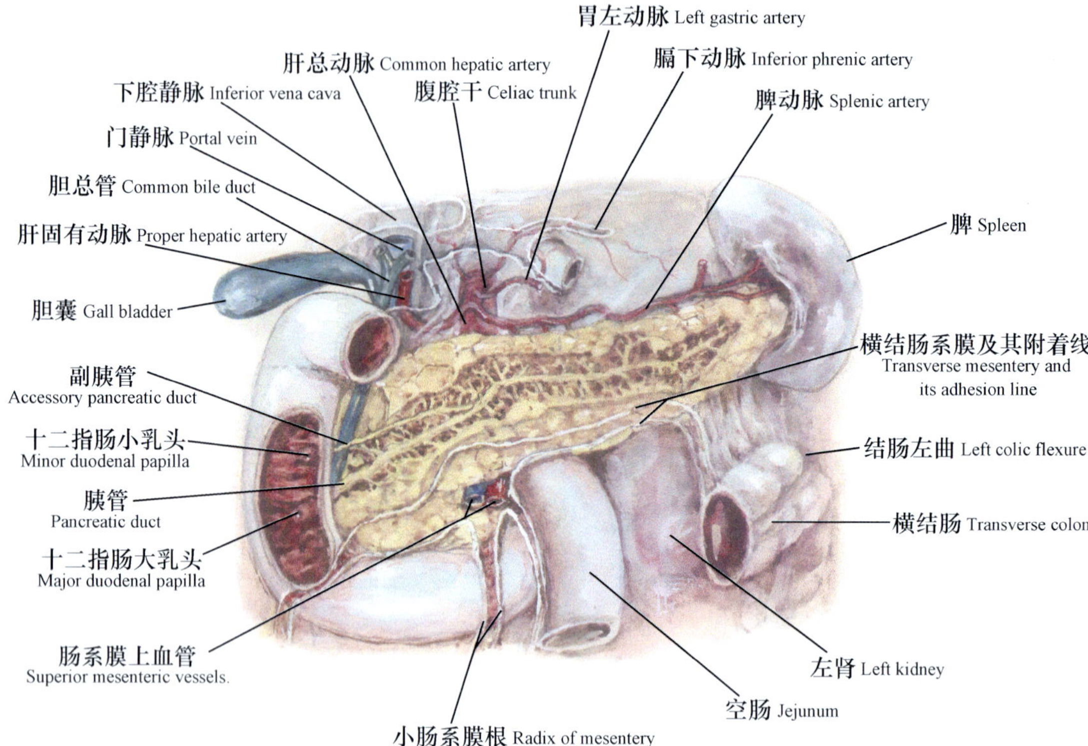

图 2-18 胰与十二指肠剖面图
Dissectied view of pancreatic and duodenal

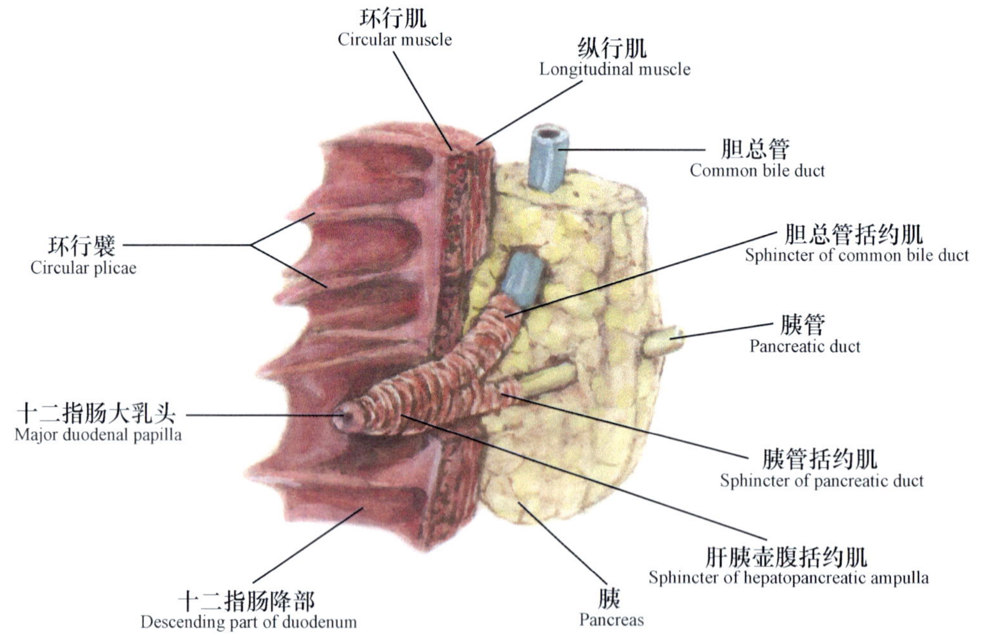

图 2-19 肝胰壶腹
Hepatopancreatic ampulla

a. 腹腔干 Celiac trunk
b. 胃左动脉 Left gastric artery
c. 脾动脉 Splenic artery
d. 肝总动脉 Common hepatic artery
e. 胃十二指肠动脉 Gastroduodenal artery
f. 胃右动脉 Right gastric artery

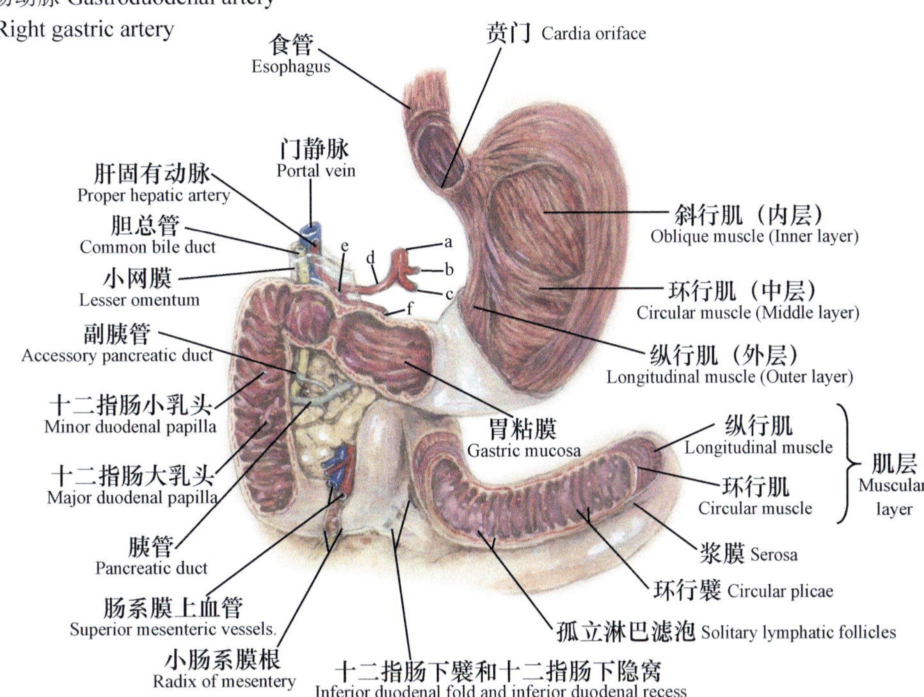

图 2-20　胃、十二指肠与空肠
Stomach, duodenum and jejunum

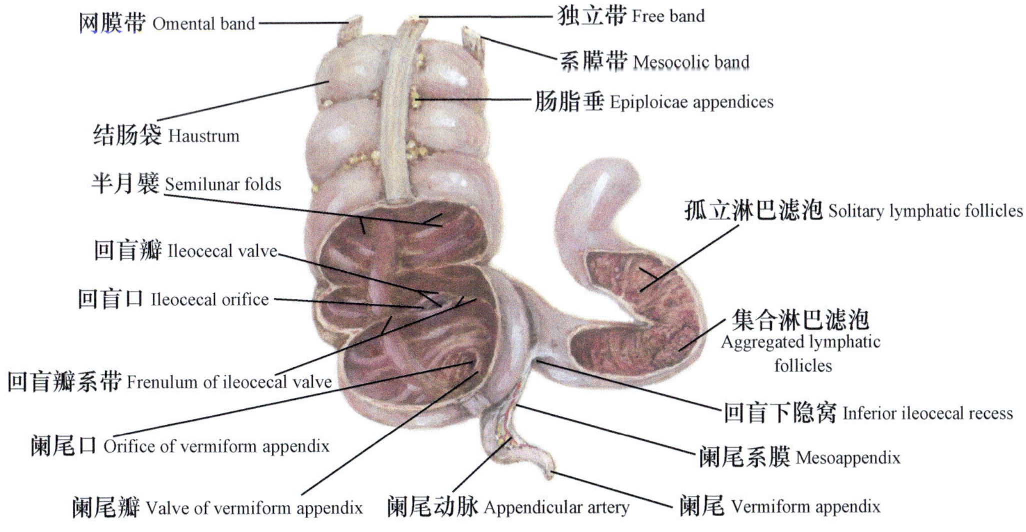

图 2-21　盲肠和阑尾
Caecum and vermiform appendix

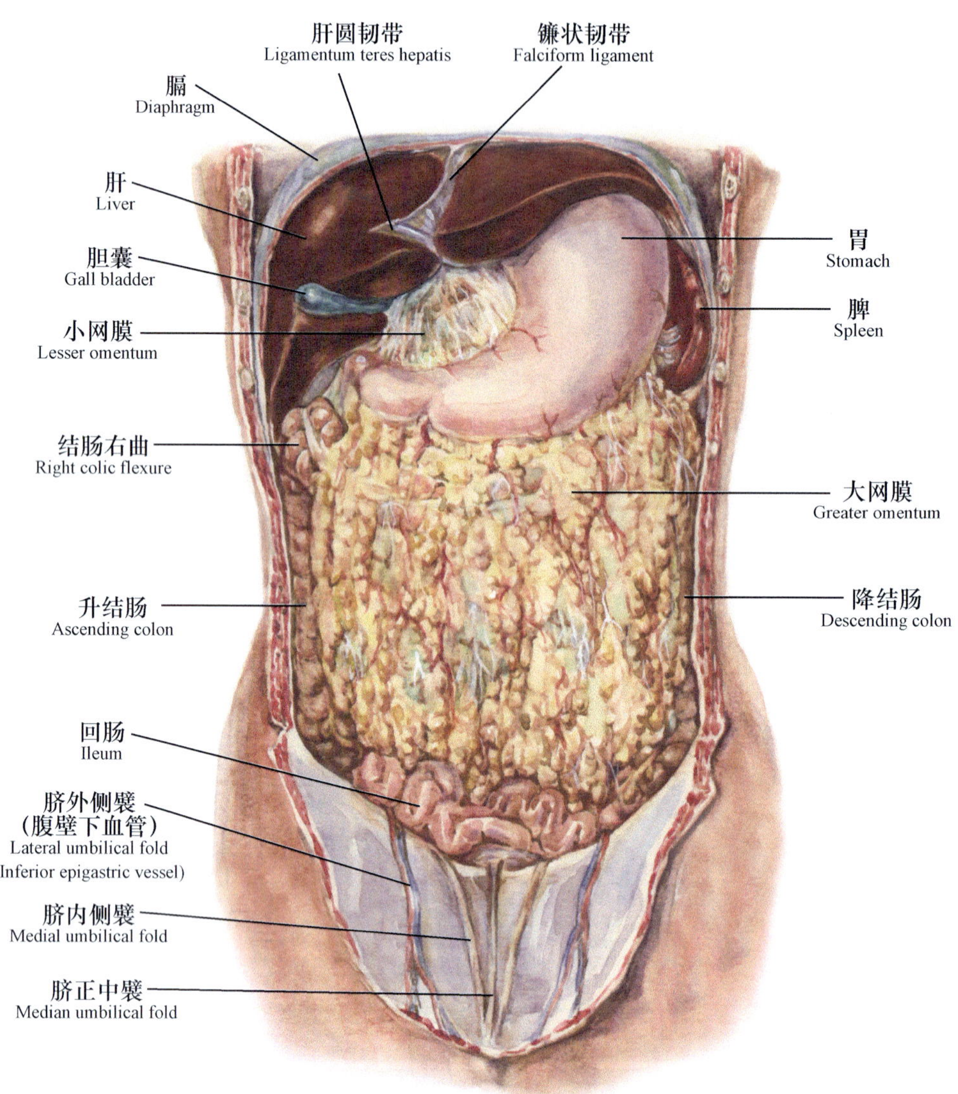

图 2-22　腹腔内脏前面观
Anterior aspect of the abdominal viscera

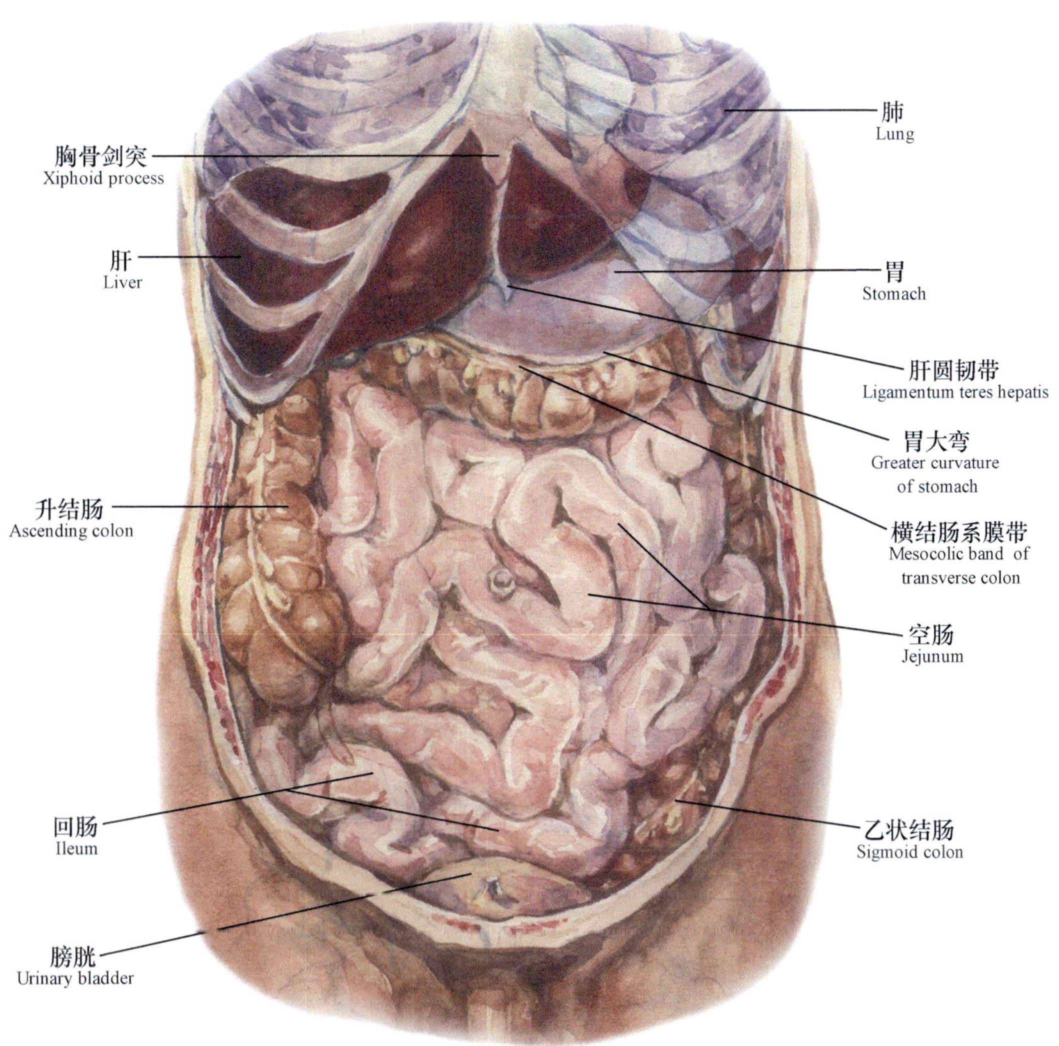

图 2-23 腹腔内脏前面观（切除大网膜）
Anterior aspect of the abdominal viscera (Remove the greater omentum)

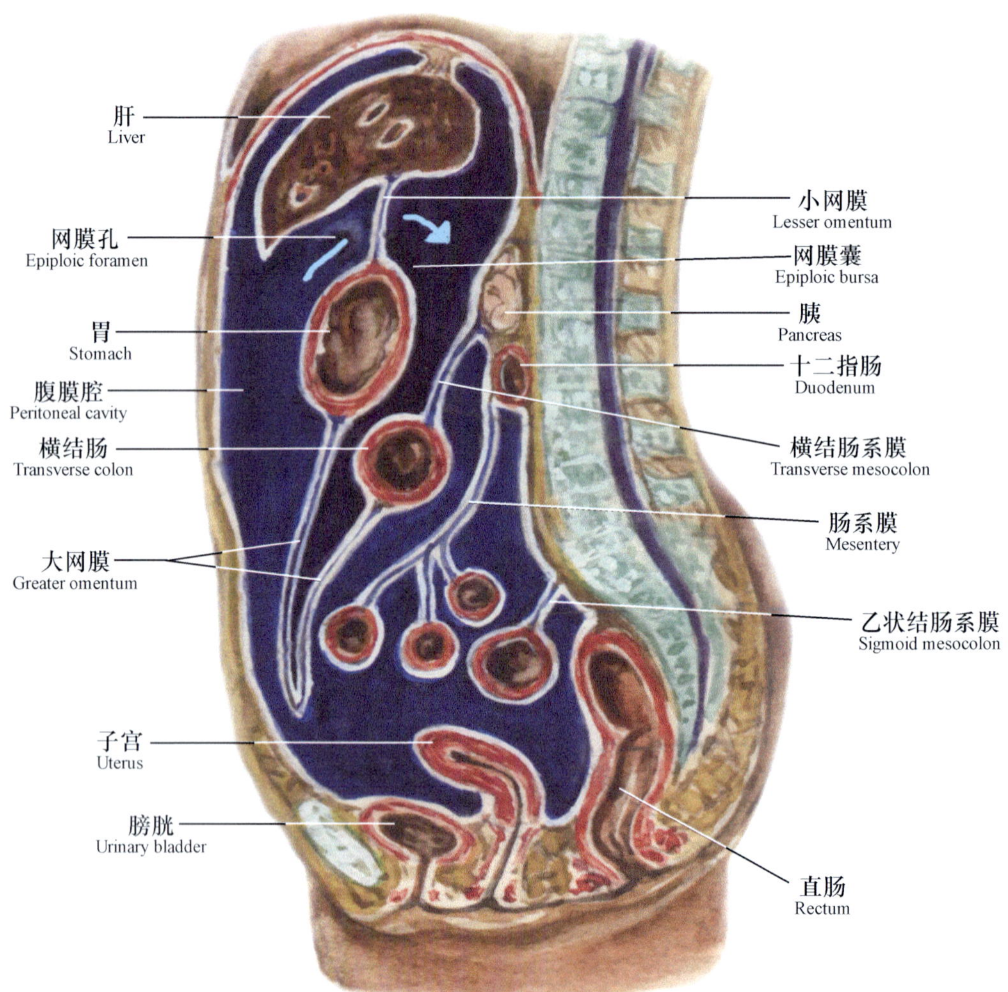

图 2-24 腹腔正中矢状切面
A median saggital section through the abdominal cavity

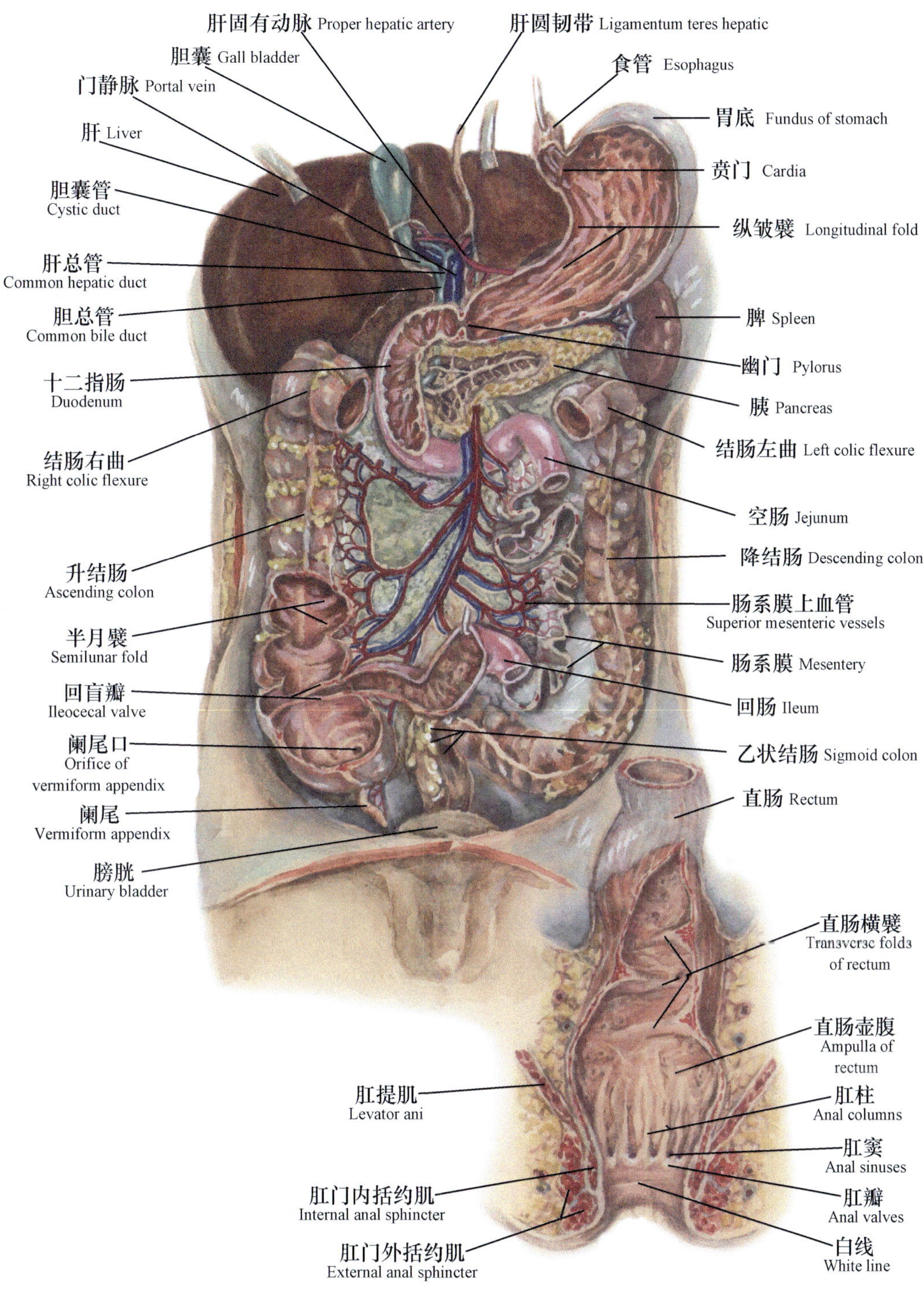

图 2-25　消化管内面观
Internal aspect of the digestive canal

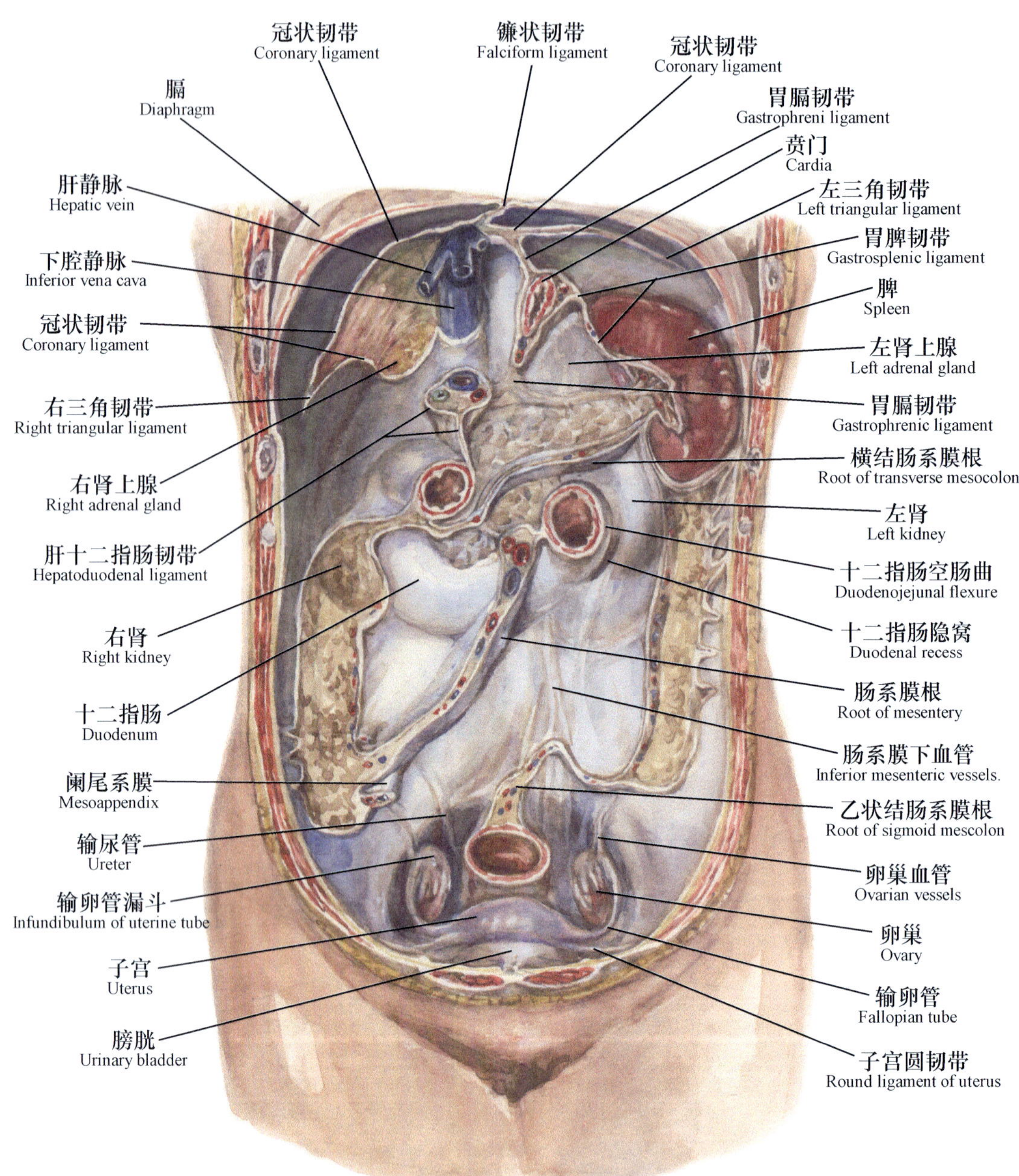

切除肝、胃和大部分肠管，以显示腹膜反转情况

After removal of the liver, stomach and most of the intestine, showing the lines of peritoneal reflexion

图 2-26 腹后壁

The posterior abdominal wall

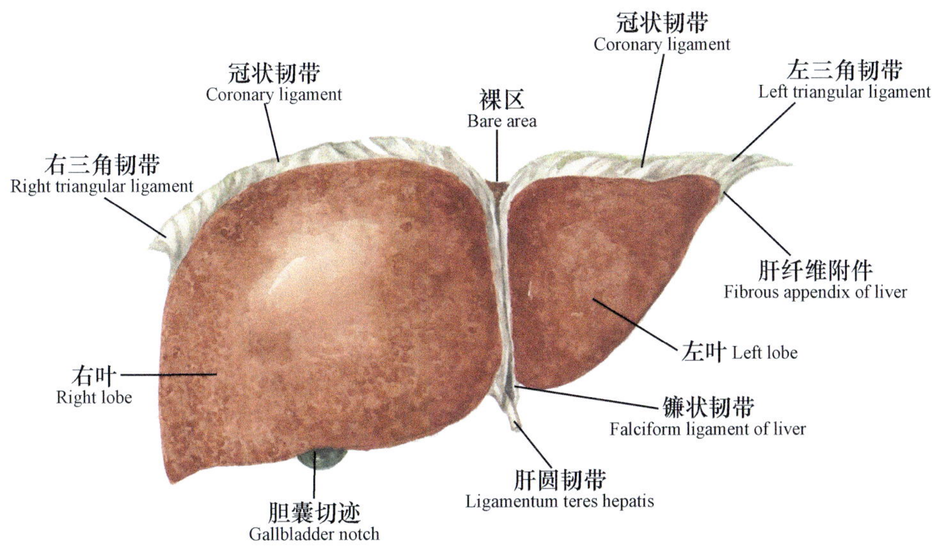

图 2-27 肝上面观
Superior aspect of liver

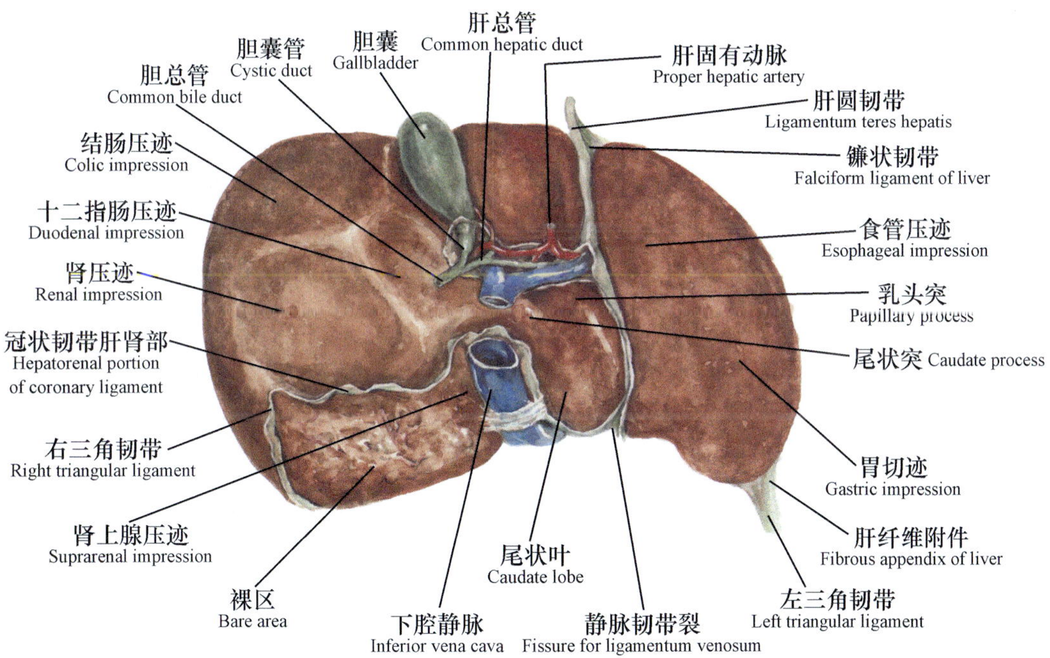

图 2-28 肝下面观
Inferior aspect of liver

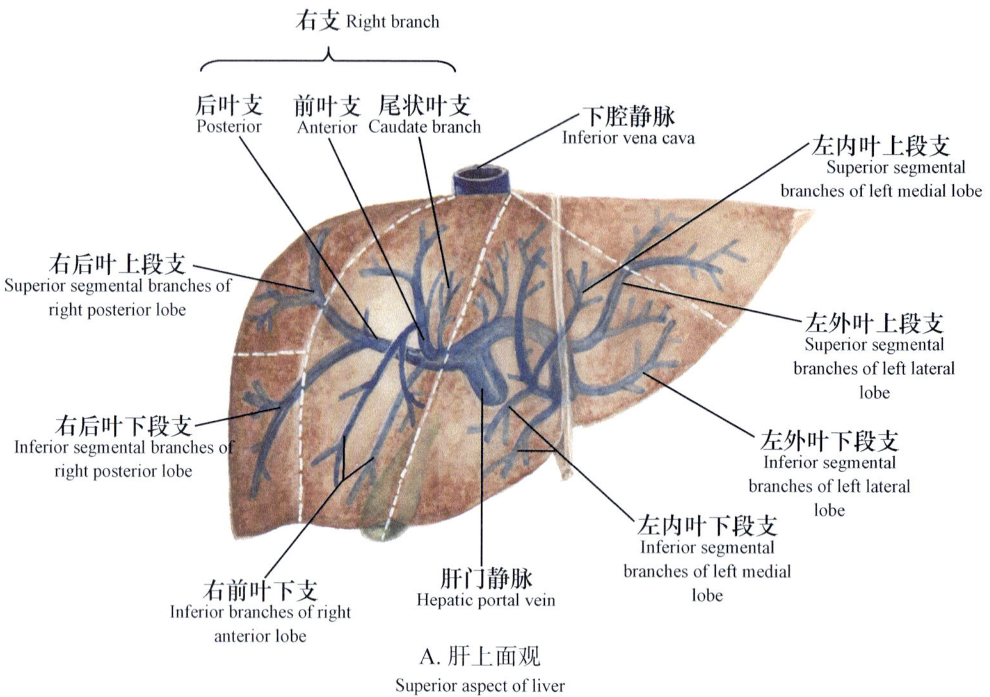

A. 肝上面观

Superior aspect of liver

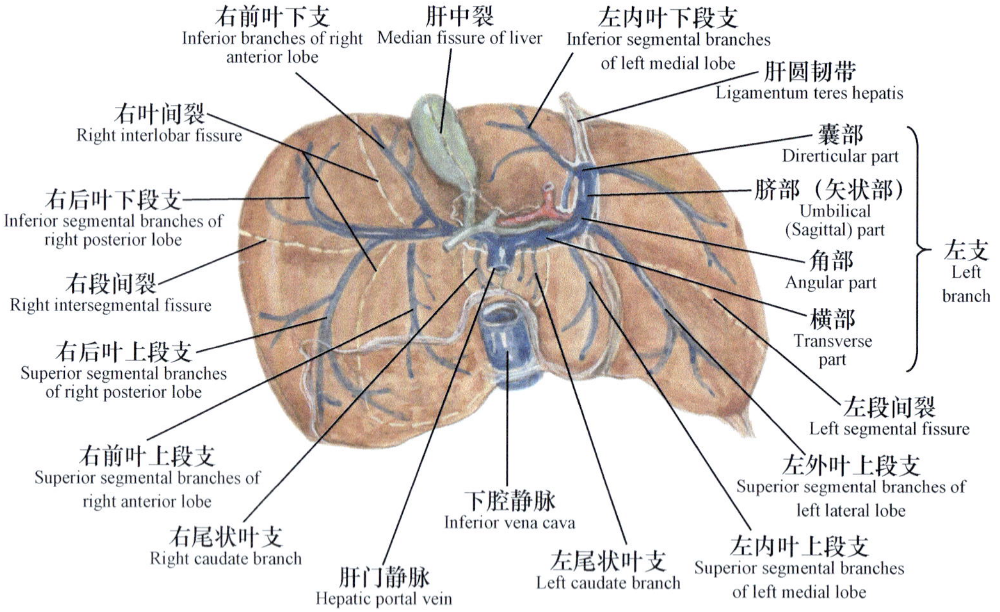

B. 肝下面观

Inferior aspect of liver

图 2-29 肝门静脉在肝内的分支

Branches of the hepatic portal vein in the liver

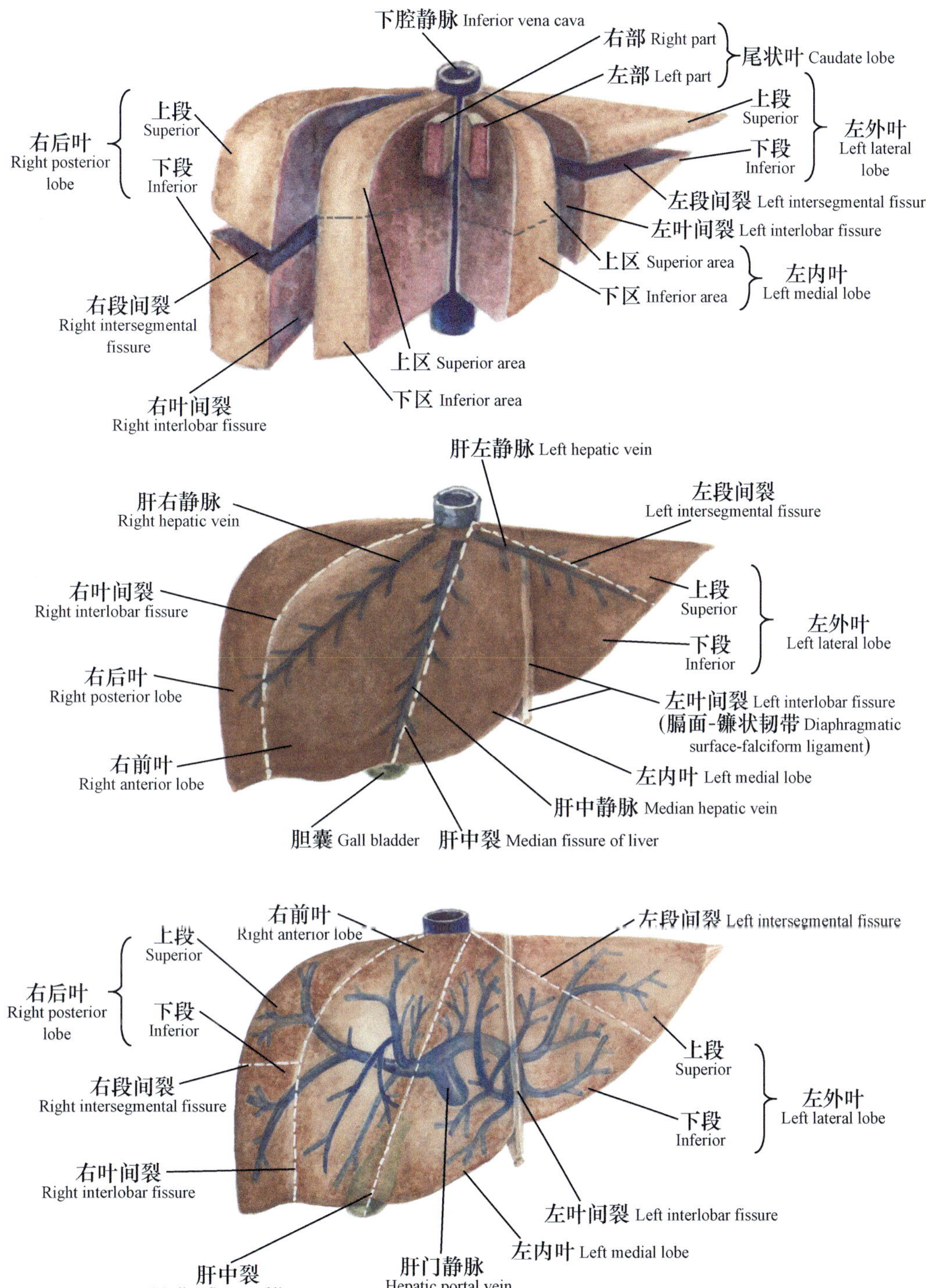

图 2-30 肝叶、肝段示意图
Scheme of the liver lobes and segments

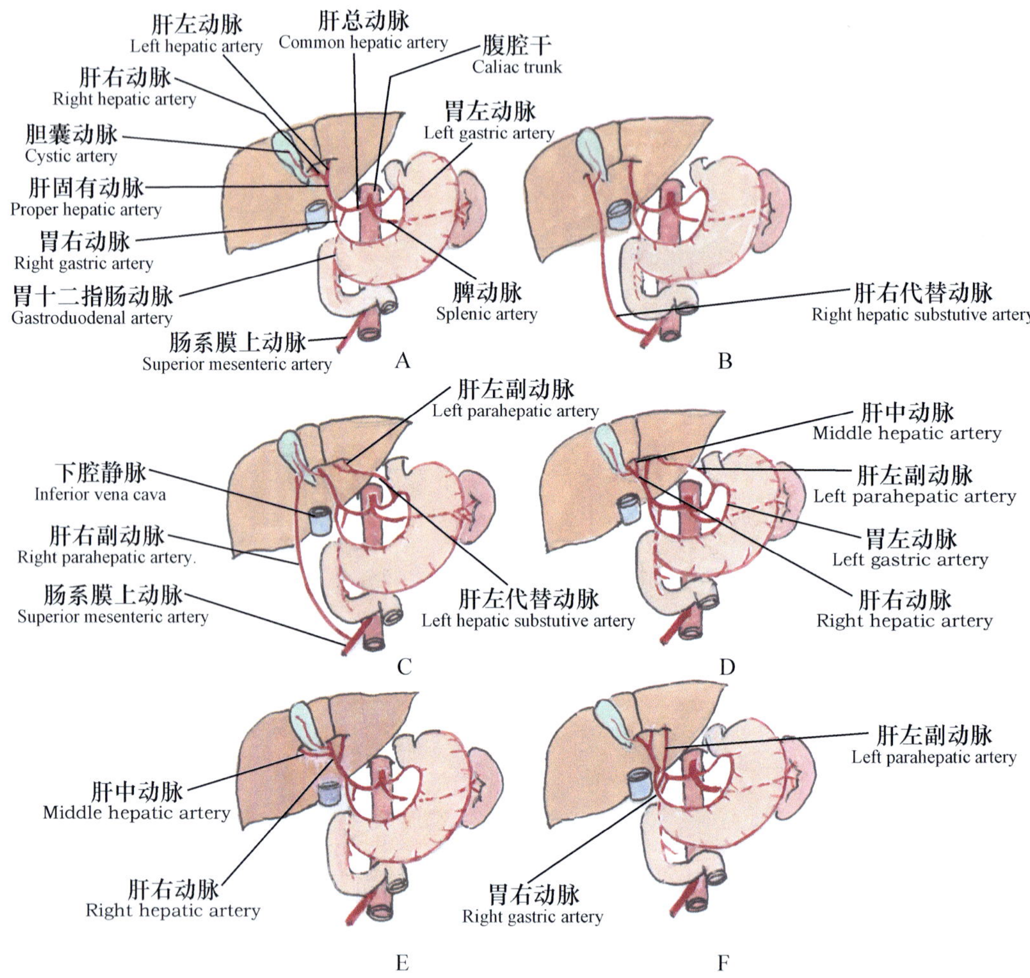

1. 肝动脉的肝外分支称肝中动脉（图 D、图 E）61/122 出现率 50%
   Branch of the hepatic artery outside the liver is called the Middle hepatic artery (Figure D,E) 61/122 occurrence rate 50%.
2. 取代正常的肝动脉的血管称肝代替动脉（图 B、图 C） 右侧 4/122 （3.3%）, 左侧 2/122 （1.6%）
   The normal hepatic artery substuted is called Hepatic substutive artery (Figure B,C) Right 4/122 (3.3%),Left 2/122 (1.6%).
3. 肝动脉之外的入肝血管称肝副动脉（图 C、图 D、图 F）, 右侧 1/122 （0.8%）， 左侧 11/122 （9.0%）
   Vessels entrancing the liver expect the hepatic artery are called Parahepatic artery (Figure C,D) Right 1/122 (0.8%),Left 11/122 (9.0%).

图 2-31　肝的动脉
The arteries of liver

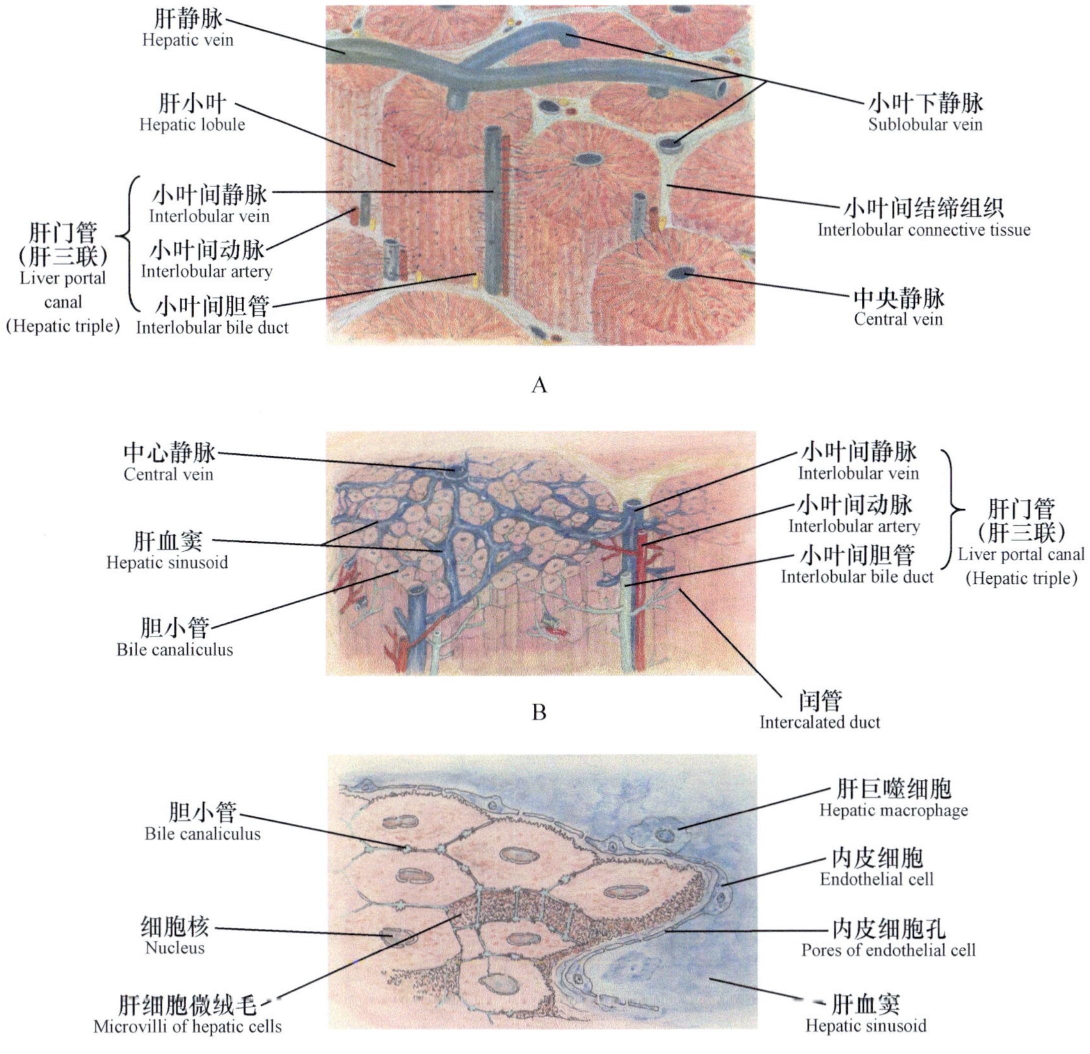

A. 肝小叶　Hepatic lobule

B. 肝板（肝索）与肝血窦　Hepatic plate (Hepatic cord) and Hepatic sinusoid

C. 电镜下的肝细胞与肝血窦　Hepatic cells and hepatic sinusoid under electron microscope

图 2-32　肝小叶模式图

Diagram of the hepatic lobule

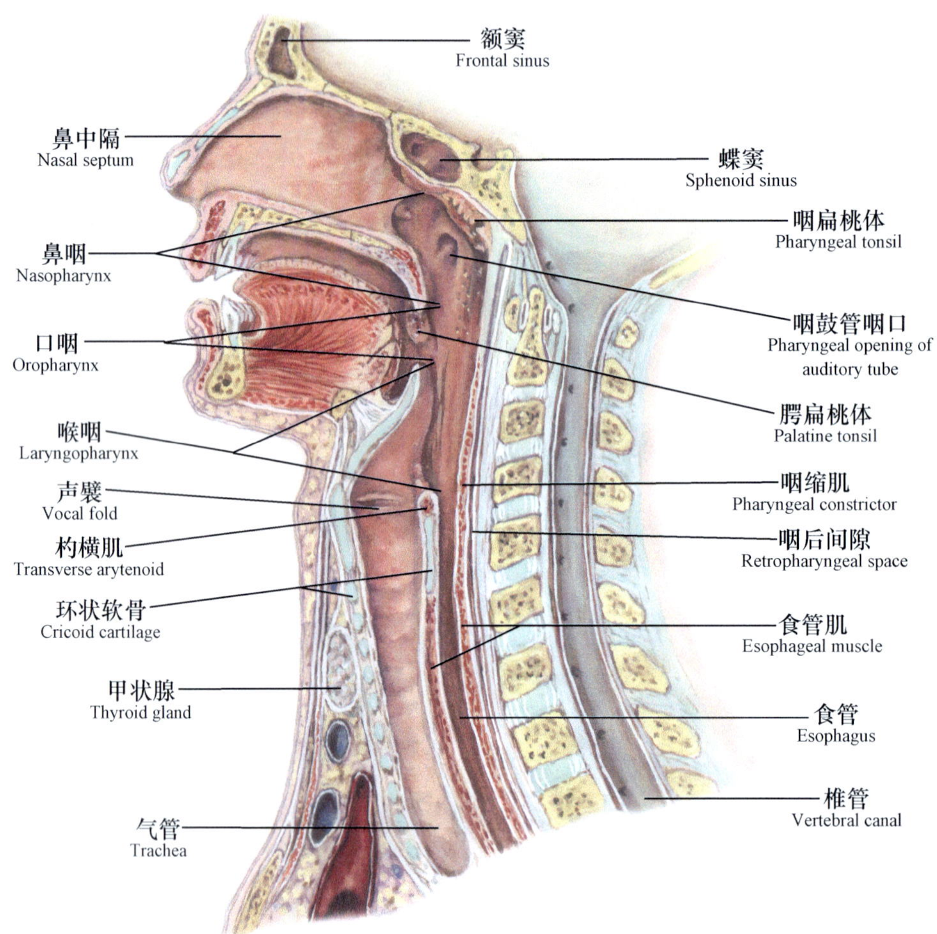

图 2-33　鼻腔与咽的正中矢状切面
Median sagittal section of the nasal cavity and pharynx

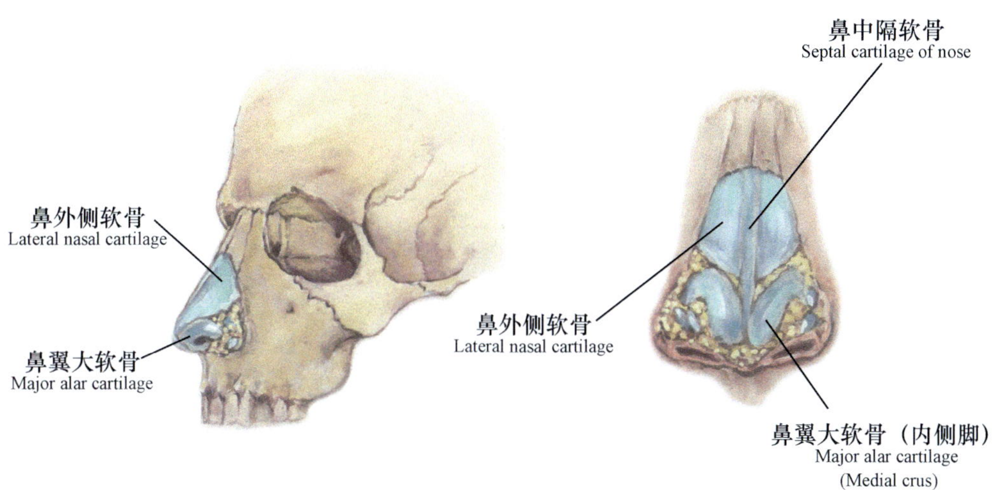

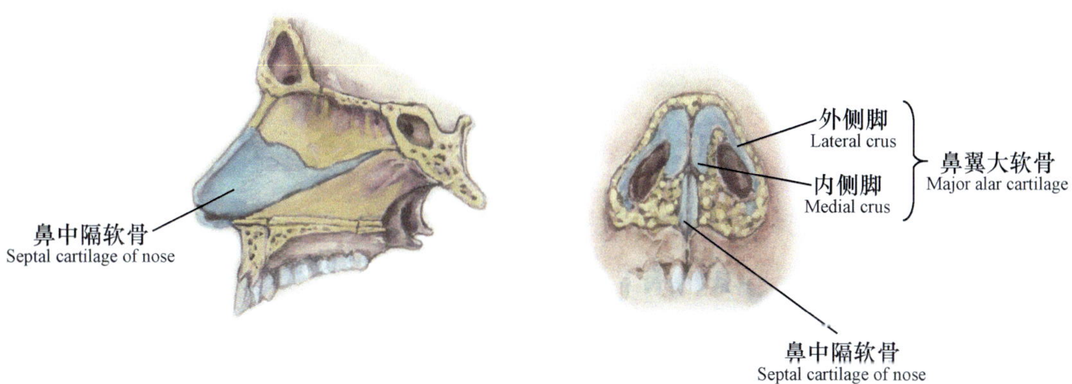

图 2-34 鼻软骨
Nasal cartilages

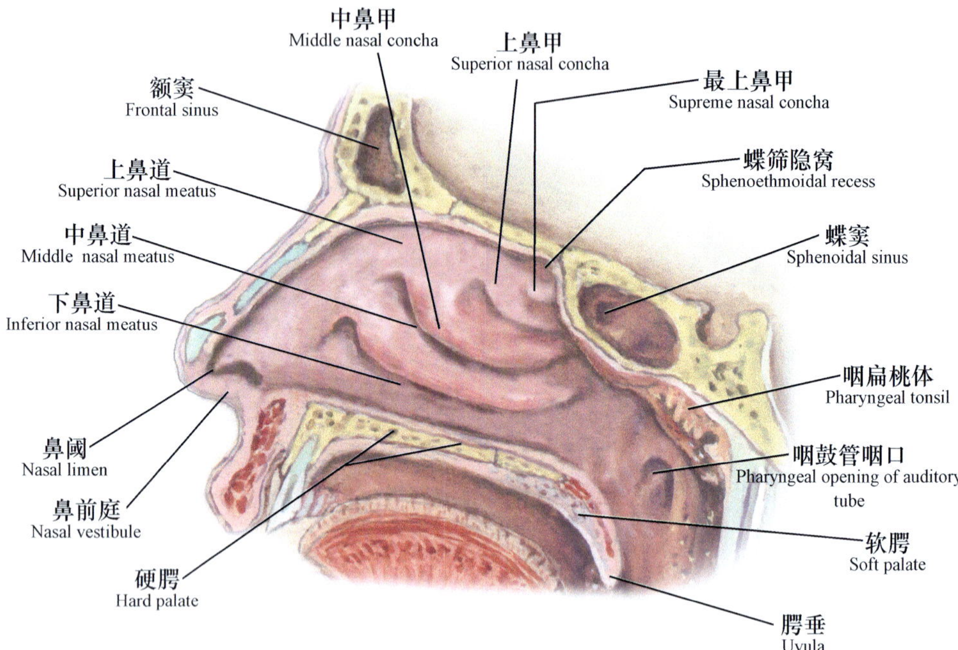

图 2-35 鼻腔右侧壁
The right wall of the nasal cavity

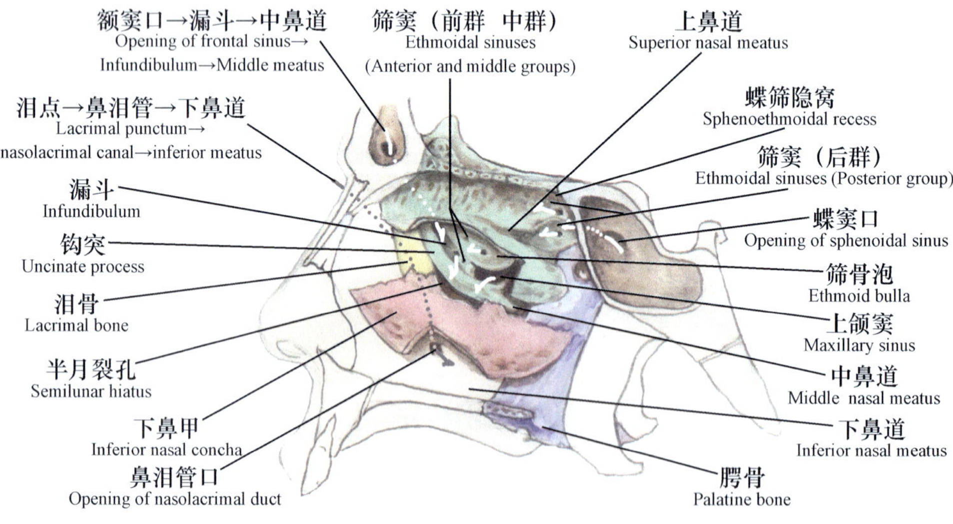

图 2-36 骨性鼻腔右侧壁显示鼻旁窦通路
The right wall of the bony nasal cavity showing openings of the paranasal sinus

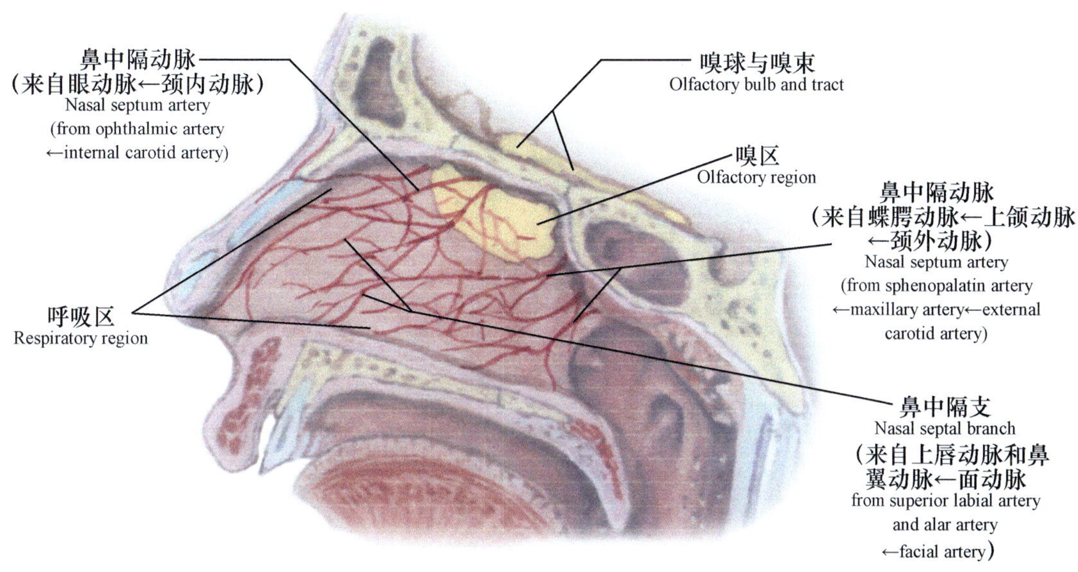

图 2-37 鼻中隔分区
Regions of the nasal septum

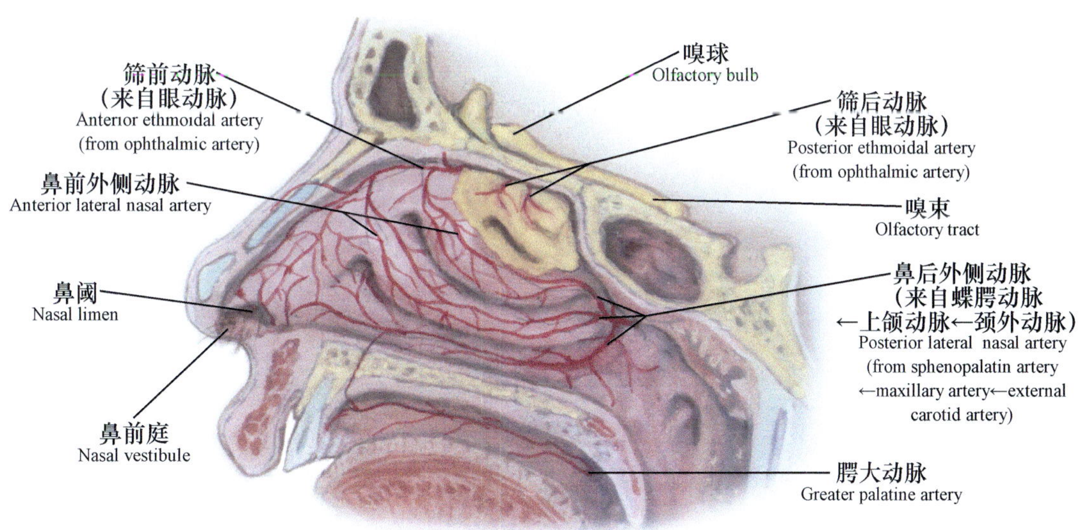

图 2-38 鼻侧壁分区
Regions of the lateral nasal cavity

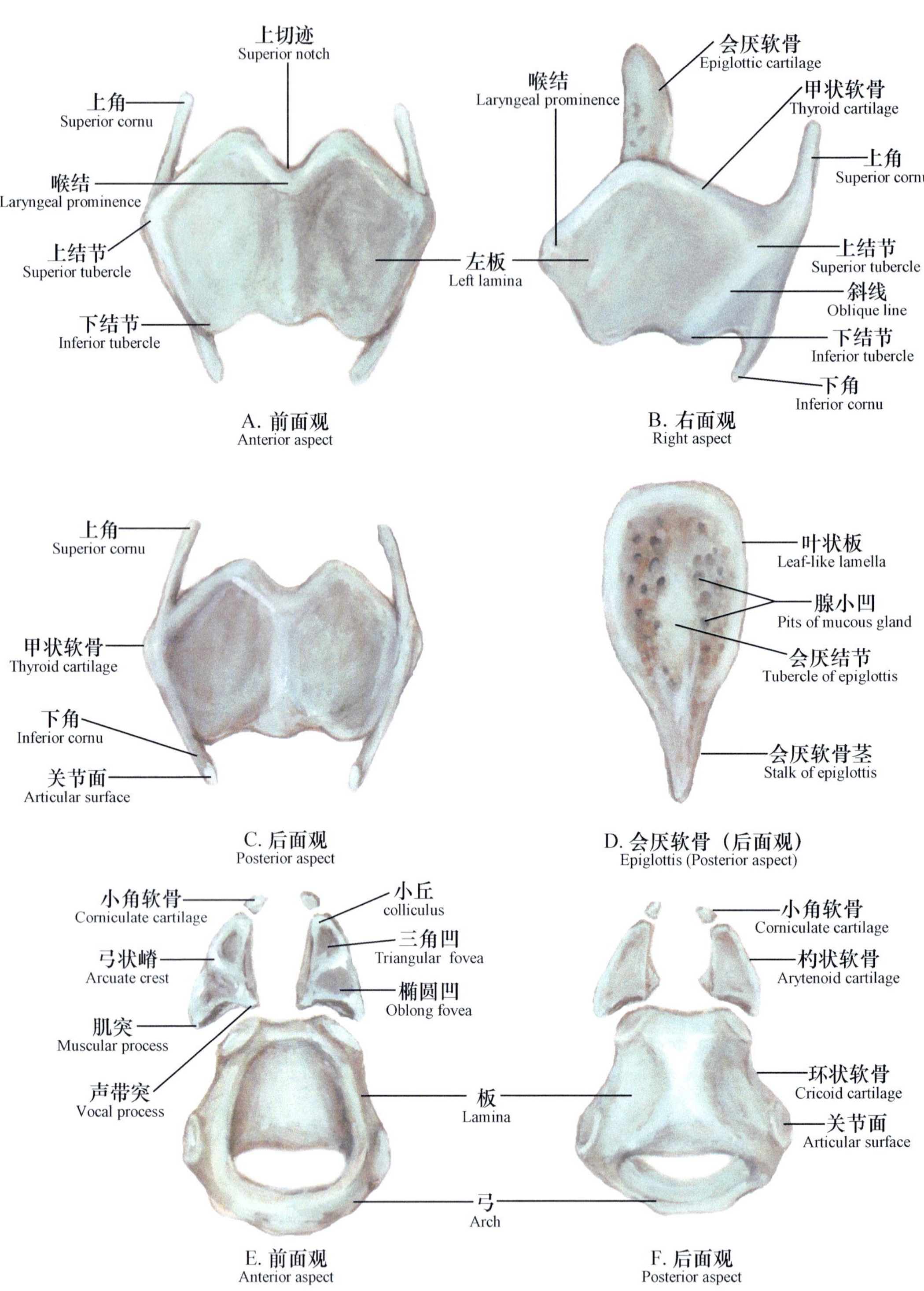

图 2-39 喉软骨
Laryngeal cartilage

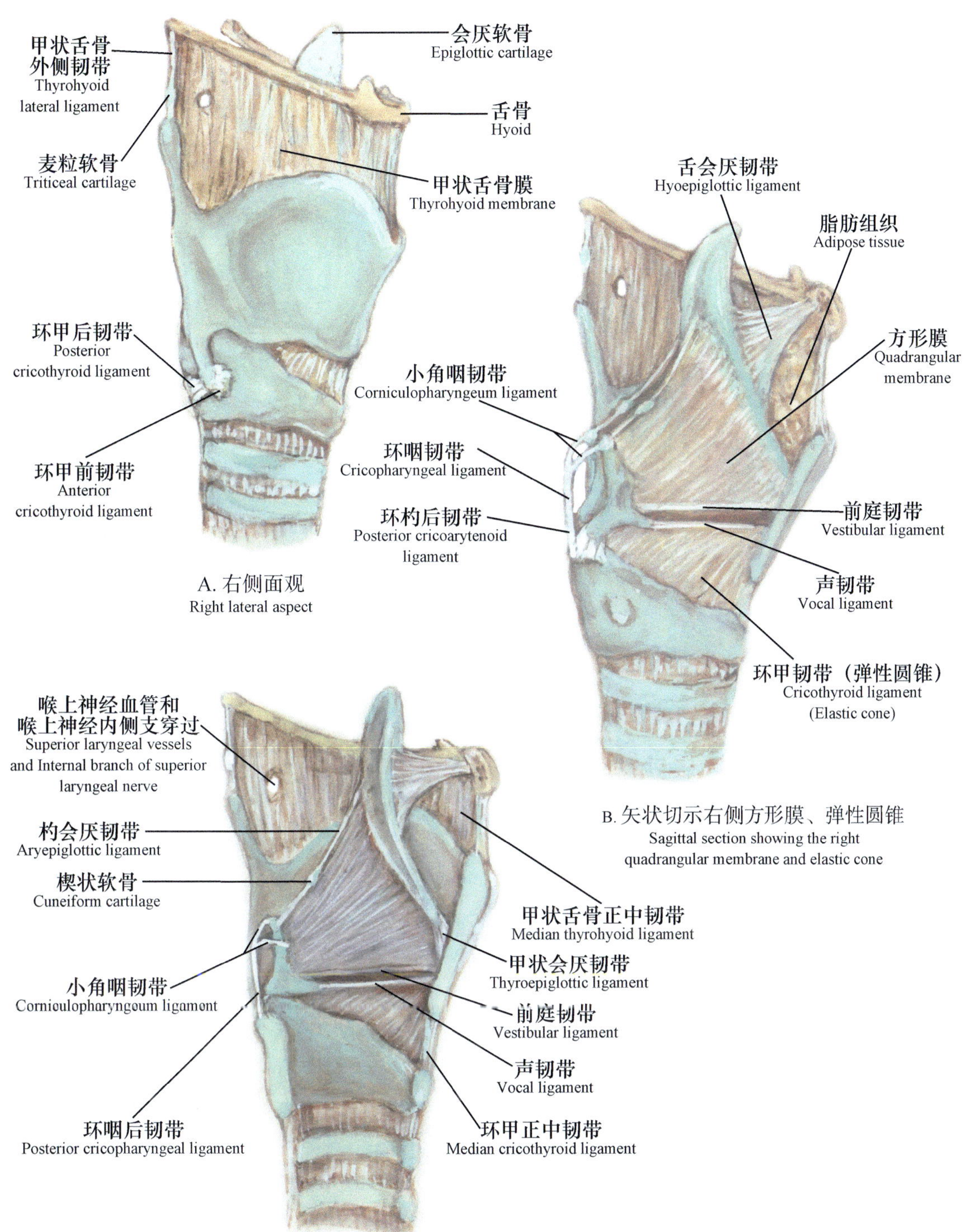

图 2-40　喉连结
Throat connection

A. 平静呼吸
Quiet respiration
声门裂膜部呈三角形软骨间部直角
The intermembranous part of the rima glottidis is triangalar and the intercardilarginous part is rectangular in shape.

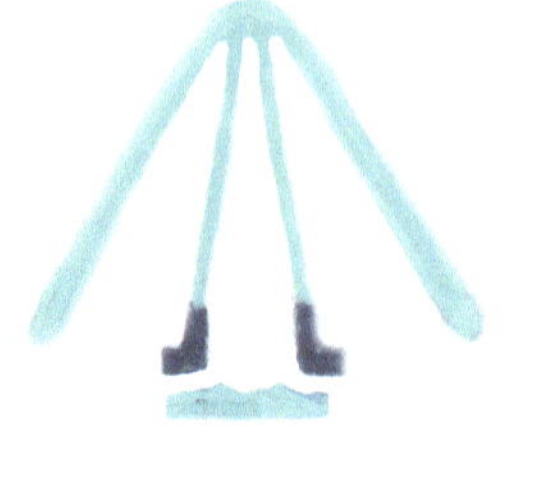

A

B. 深呼吸
Forced respiration
声门裂的二部均呈三角形
Both of the rima glottidis are triangalar in shape.

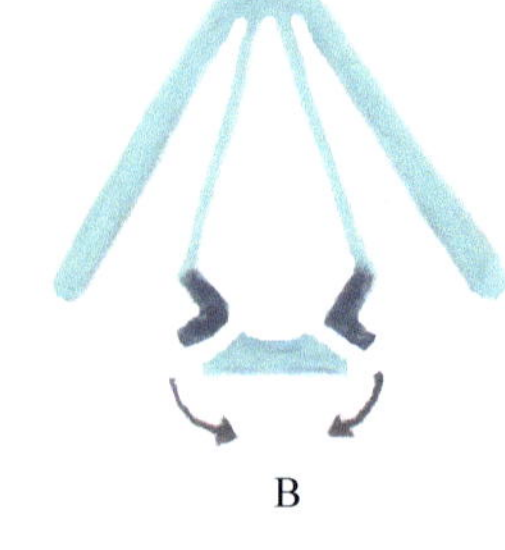

B

C. 声带内收
Adduction of the vocal folds
环杓外侧肌牵引杓状软骨内旋，从而使声带内收
The lateral criarytenoid muscles pull the arytenoid cartilage medially rotated and the vocal folds adducted.

C

D. 声门闭合
Closure of the glottis
杓横机牵引声带和杓状软骨内收，但无软骨内旋动作
The transverse arytenoid muscles pull both the vocal folds and the arytenoid cartilages, but there is no rotation of the cartilages.

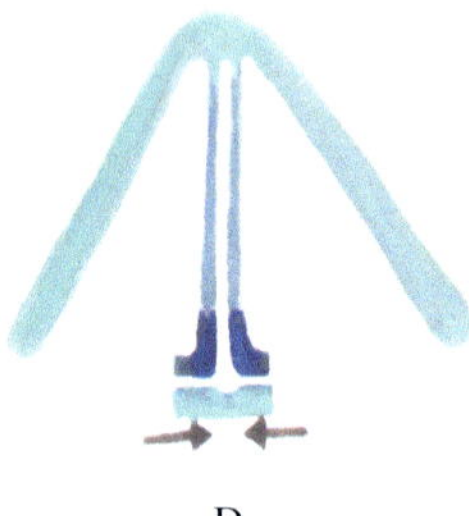

D

E. 声带紧张
Tension of the vocal folds
环甲收缩使环状软骨前部斜向上倾，导致杓状软骨后移
The cricothyroid muscles tilt the anterior part of the cricoid cartilage cranially and so carry the arytenoid cartilages dorsally.

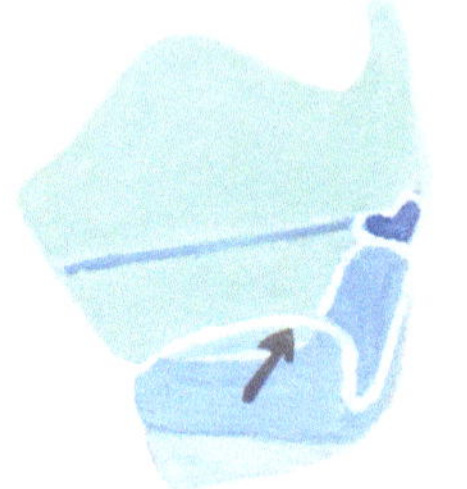

E

F. 声带松弛
Relaxation of the vocal folds
甲杓肌向前牵引杓状软骨所致
This is produces by the thyroarytenoid muscles which draw the arytenoid cartrlages ventrally.

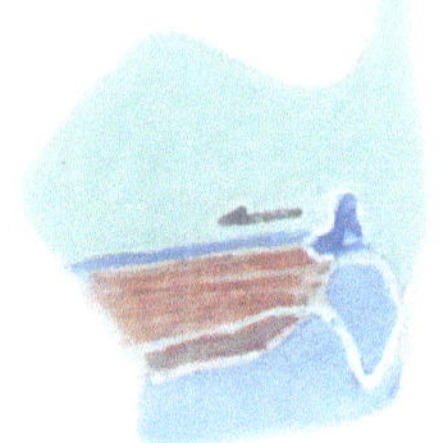

F

图 2-41　发音
Pronunciation

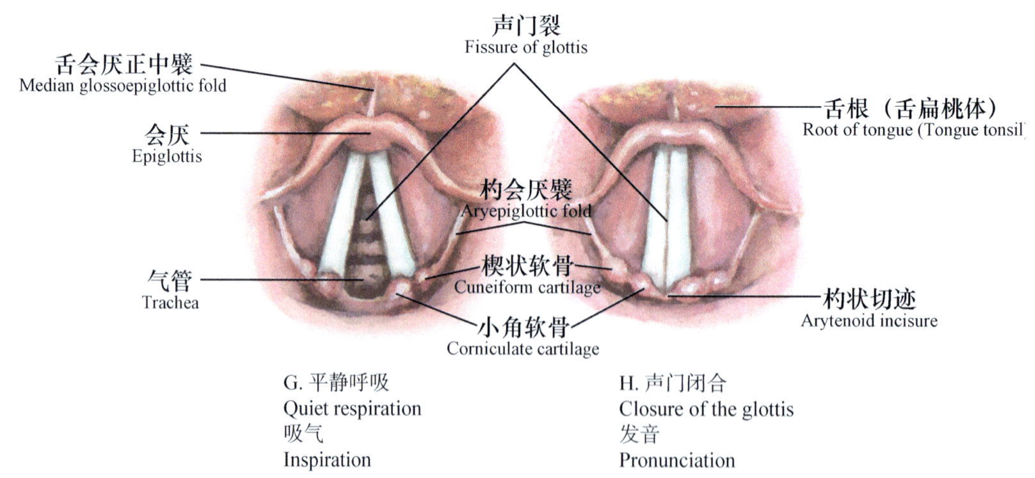

G. 平静呼吸
Quiet respiration
吸气
Inspiration

H. 声门闭合
Closure of the glottis
发音
Pronunciation

图 2-42　喉口（上面观）
Aperture of larynx (Superior aspect)

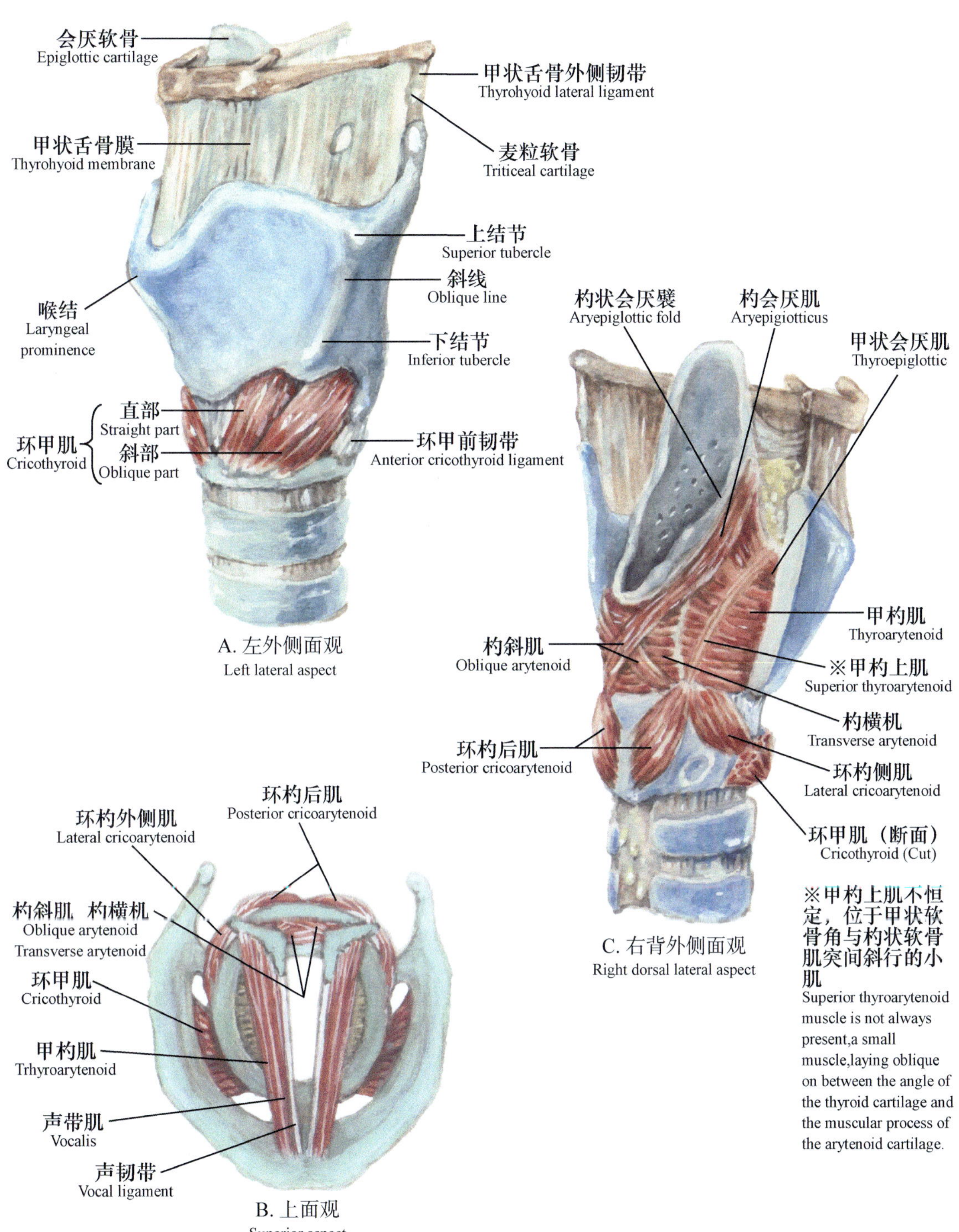

图 2-43 喉肌（1）
Laryngeal muscle (1)

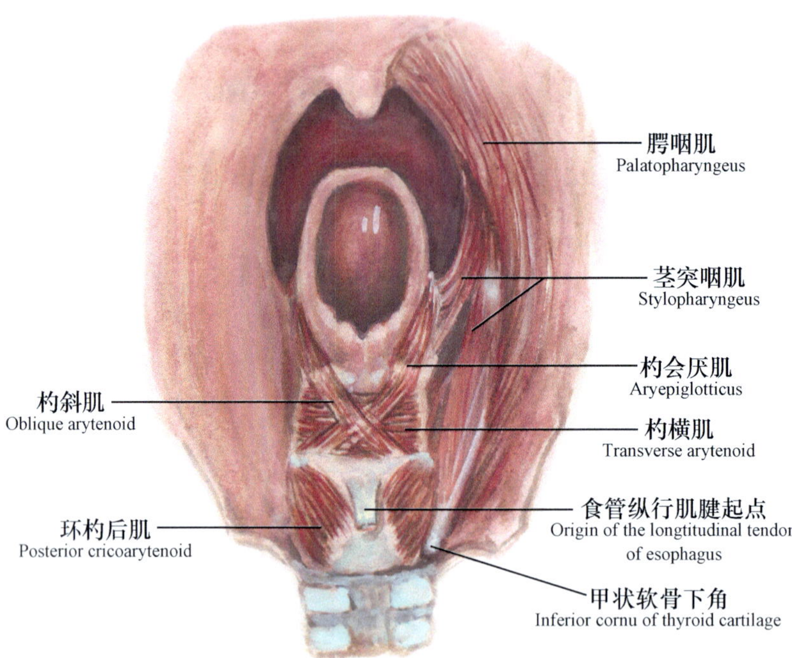

图 2-44 喉肌（2）
Laryngeal muscle (2)

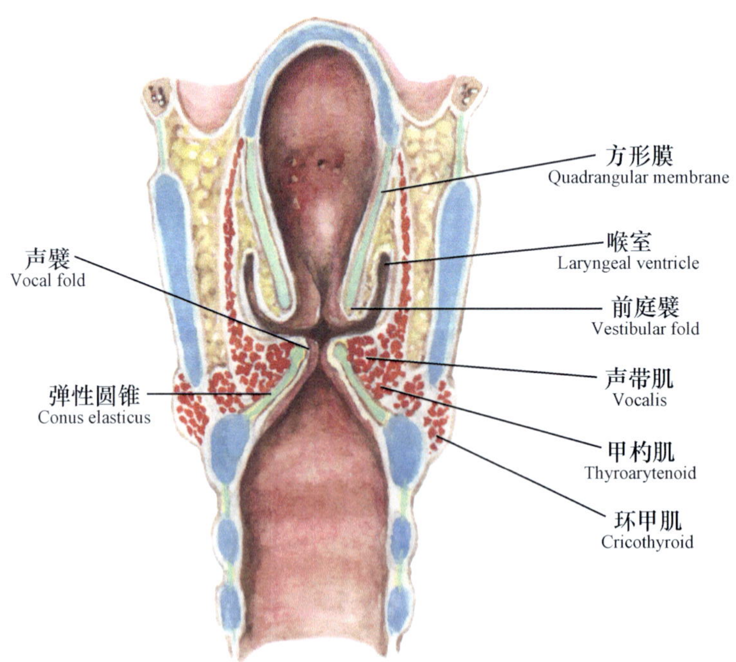

图 2-45 喉的冠状切面
Coronal section through the larynx

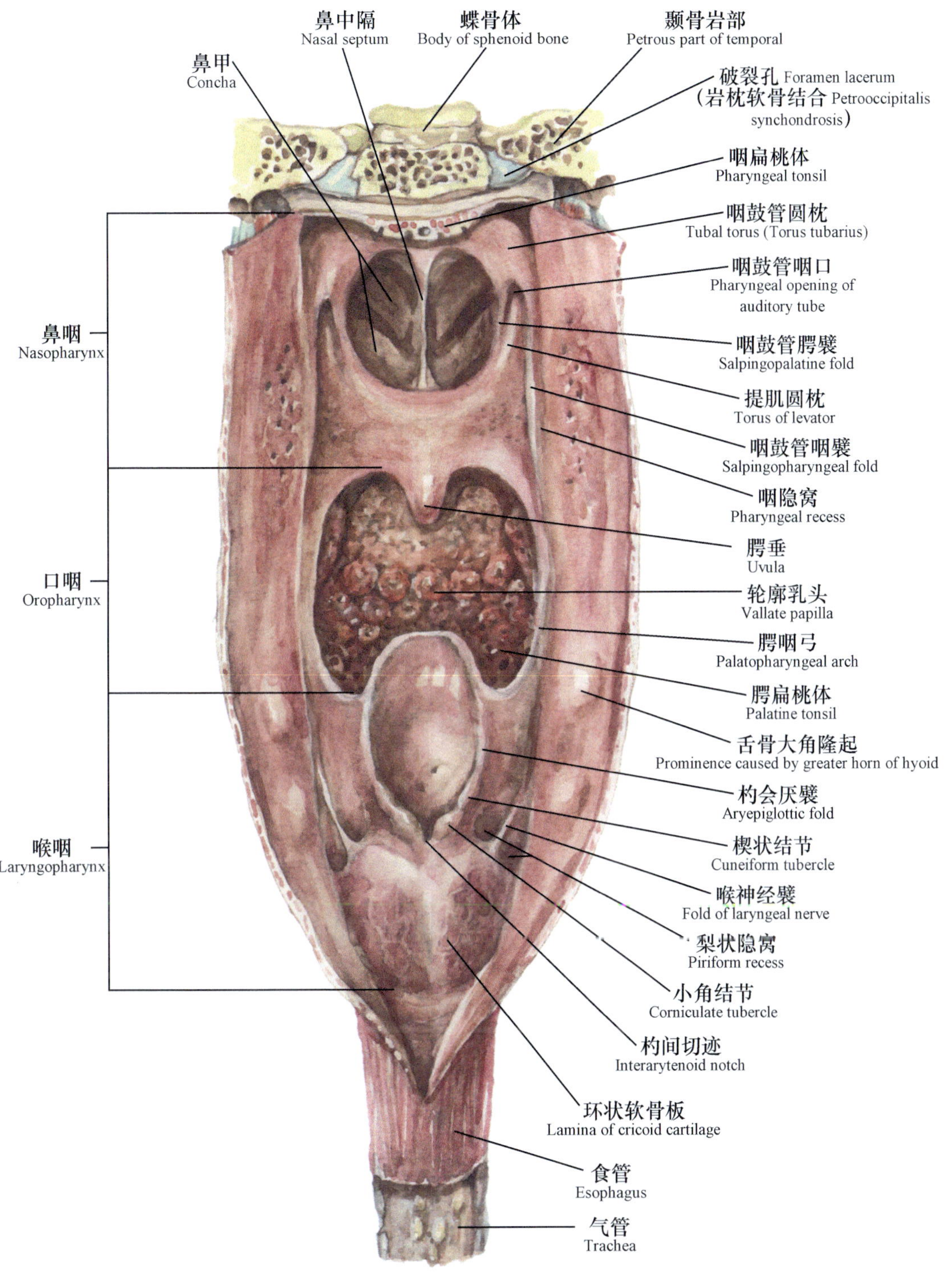

图 2-46　咽黏膜背侧观
The dorsal aspect of pharyngeal mucosa

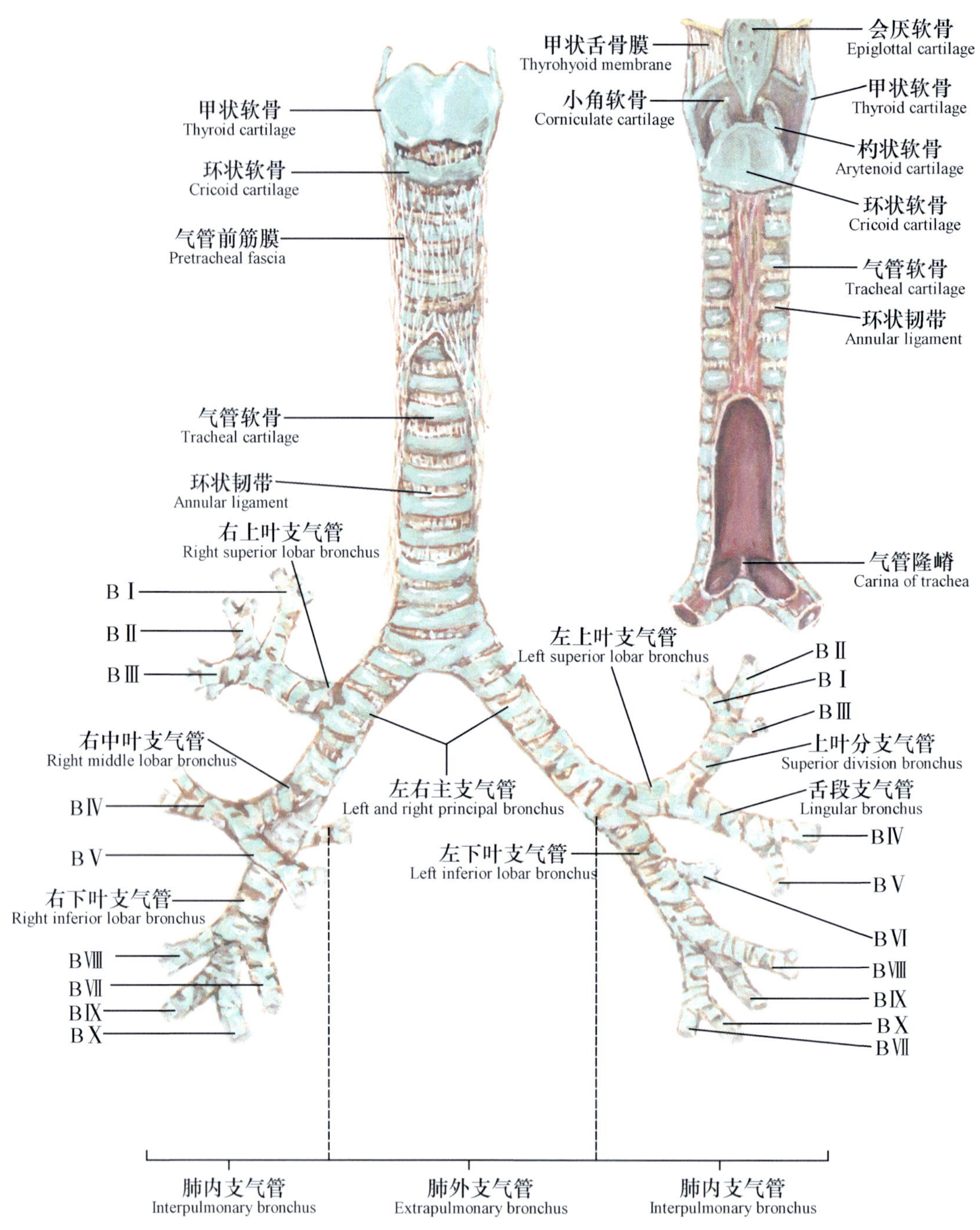

图 2-47 气管、支气管和支气管肺段
Trachea,bronchi and bronchopulmonary segment

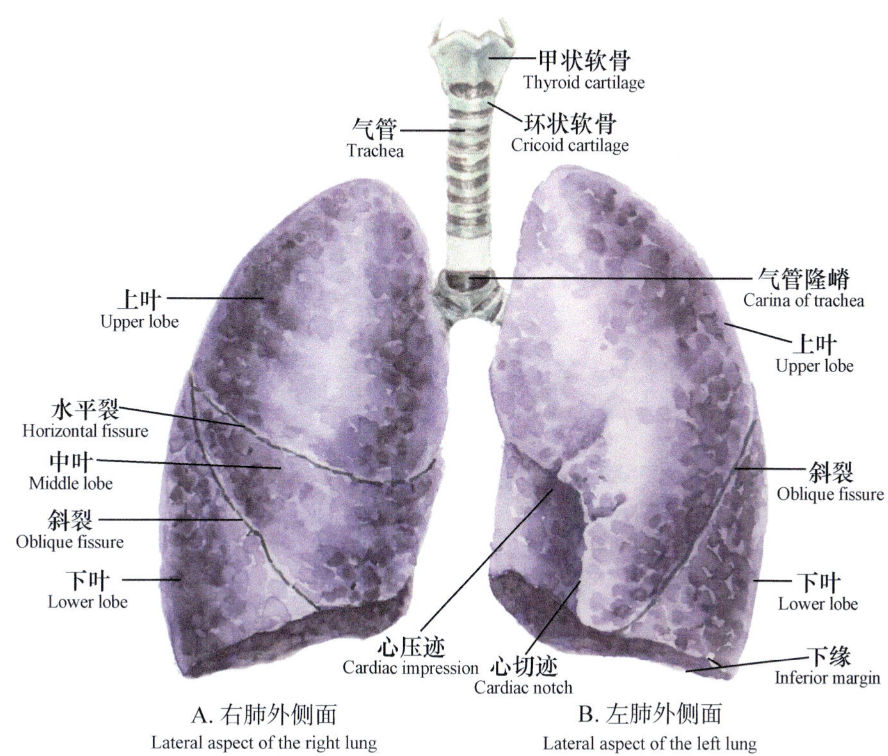

A. 右肺外侧面
Lateral aspect of the right lung

B. 左肺外侧面
Lateral aspect of the left lung

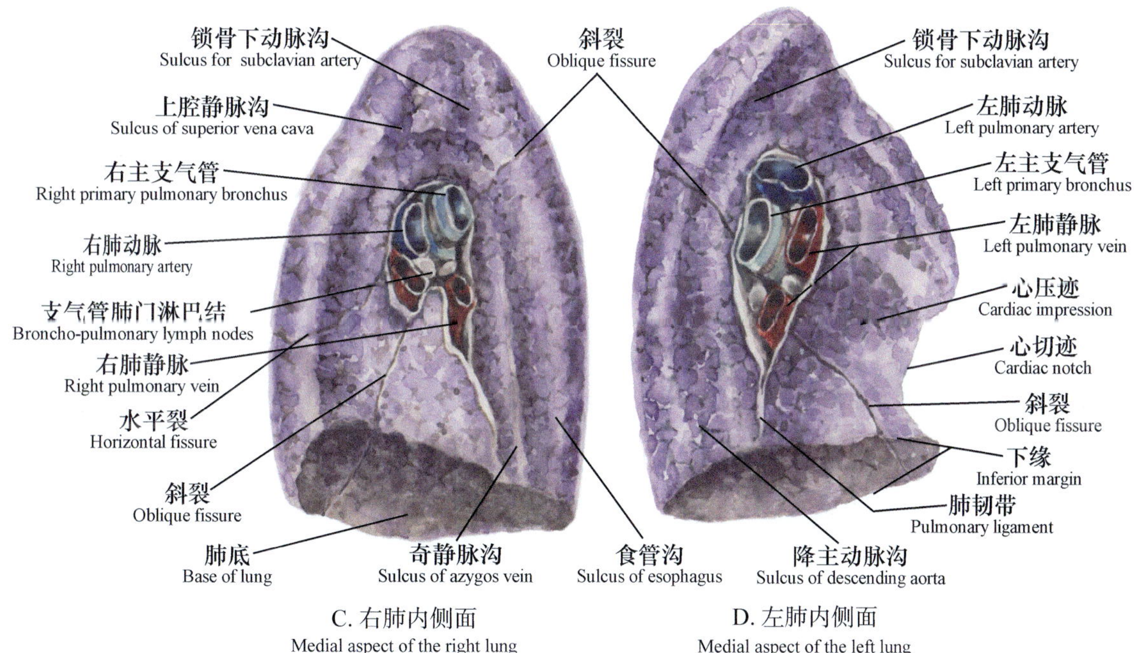

C. 右肺内侧面
Medial aspect of the right lung

D. 左肺内侧面
Medial aspect of the left lung

图 2-48 肺
Lung

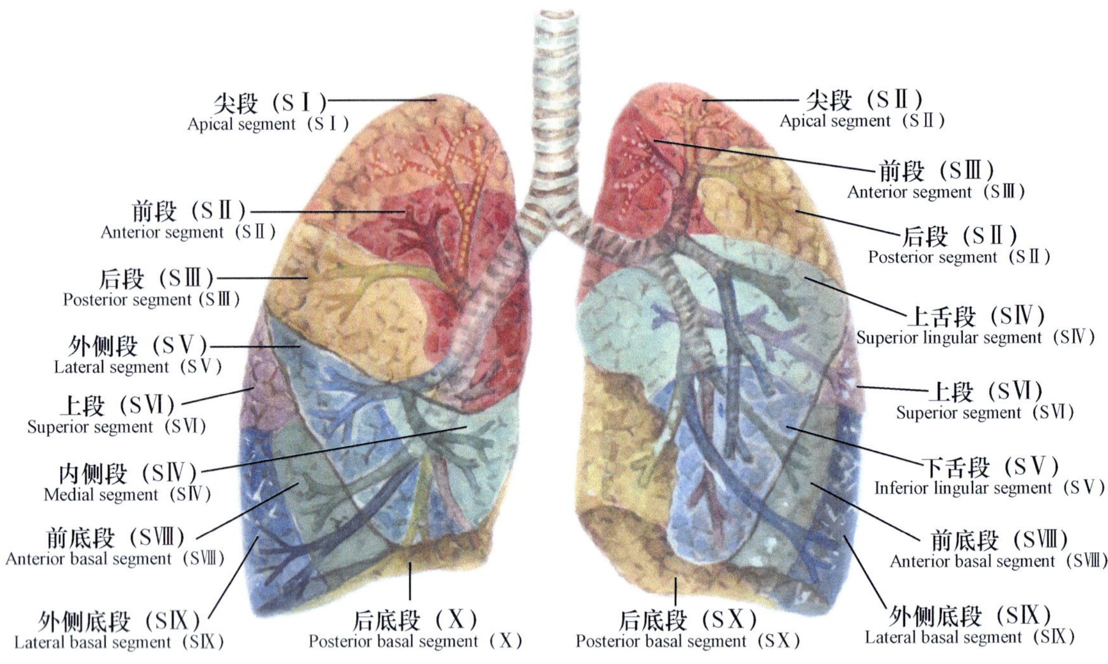

A. 前面观
Anterior aspect

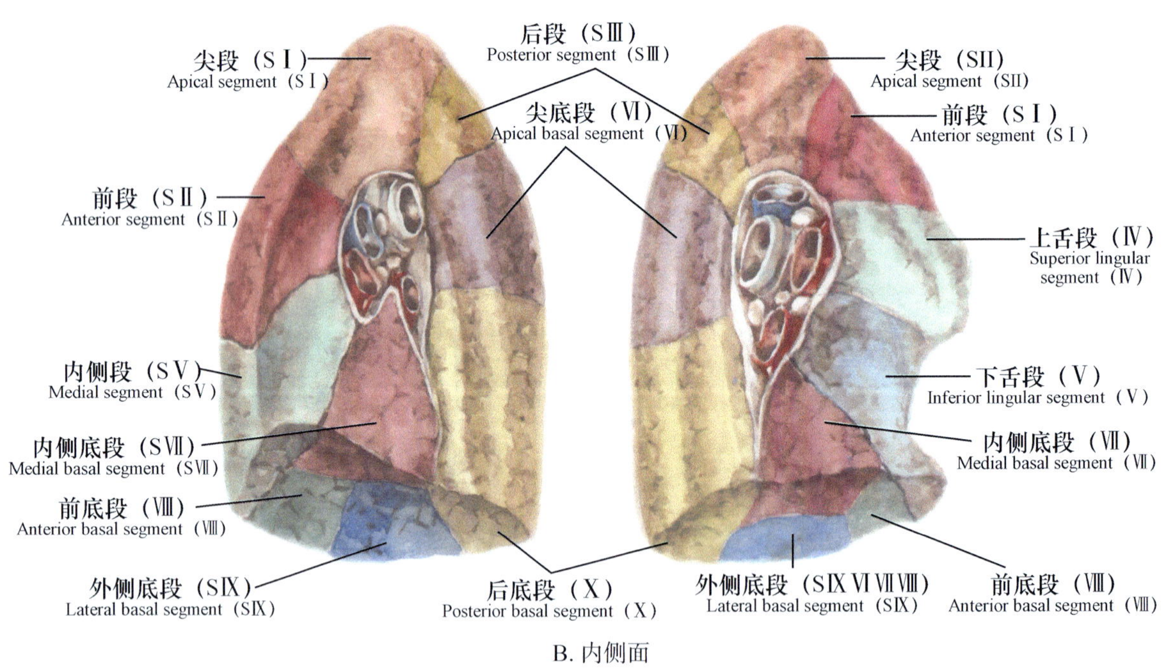

B. 内侧面
Medial aspect

图 2-49 支气管肺段
Bronchopulmonary segment

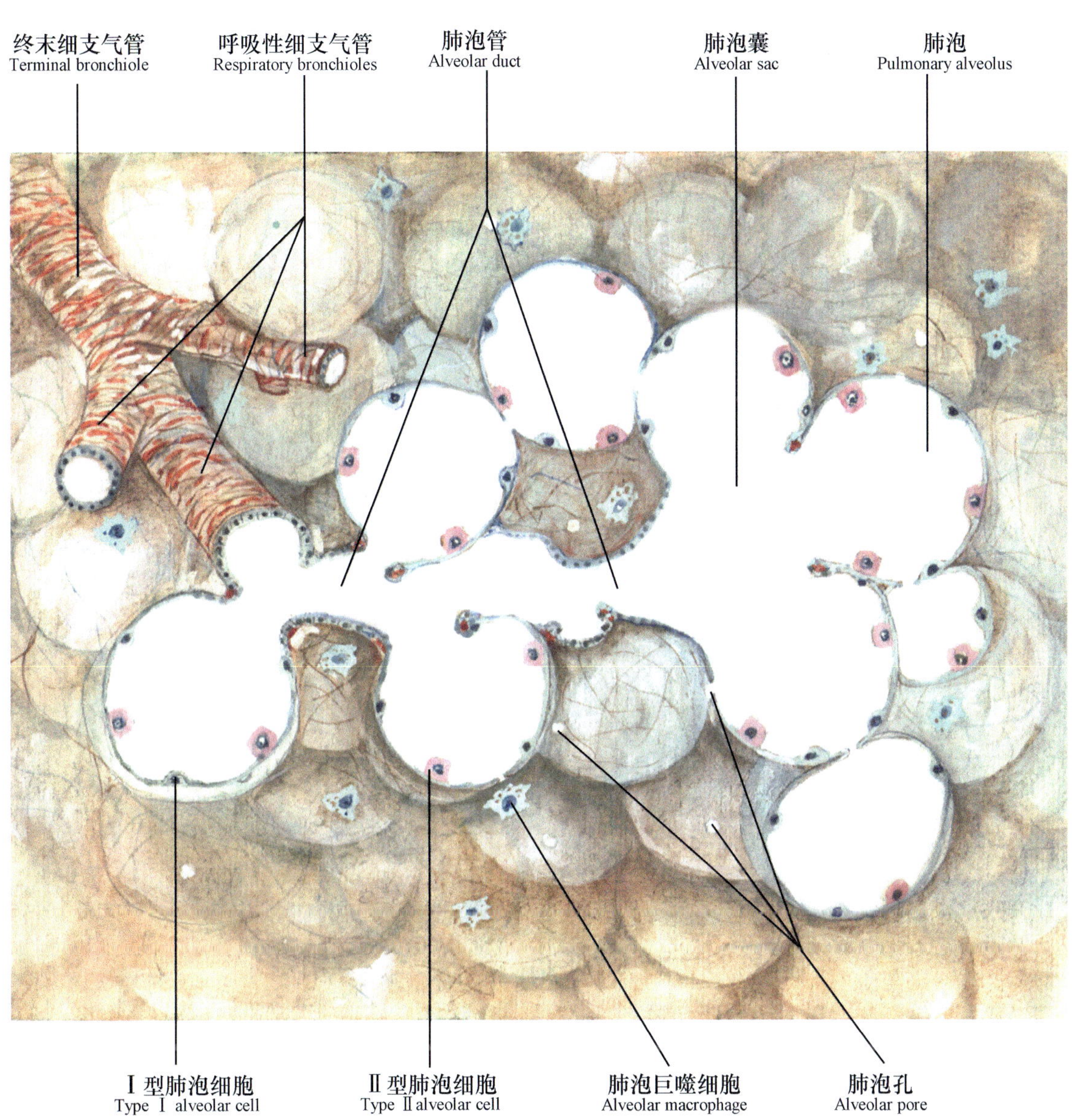

图 2-50　肺呼吸部模式图
Scheme of the respiratory part of the lung

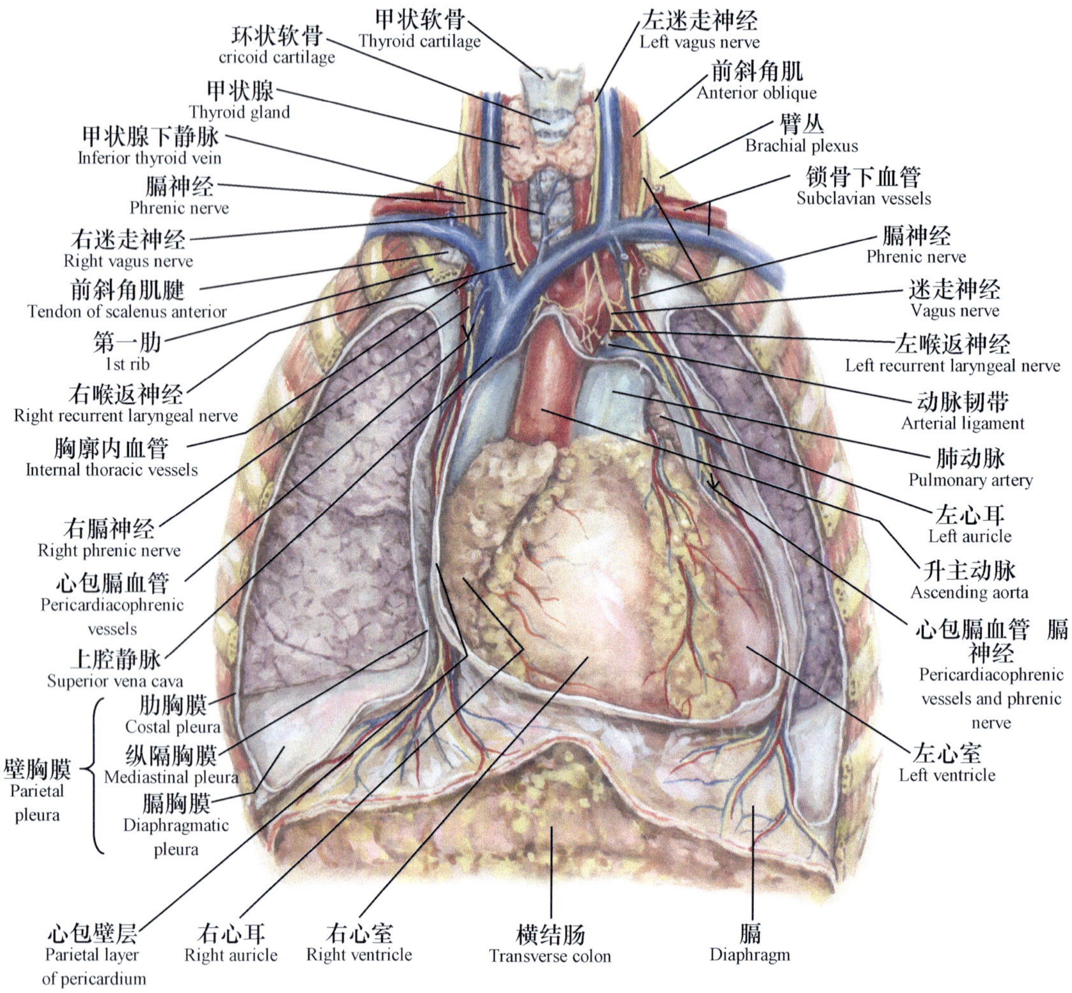

甲状软骨 Thyroid cartilage
环状软骨 cricoid cartilage
甲状腺 Thyroid gland
甲状腺下静脉 Inferior thyroid vein
膈神经 Phrenic nerve
右迷走神经 Right vagus nerve
前斜角肌腱 Tendon of scalenus anterior
第一肋 1st rib
右喉返神经 Right recurrent laryngeal nerve
胸廓内血管 Internal thoracic vessels
右膈神经 Right phrenic nerve
心包膈血管 Pericardiacophrenic vessels
上腔静脉 Superior vena cava
壁胸膜 Parietal pleura
肋胸膜 Costal pleura
纵隔胸膜 Mediastinal pleura
膈胸膜 Diaphragmatic pleura
左迷走神经 Left vagus nerve
前斜角肌 Anterior oblique
臂丛 Brachial plexus
锁骨下血管 Subclavian vessels
膈神经 Phrenic nerve
迷走神经 Vagus nerve
左喉返神经 Left recurrent laryngeal nerve
动脉韧带 Arterial ligament
肺动脉 Pulmonary artery
左心耳 Left auricle
升主动脉 Ascending aorta
心包膈血管 膈神经 Pericardiacophrenic vessels and phrenic nerve
左心室 Left ventricle
心包壁层 Parietal layer of pericardium
右心耳 Right auricle
右心室 Right ventricle
横结肠 Transverse colon
膈 Diaphragm

图 2-51 肺与纵隔结构（前面观）
Structures of lungs and mediastinum (Anterior aspect)

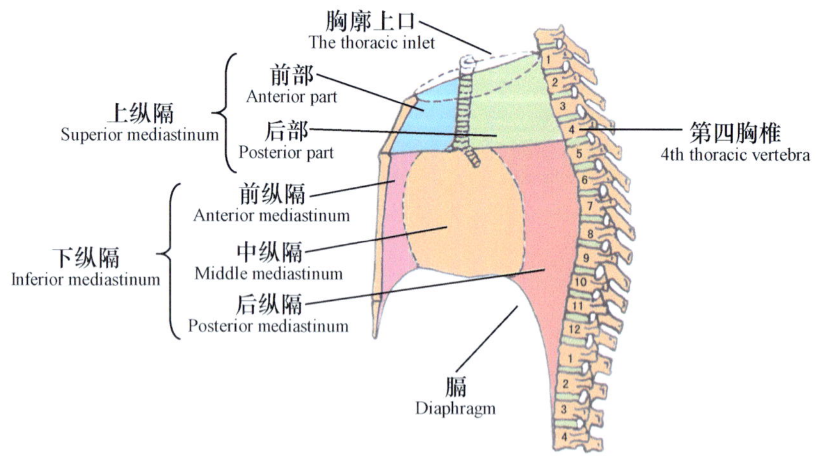

图 2-52 纵隔示意图
A diagram of the mediastinum

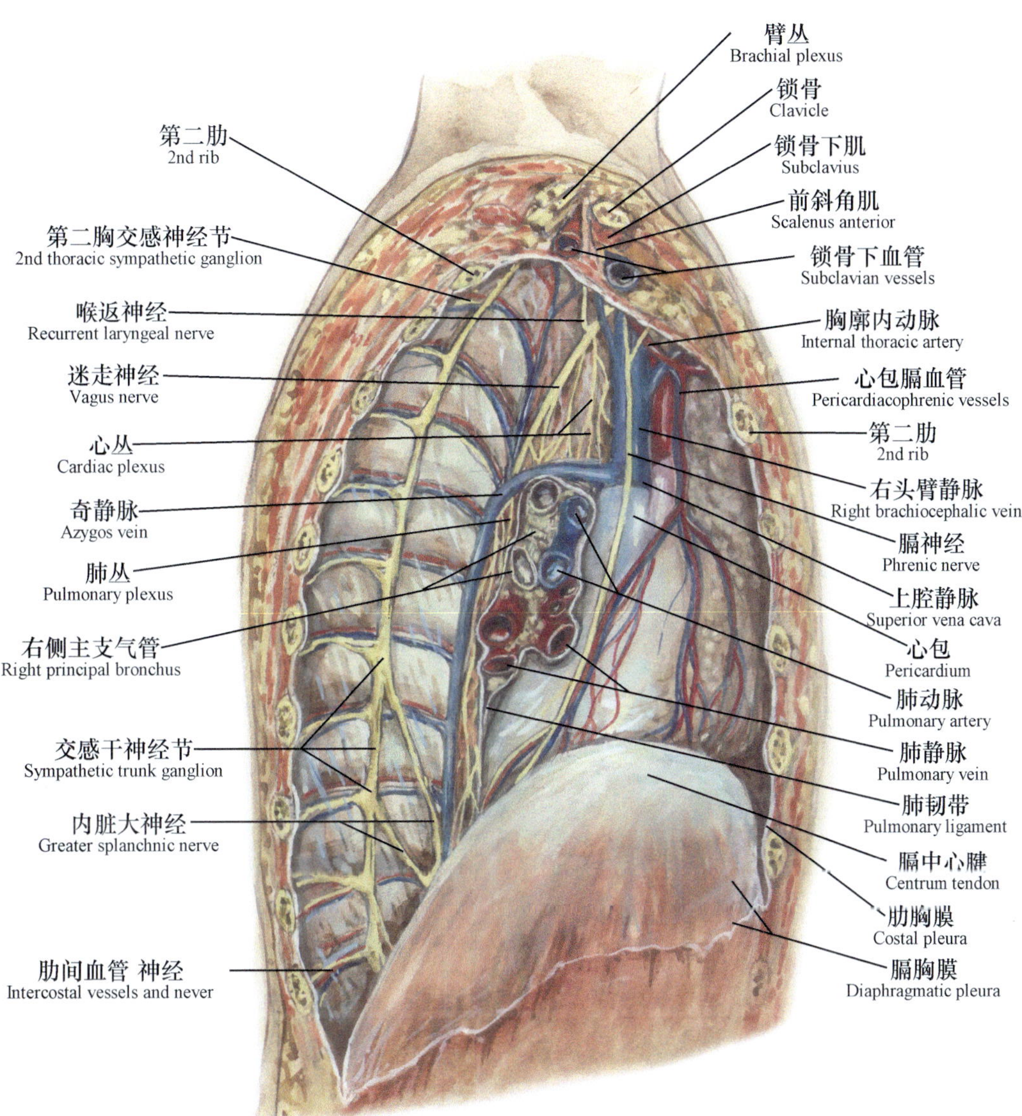

图 2-53　纵隔（右侧观）
The mediastinum (Right aspect)

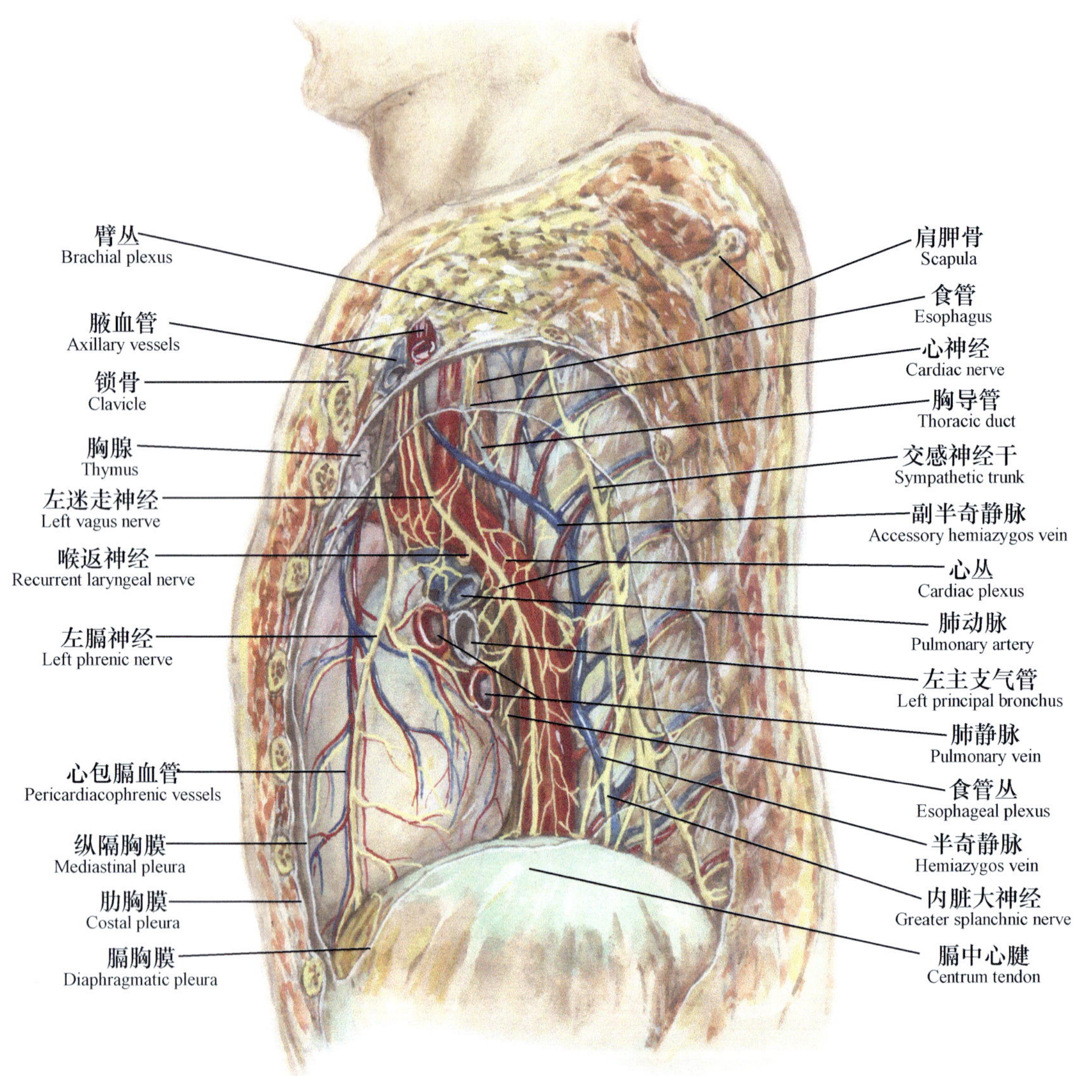

图 2-54 纵隔（左侧观）
The mediastinum (Left aspect)

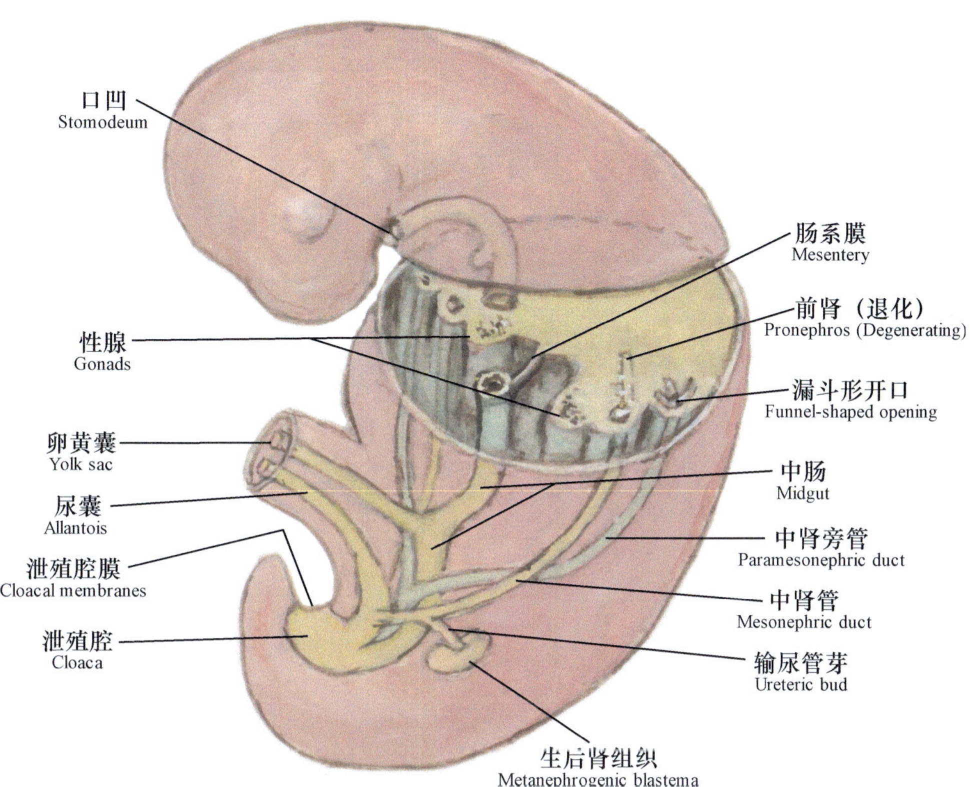

早期（5—8周）发生示意图
Diagrammatic sketch illustrating the early developing (5-8 weeks)

图2-55 胎儿泌尿生殖系统（1）
The urogenital system of fetus (1)

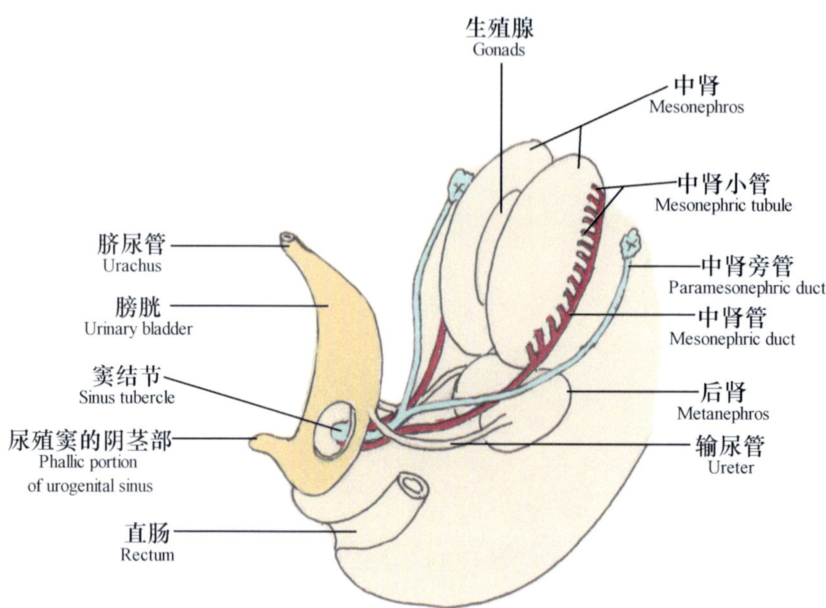

第九周胎儿侧面观（示窦结节）
Lateral aspect of a nine-week fetus (Showing the sinus tubercle)

图 2-55 胎儿泌尿生殖系统（2）
The urogenital system of fetus (2)

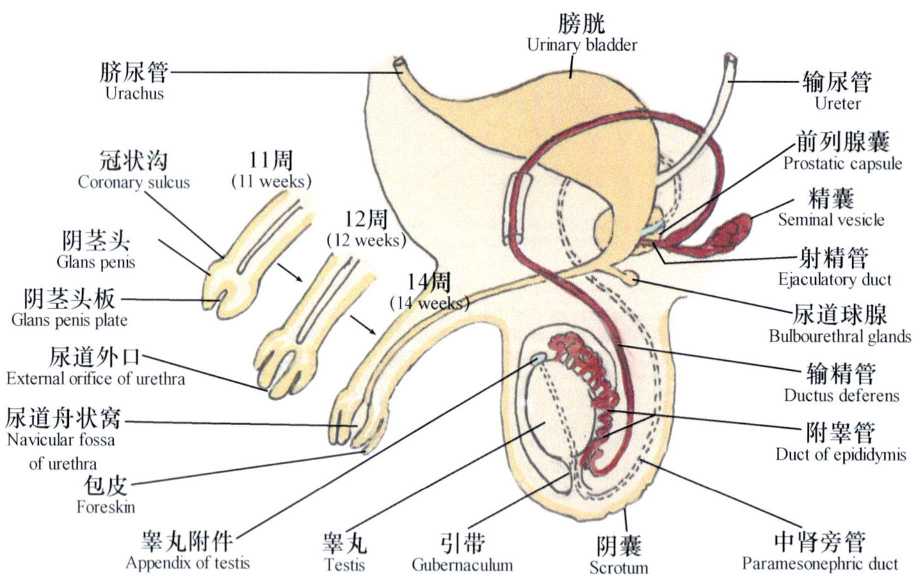

图 2-56 男性出生时的生殖系统器官及其遗迹示意图
A sketch illustrating the development of the reproductive organs and their vestigial structures in a newborn male

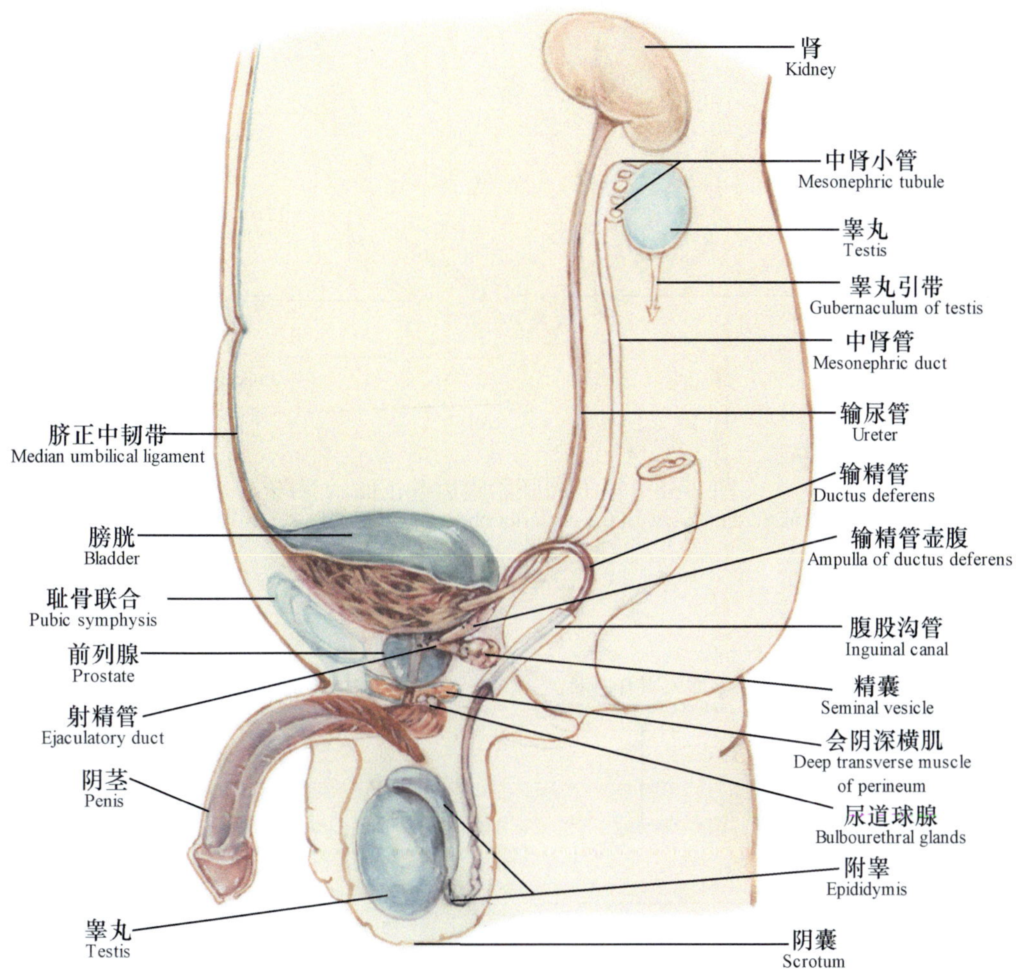

图 2-57 男性生殖器官及其胚胎遗迹示意图
A sketch showing the male reproductive organs and their vestigial structures

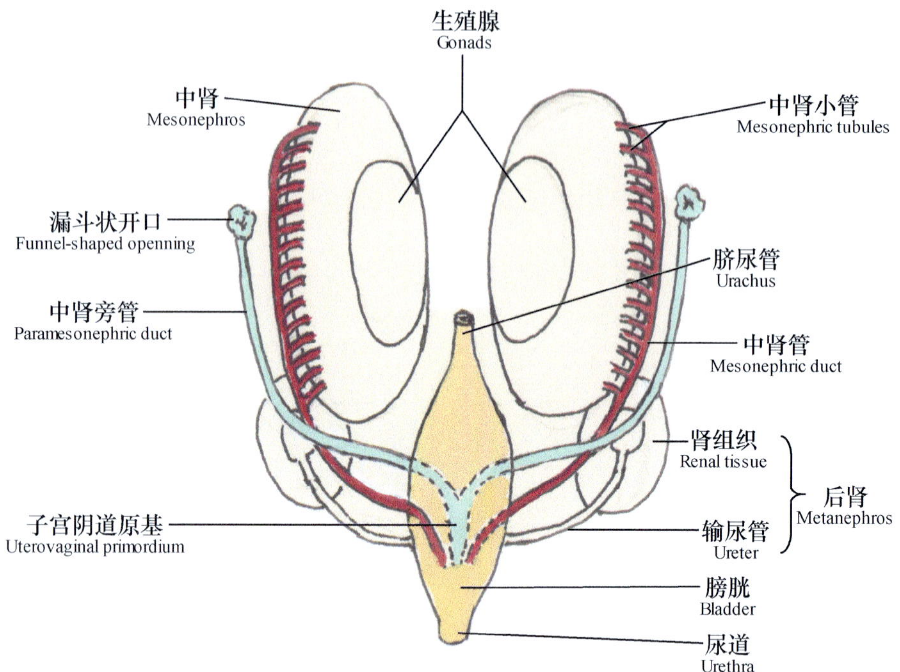

图 2-58　第七周胚胎腹后壁正面示意图
Sketch of a frontal view of the posterior abdominal wall of a seven-week fetus

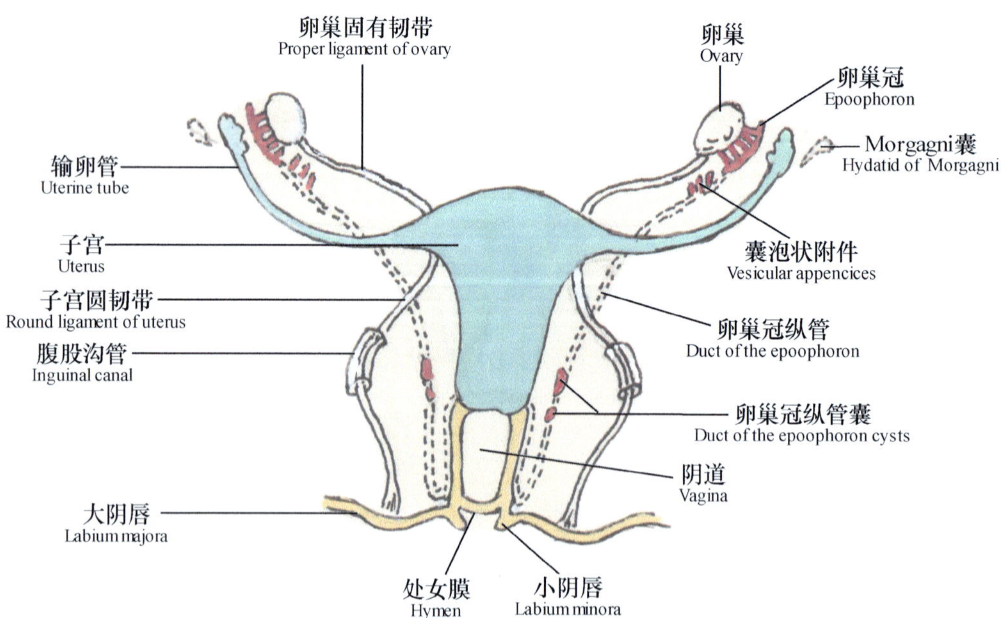

图 2-59　女性出生时的生殖系统器官及其遗迹示意图
Schematic drawing illustrating development of the reproductive organs in a newborn female,vestigial structures are also shown

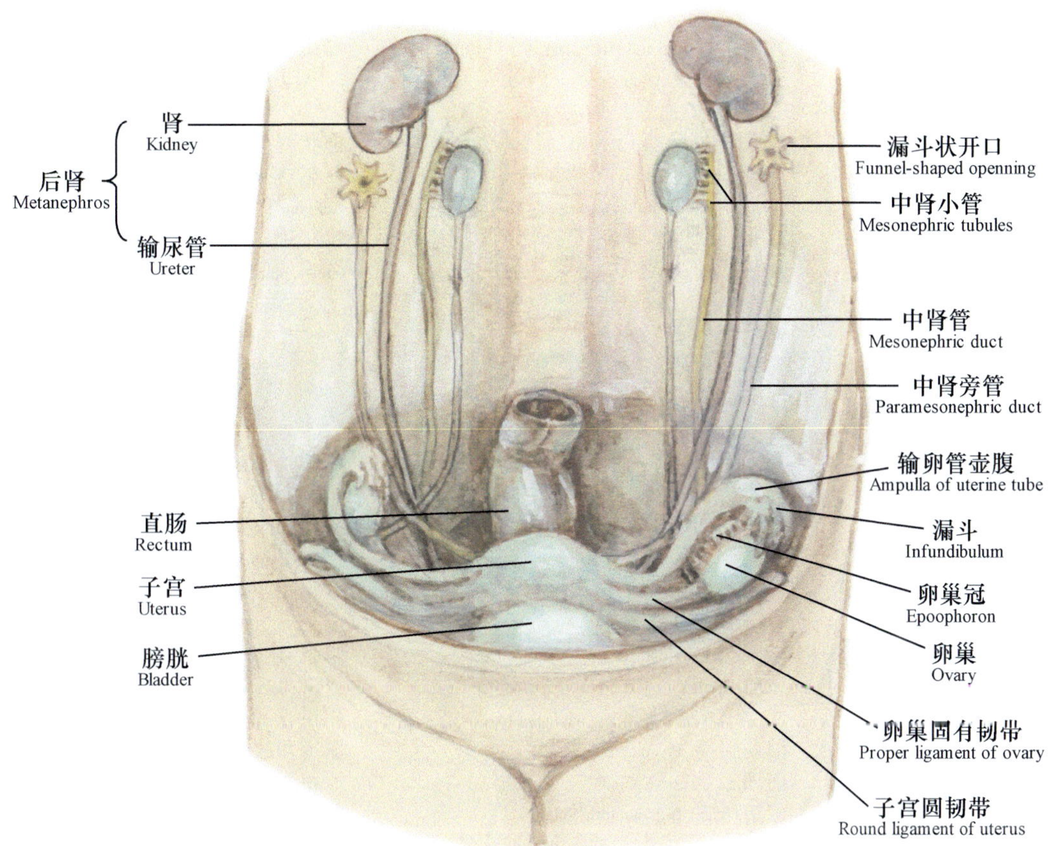

图 2-60 女性生殖器官及其胚胎遗迹示意图
A sketch showing the female reproductive organs and their vestigial structures

胚胎泌尿生殖系统的衍生物与残余物

Adult Derivatives and Vestigial Remans of Embryonic Urogenic Structures

胚胎结构 Embryonic Structure	男性 Male	女性 Female
未分化生殖腺 Indifferent gonad 皮质 Cortex 髓质 Medulla	睾丸 Testis 精曲小管 Contorted Seminiferous tubules 睾丸网 Rete testis	卵巢 Ovary 卵泡 Ovarian follicles 髓质 Medulla 卵巢网 Rete ovarii
引带 Gubernaculum	睾丸引带 Gubernaculum of testis	卵巢固有韧带 Proper ligamgnt of Ovary 子宫圆韧带 Round ligament of uterus
中肾小管 Mesonephric tubules	输出小管 Ductuli efferentes 旁睾 Paradidymis	卵巢冠 Epoophoron 卵巢旁体 Paroophoron
中肾管 Mesonephric duct	附睾管 Ductus epididymis 附睾附件 Appendix of epididymis 输尿管 肾盂 肾盏 集合管 Ureter, renal pelvis, renal calyces and collecting tubules 输精管 Ductus deferens 射精管和精囊 Ejaculatory duct and seminal vesicle	泡状附件 Appendix vesiculosa 卵巢冠导管 Duct of epoophoron Gartner 管 Duct of Gartner 输尿管 肾盂 肾盏 集合管 Ureter, renal pelvis, renal calyces and collecting tubules
中肾旁管 Paramesonephric duct	睾丸附件 Appendix of testis	输卵管 Uterine tube 子宫 Uterus 阴道纤维肌壁 Fibromuscular wall of vagina Morgagni 水囊 Hydatid of Morgagni
尿生殖窦 Urogenital sinus	膀胱 Urinary bladder 尿道 Urethra （除外舟状窝）(except navicular fossa) 前列腺囊 Prostatic utricle 前列腺 Prostate gland 尿道球腺 Bulbourethral glands	膀胱 Urinary bladder 尿道 Urethra 阴道 Vagina 尿道和尿道旁腺 Urethra and paraurethral glands 前庭大腺 Greater vestibular glands
窦结节 Sinus tubercle	精阜 Seminal colliculus	处女膜 Hymen
初阴 Phallus	阴茎 Penis 阴茎头 Glans penis 阴茎海绵体 Corpora cavernosa penis 尿道海绵体 Corpora spongiosum urethra	阴蒂 Clitoris 阴蒂头 Glans clitoridis 阴蒂海绵体 Corpora cavernosa clitoridis 前庭球 Bulb of vestibule
尿生殖褶 Urogenital folds	阴茎腹侧面 Ventral aspect of penis	小阴唇 Labia minora
阴唇阴囊隆突 Labioscrotal swellings	阴囊 Scrotum	大阴唇 Labia majora

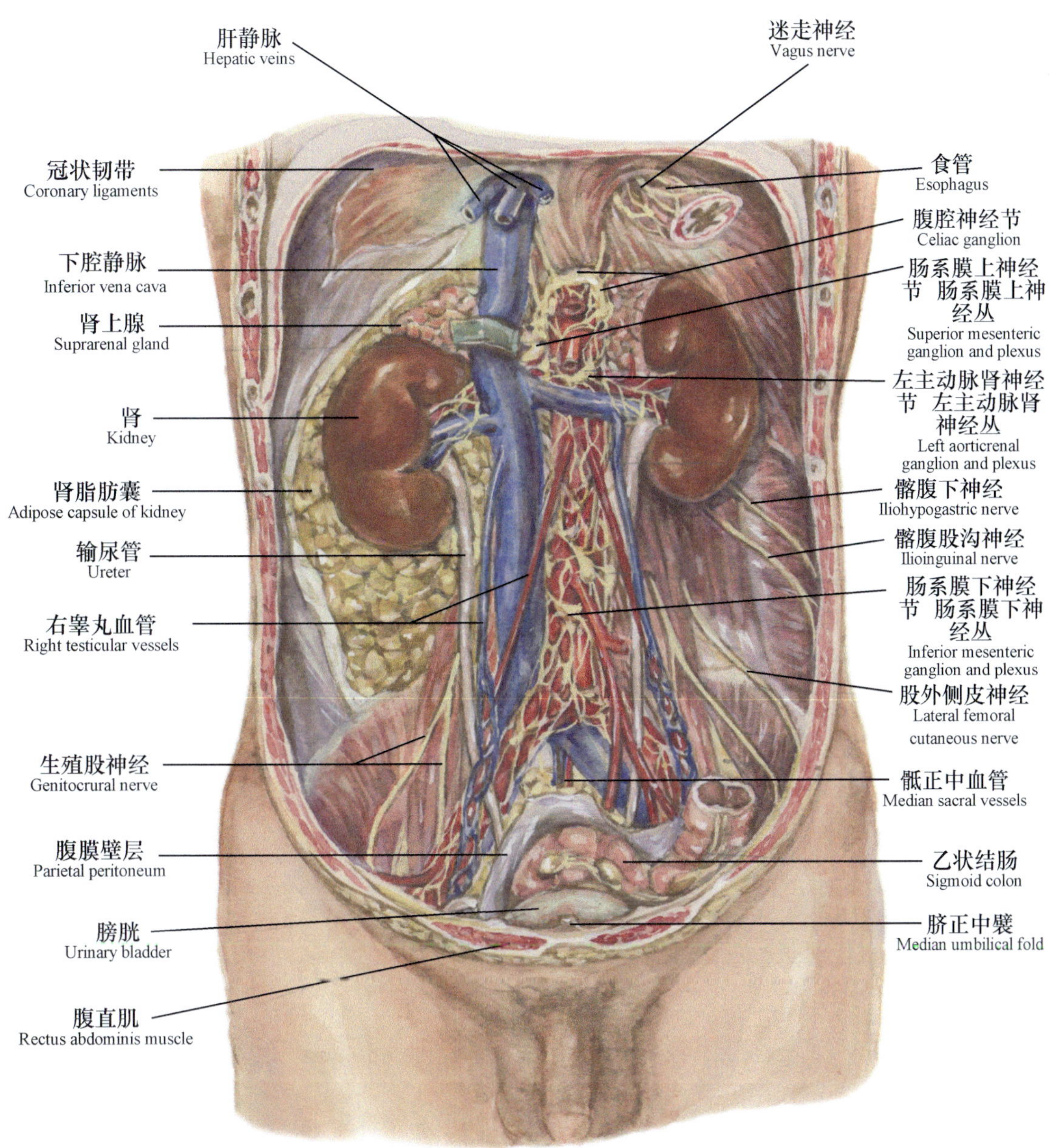

图 2-61 腹后壁示泌尿系统和神经、血管
The urinary system, nerves, and vessels of the posterior abdominal wall

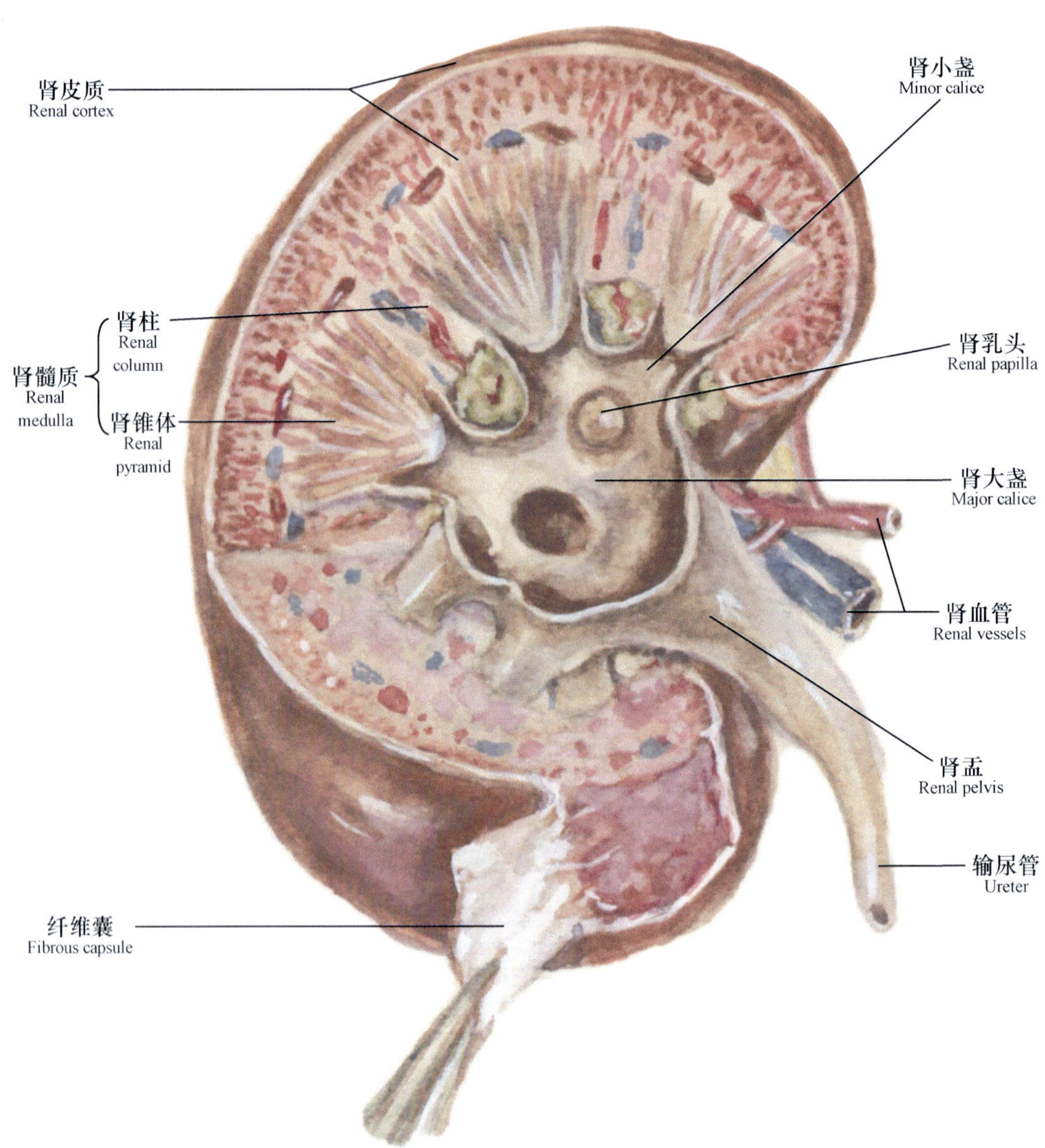

图 2-62 右肾冠状与水平切面
Right kidney sectioned in coronary and horizontal planes

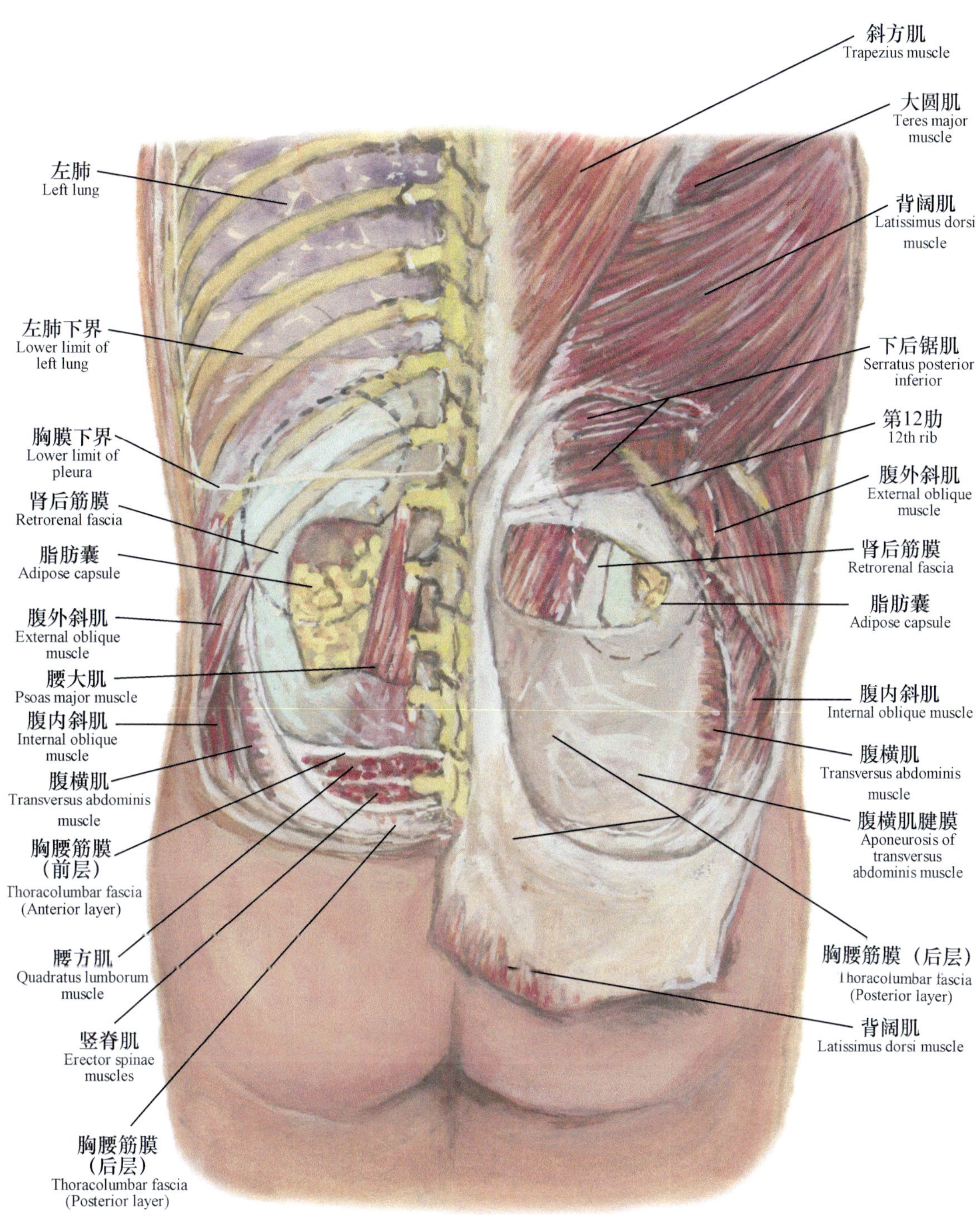

图 2-63　腹后壁示肾背侧的毗邻关系（1）
Posterior abdominal wall shows the relationship of the dorsal kidney (1)

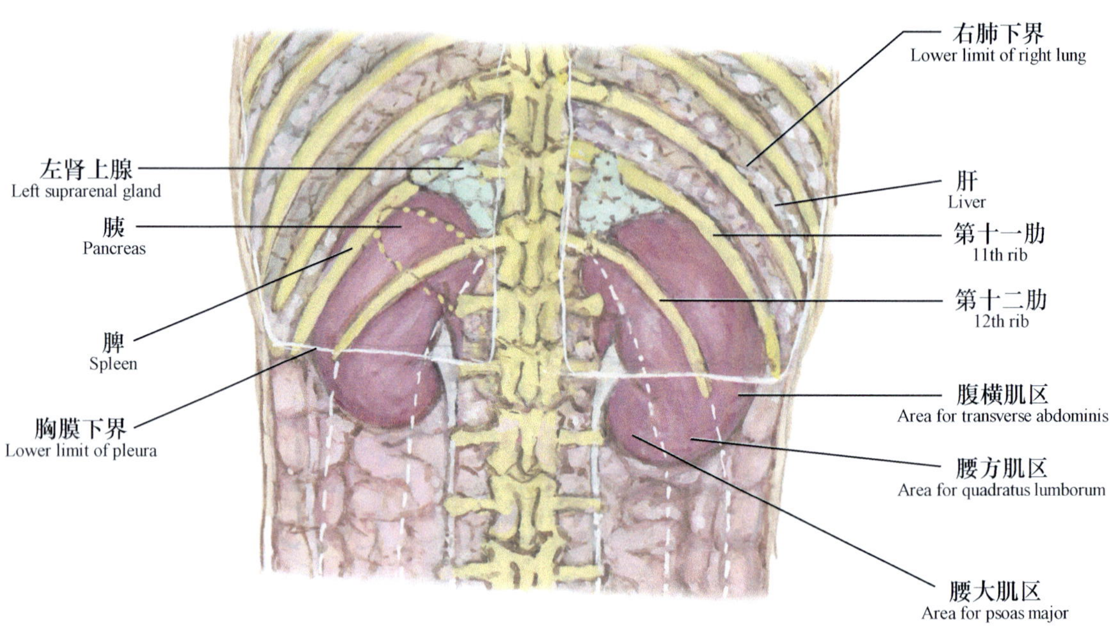

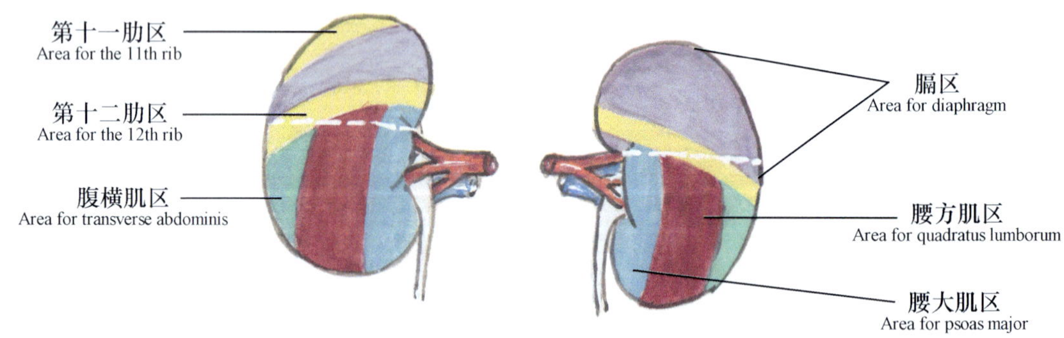

图 2-64 腹后壁示肾背侧的毗邻关系（2）
The posterior abdominal wall shows the relationship of the dorsal kidney (2)

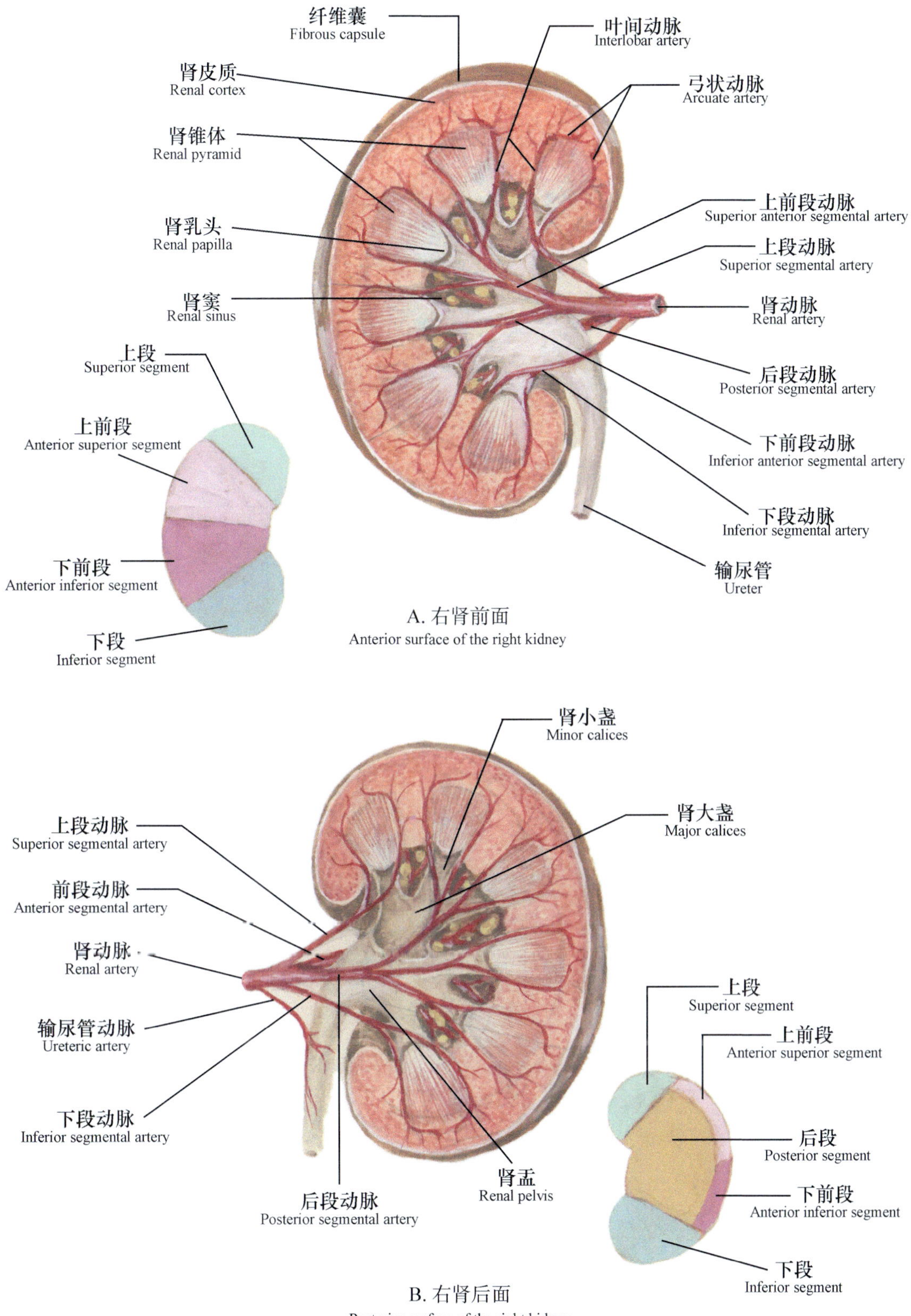

图 2-65　肾动脉及肾段（右肾）
Renal artery and renal segment (Right renal)

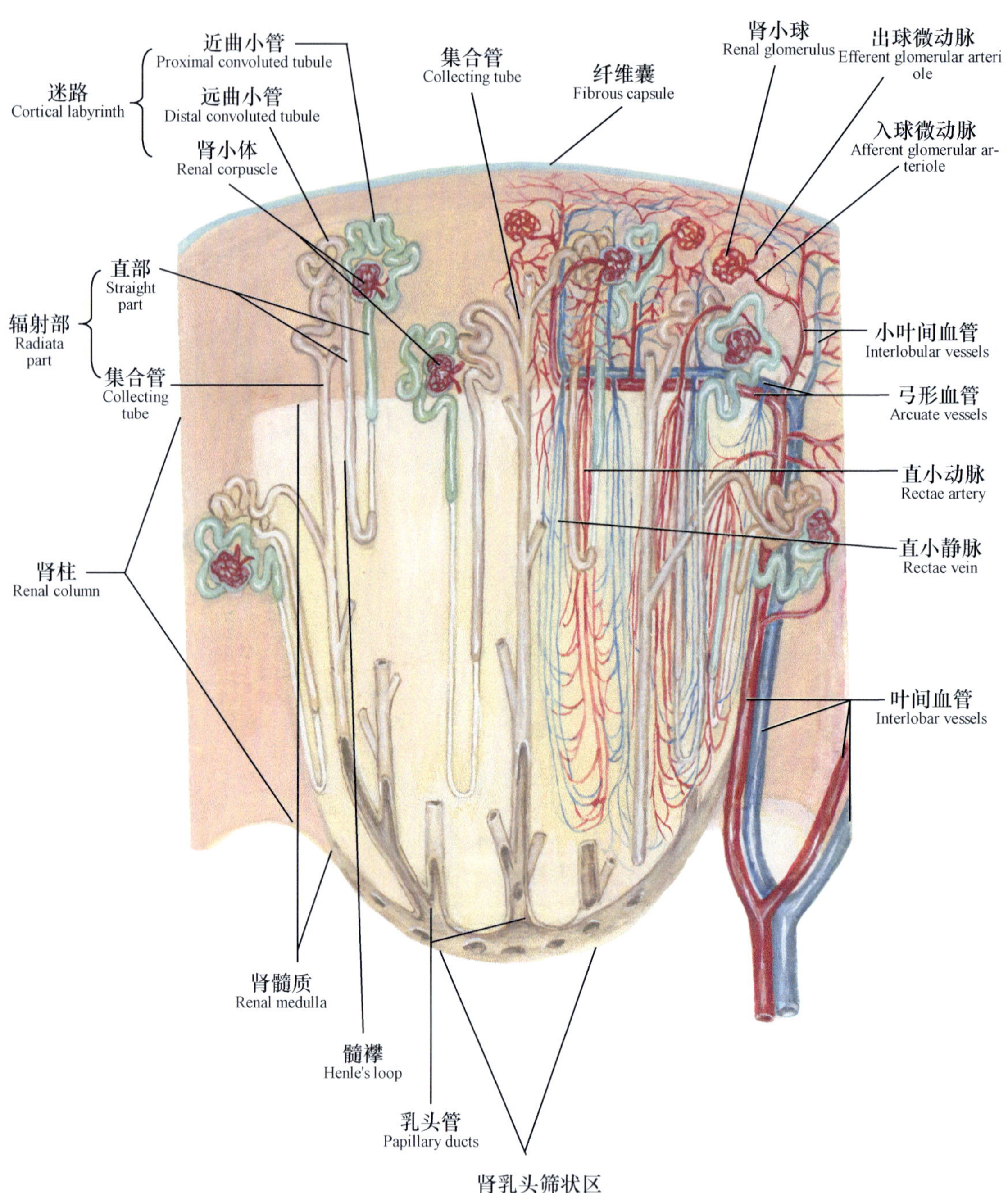

图 2-66 肾单位示意图
Schema for nephron

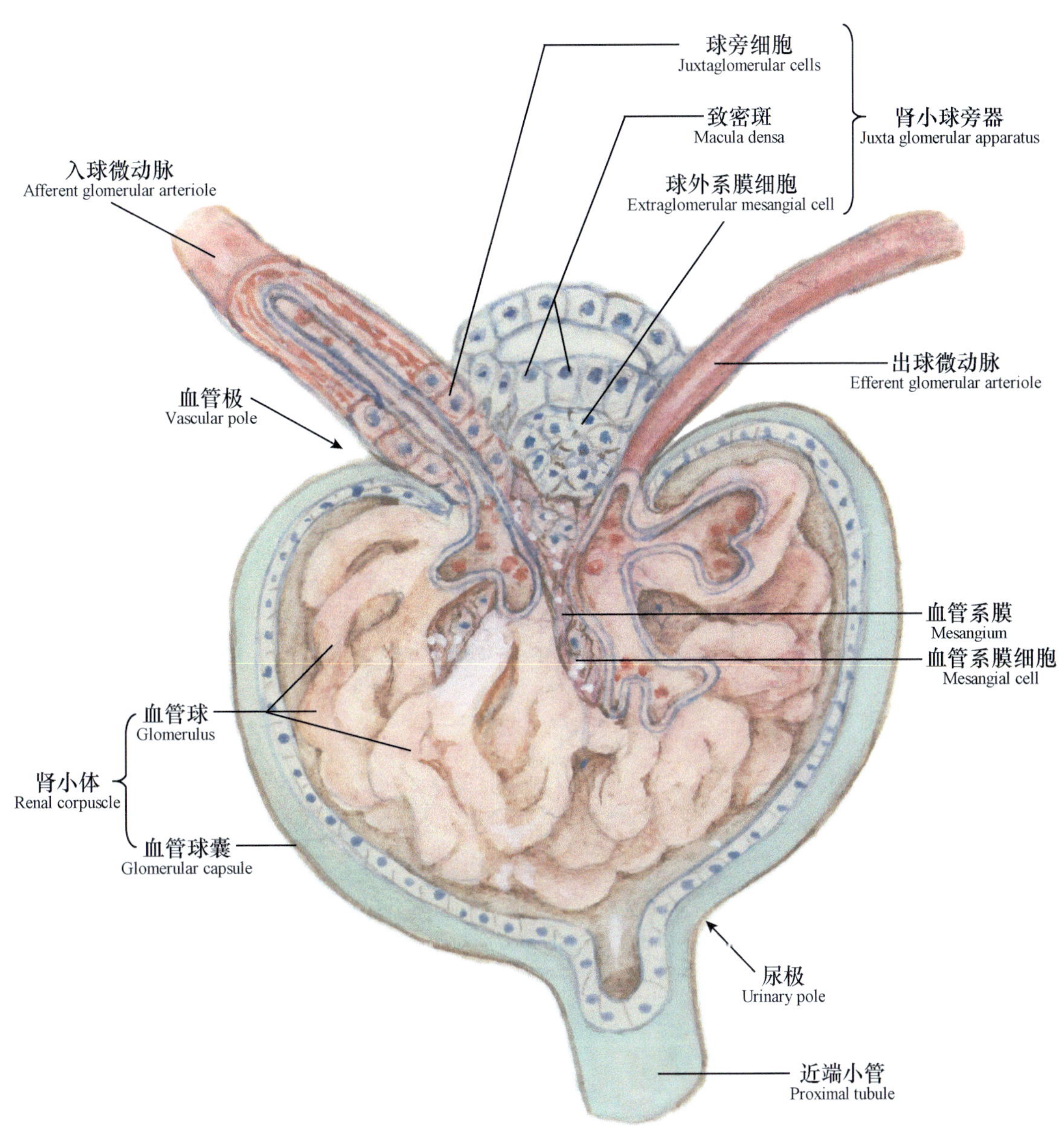

图 2-67　肾小体和球旁器模式图
Pattern of renal corpuscle and parabulbar organs

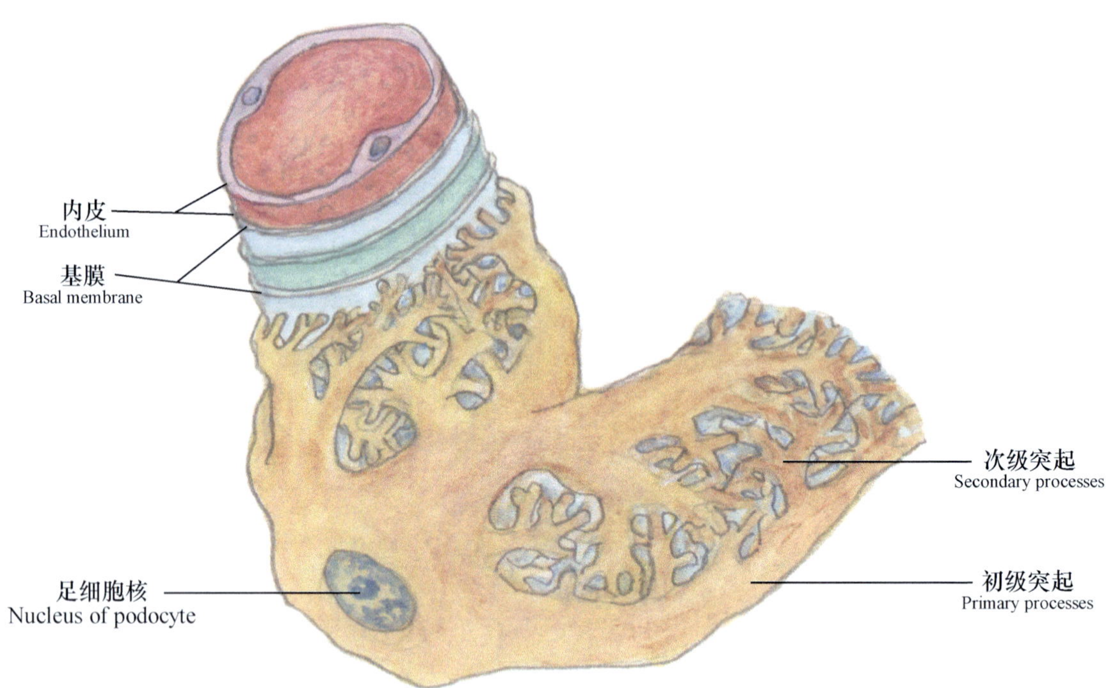

图 2-68　足细胞超微结构模式图
Ultrastructural pattern of podocytes

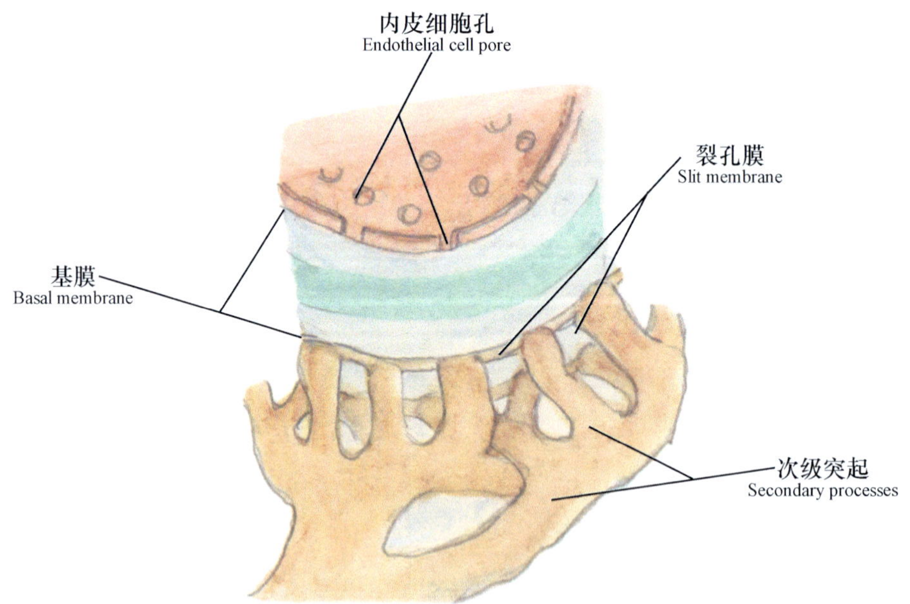

图 2-69　滤过膜超微结构模式图
Ultrastructure pattern of the membrane

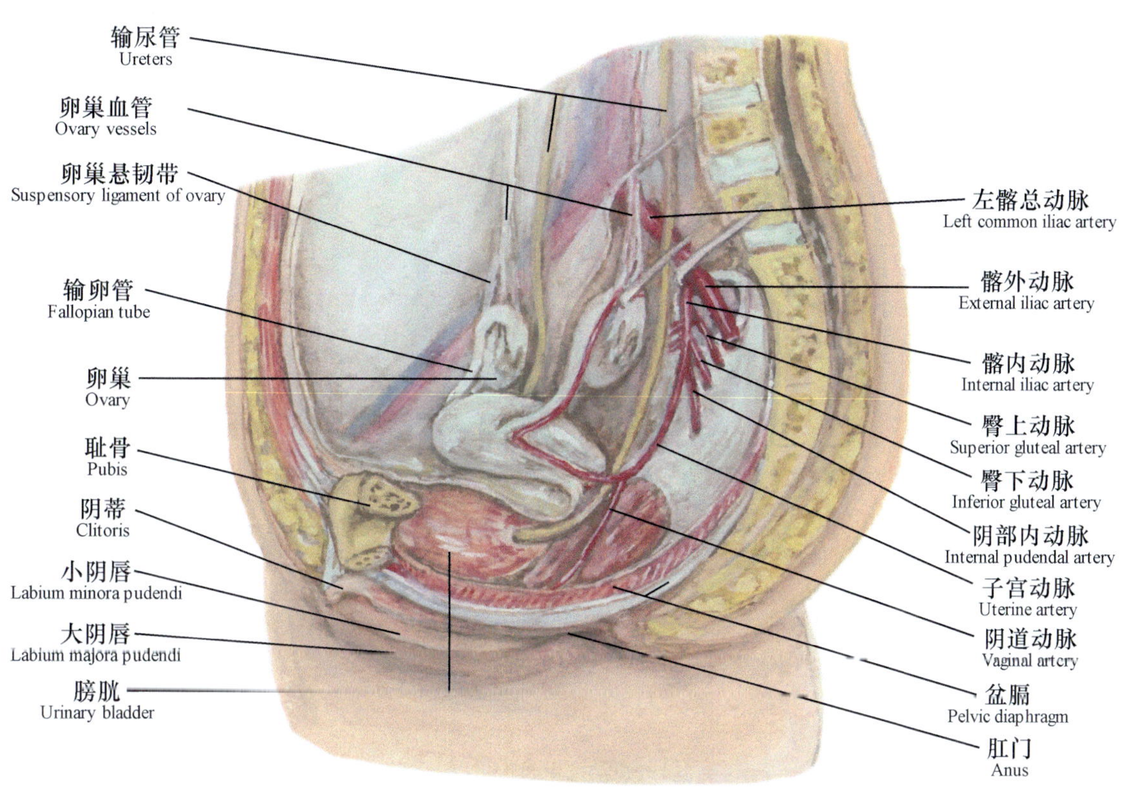

图 2-70 女性生殖器官与子宫动脉
Productive organs of female and uterine artery

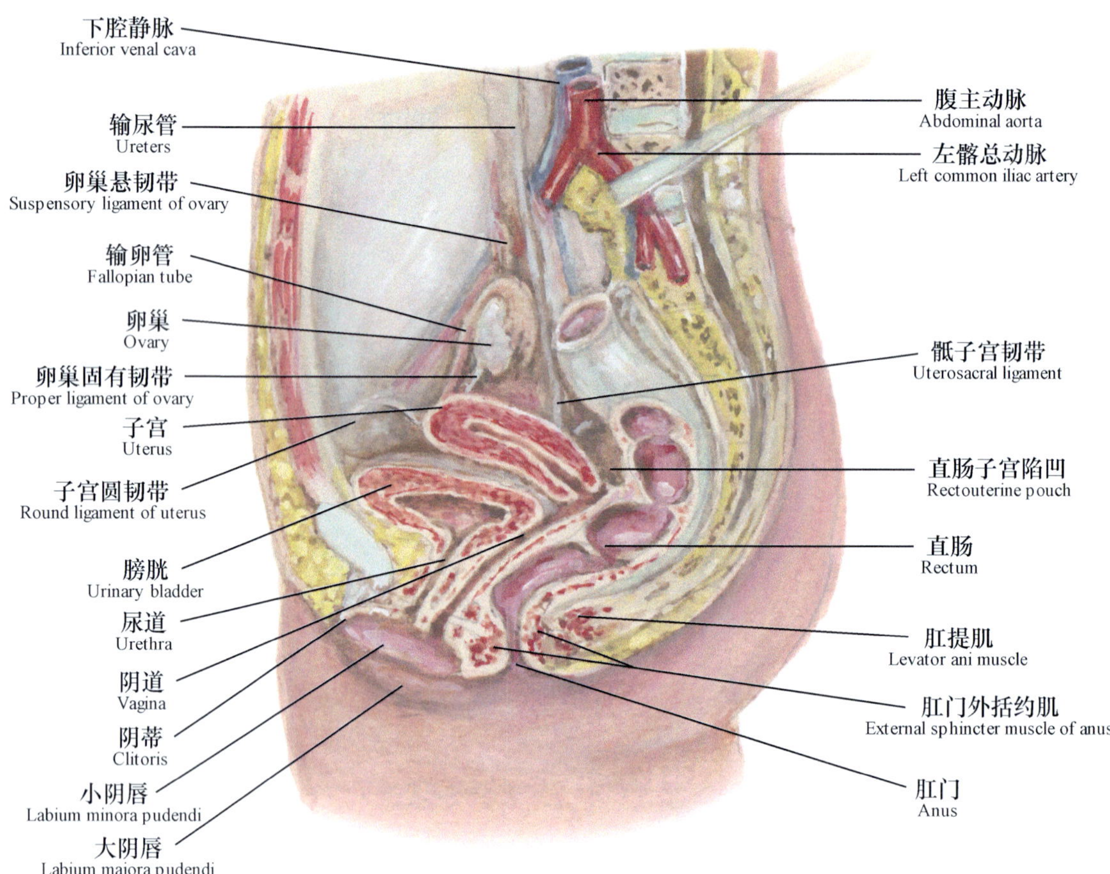

图 2-71 女性盆腔器官
Pelvic Organs of female

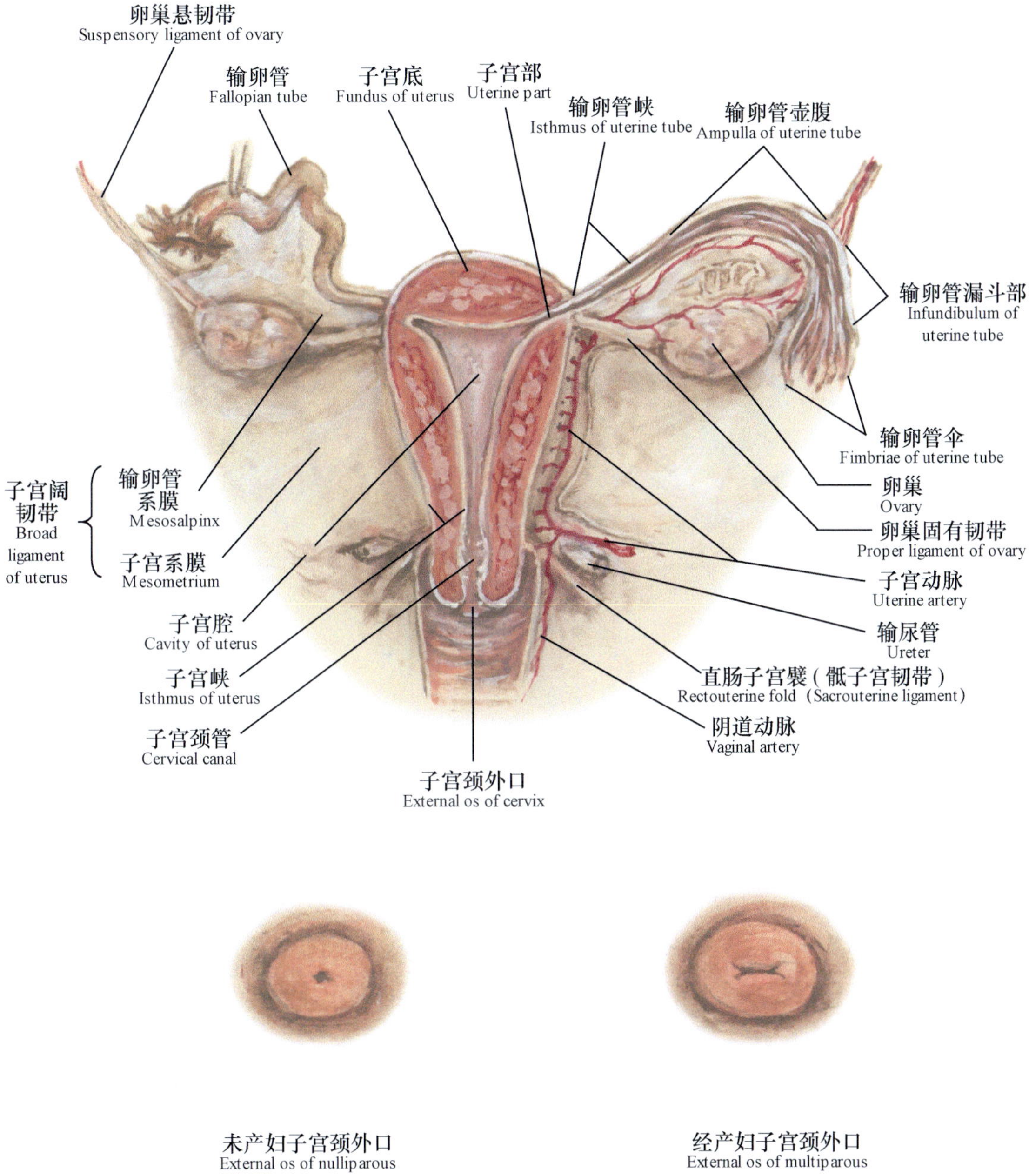

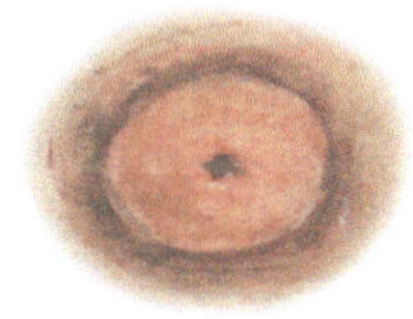

图 2-72　子宫冠状切面及其附件
Coronal section of uterus and its adnexa

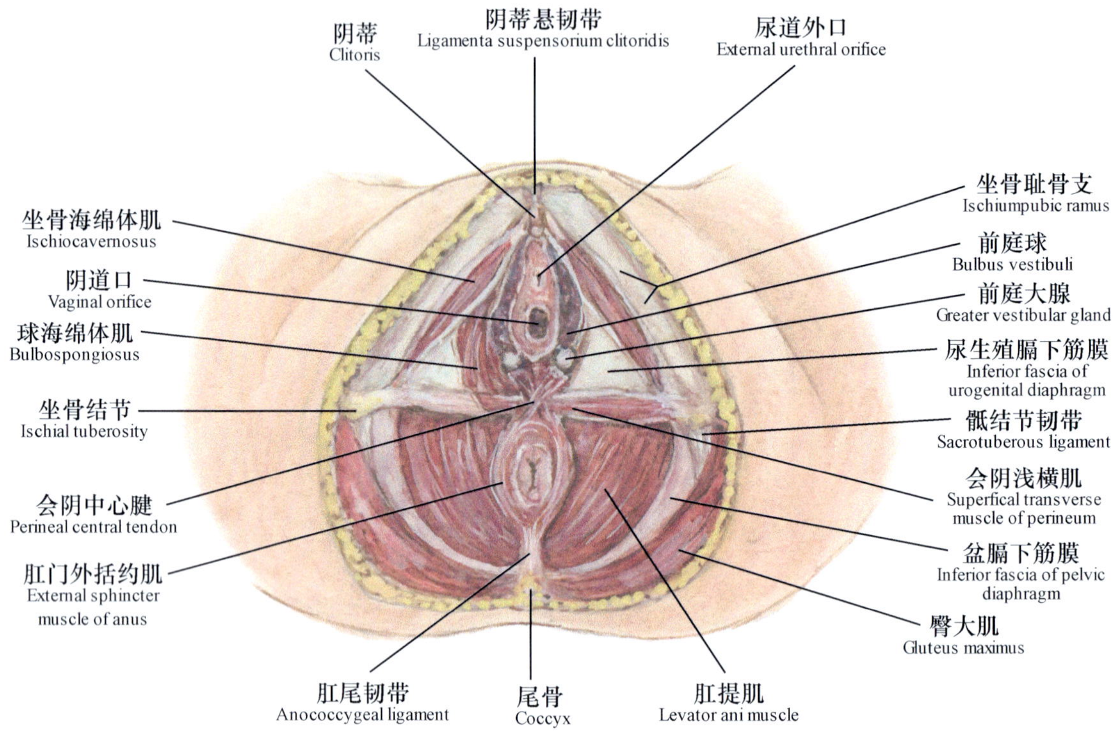

图 2-73 女性会阴
Female perineum

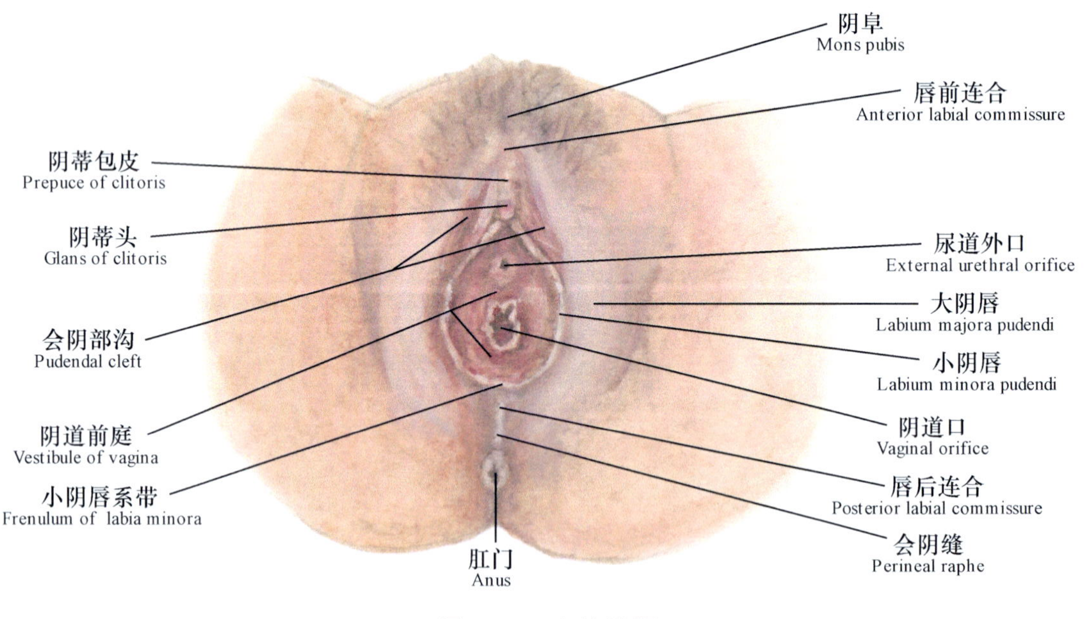

图 2-74 女性外阴
Vulva

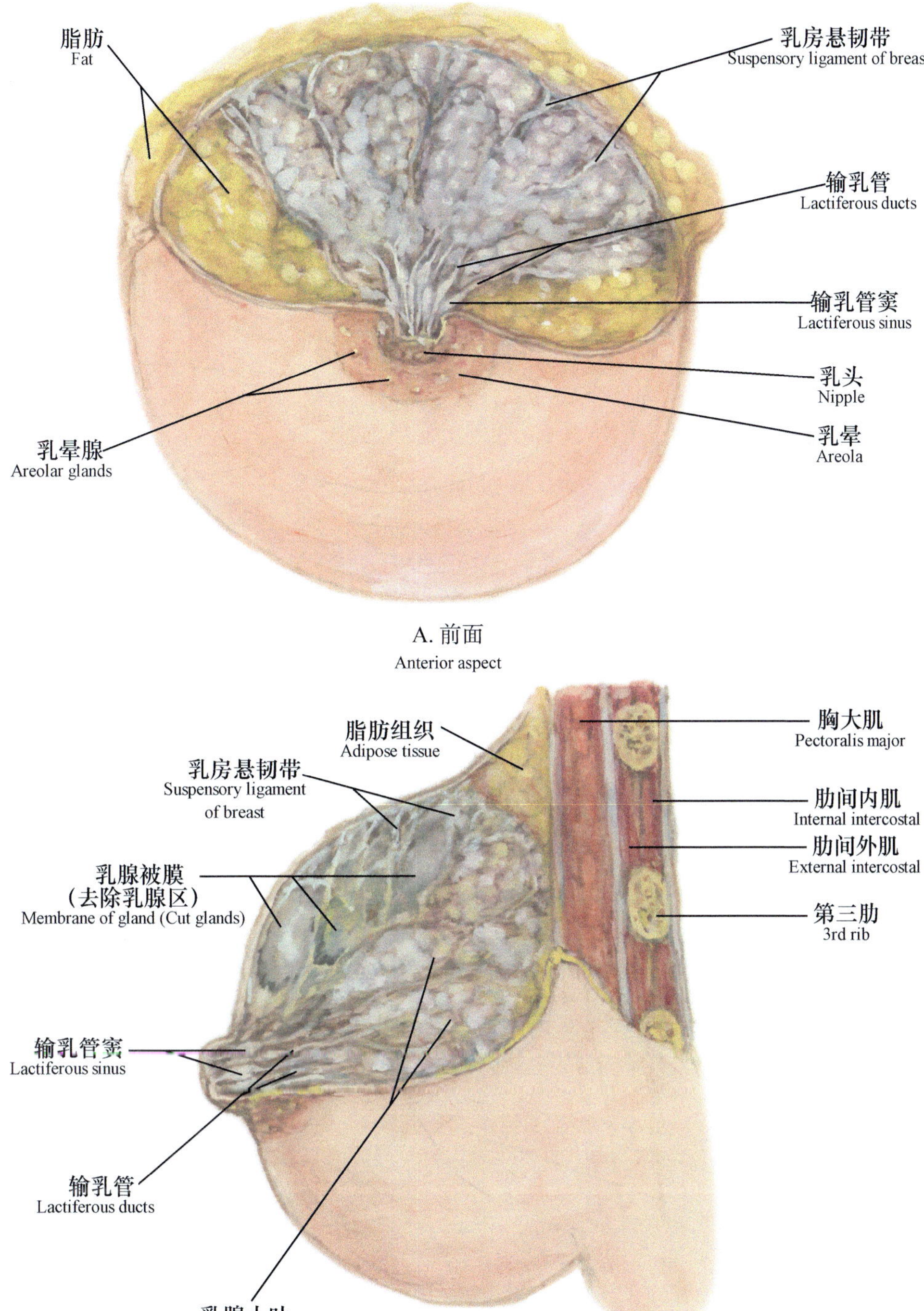

图 2-75 乳房
Mamma (Papillary gland)

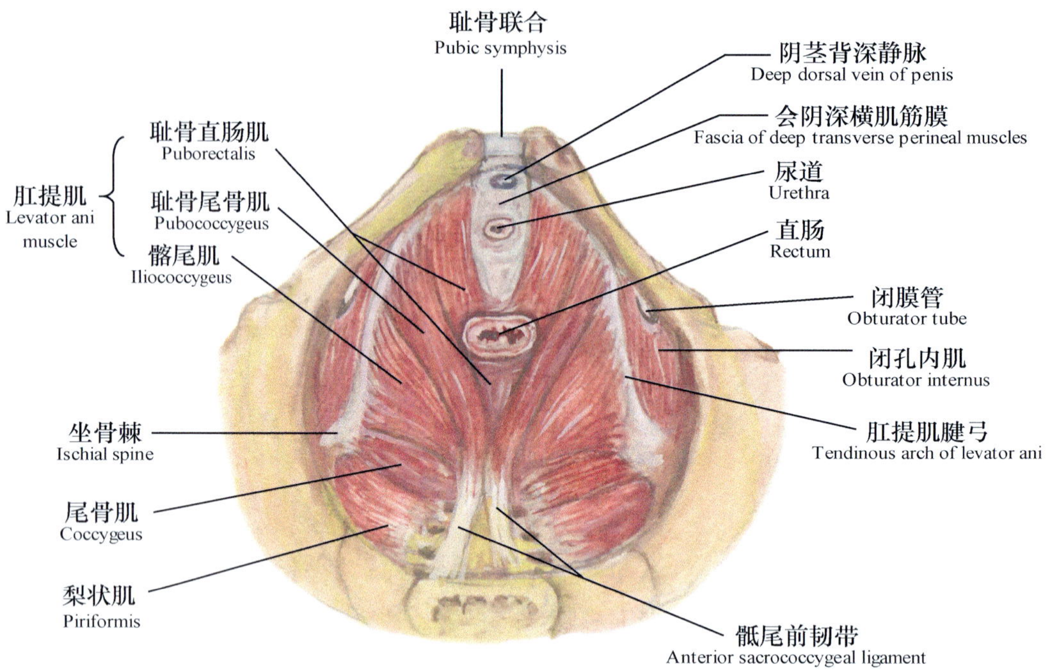

图 2-76 男性盆膈（上面观）

Pelvic diaphragm of male (Superior aspect)

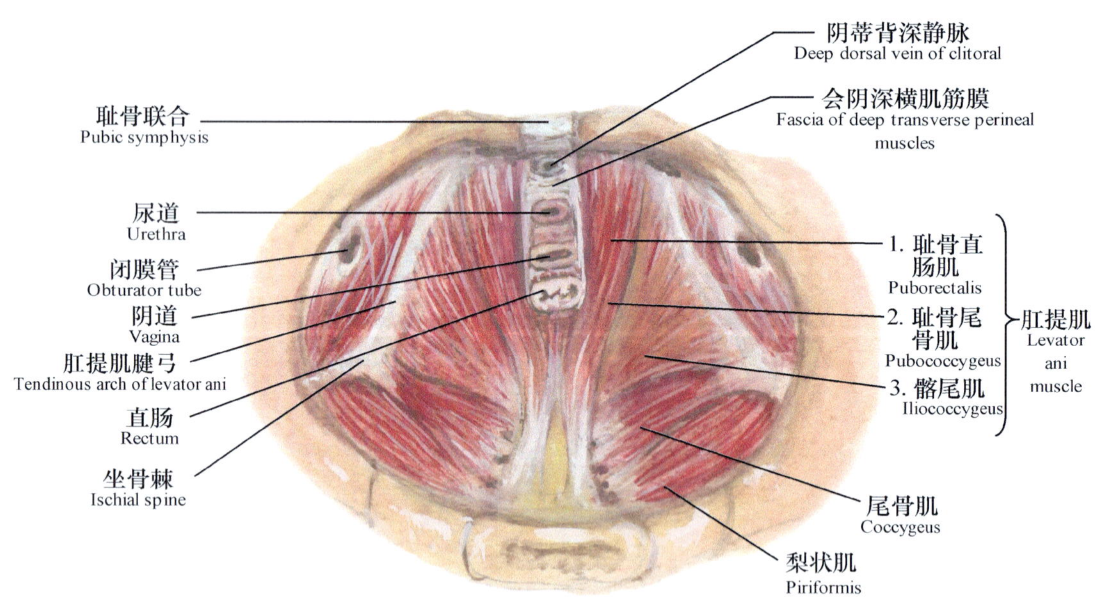

图 2-77 女性盆膈（上面观）

Pelvic diaphragm of female (Superior aspect)

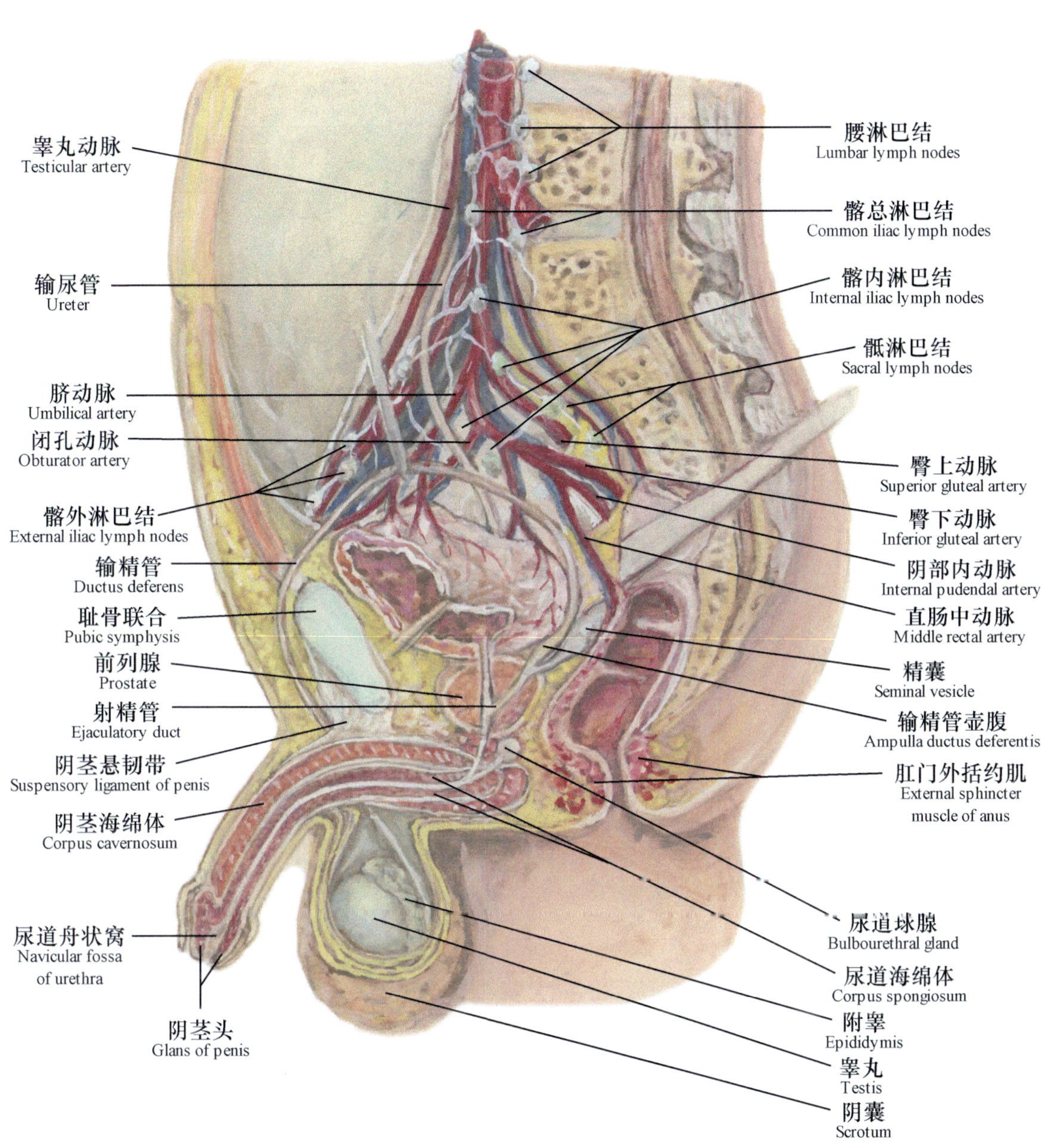

图 2-78 男性盆腔器官
Pelvic viscera of the male

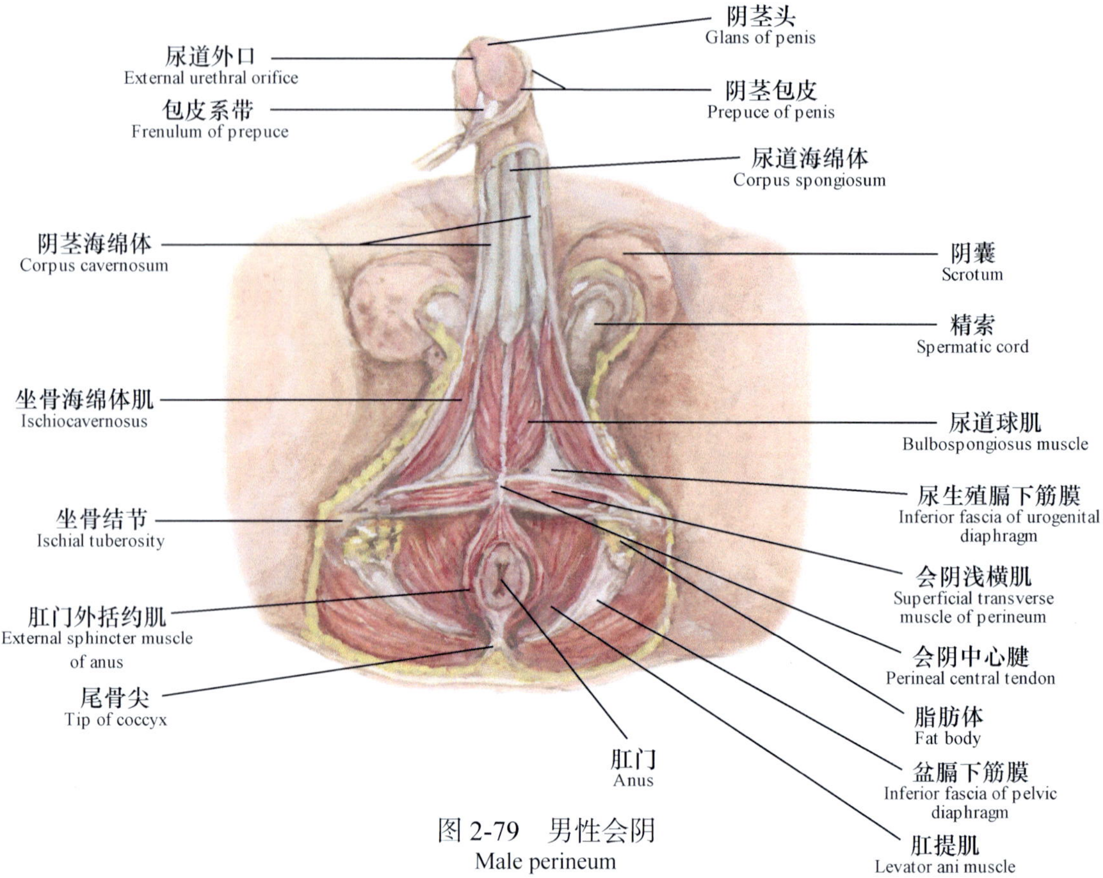

阴茎头
Glans of penis
尿道外口
External urethral orifice
阴茎包皮
Prepuce of penis
包皮系带
Frenulum of prepuce
尿道海绵体
Corpus spongiosum
阴茎海绵体
Corpus cavernosum
阴囊
Scrotum
精索
Spermatic cord
坐骨海绵体肌
Ischiocavernosus
尿道球肌
Bulbospongiosus muscle
尿生殖膈下筋膜
Inferior fascia of urogenital diaphragm
坐骨结节
Ischial tuberosity
会阴浅横肌
Superficial transverse muscle of perineum
肛门外括约肌
External sphincter muscle of anus
会阴中心腱
Perineal central tendon
尾骨尖
Tip of coccyx
脂肪体
Fat body
肛门
Anus
盆膈下筋膜
Inferior fascia of pelvic diaphragm
肛提肌
Levator ani muscle

图 2-79 男性会阴
Male perineum

阴茎背动脉 阴茎背神经
Dorsal artery and nerve of penis
阴茎背浅静脉
Superficial dorsal vein of penis
阴茎背深静脉
Deep dorsal vein of penis
皮肤
Skin
外侧浅静脉
Lateral superficial vein
阴茎浅筋膜
Superficial fascia of penis
阴茎深动脉
Deep artery of penis
阴茎海绵体
Corpus cavernosum
阴茎深筋膜
Deep fascia of penis
尿道海绵体
Corpus spongiosum
白膜
Tunica albuginea
尿道
Urethra

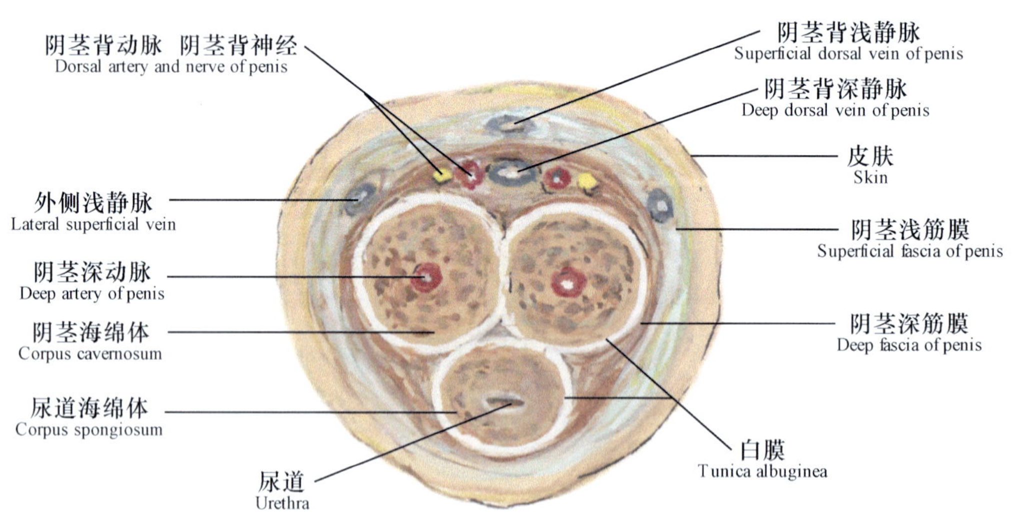

图 2-80 阴茎断面
Section through body of penis

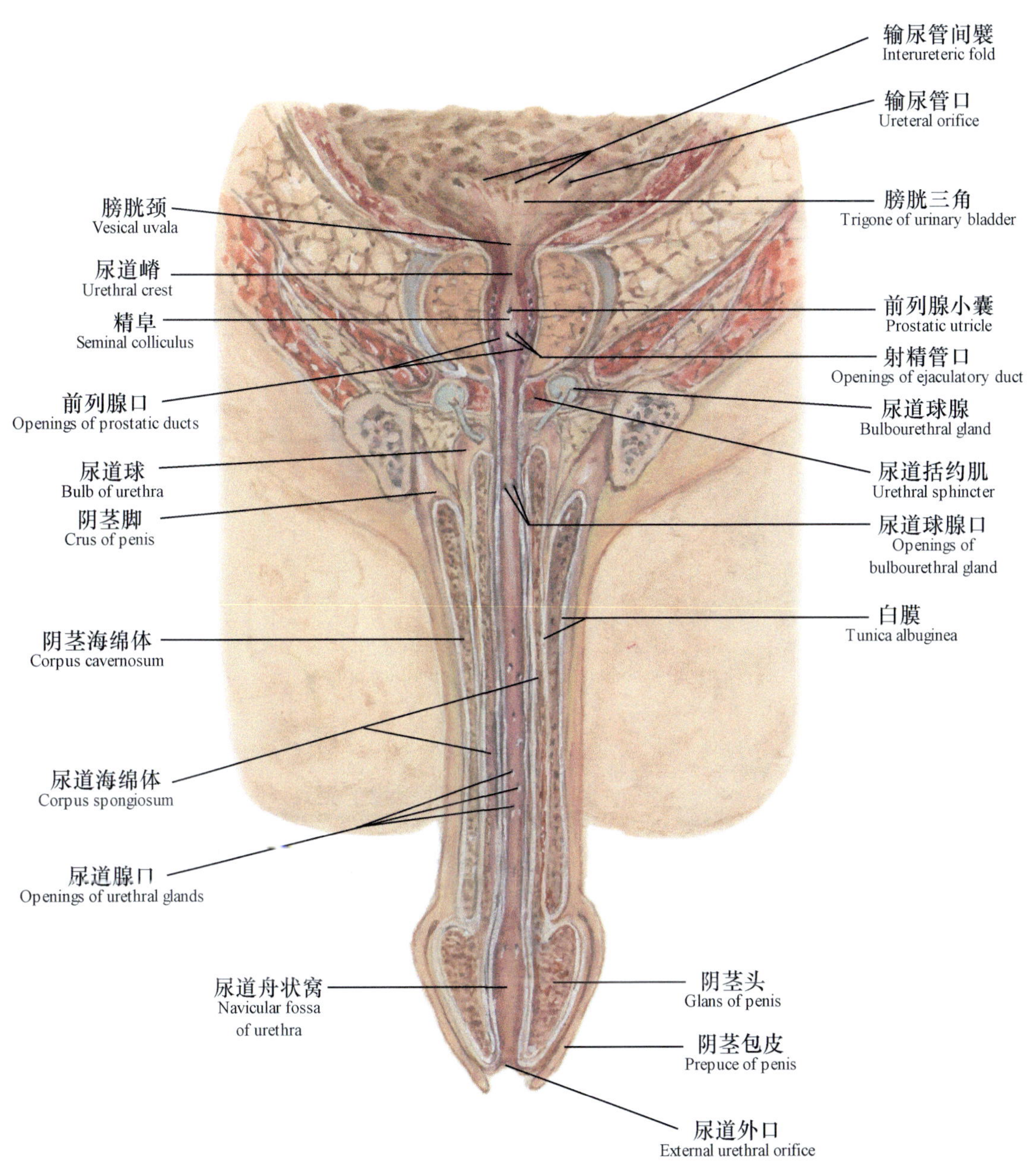

图 2-81 男性尿道
The male urethra

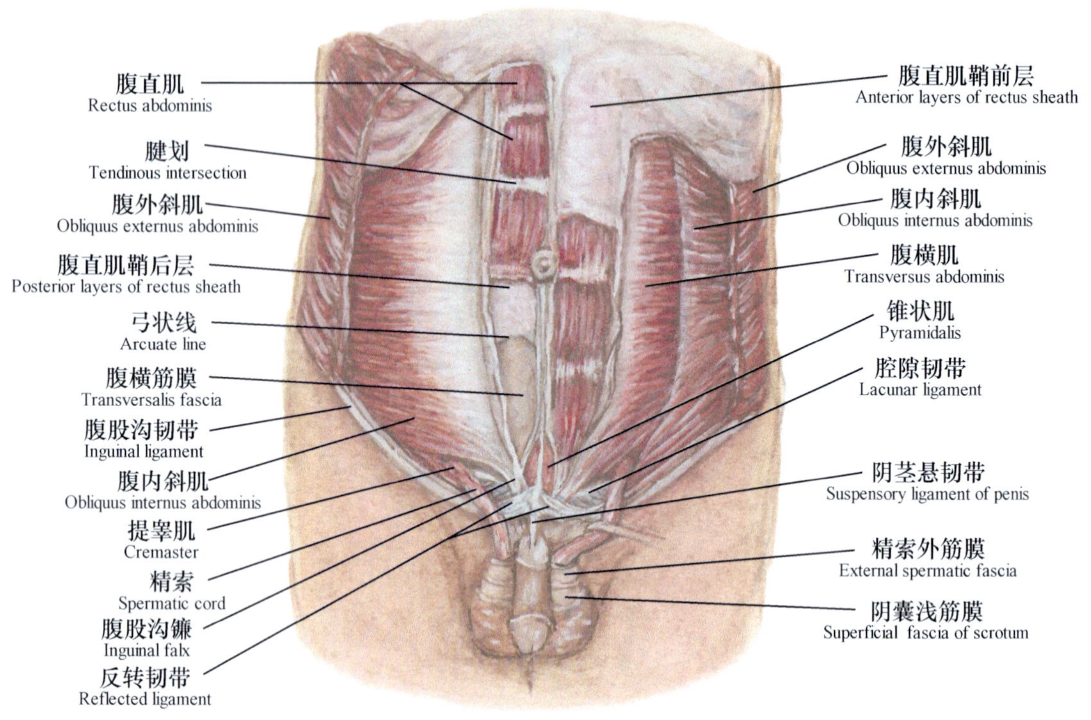

图 2-82 腹前壁与腹股沟区
Anterior abdominal wall and its inguinal area

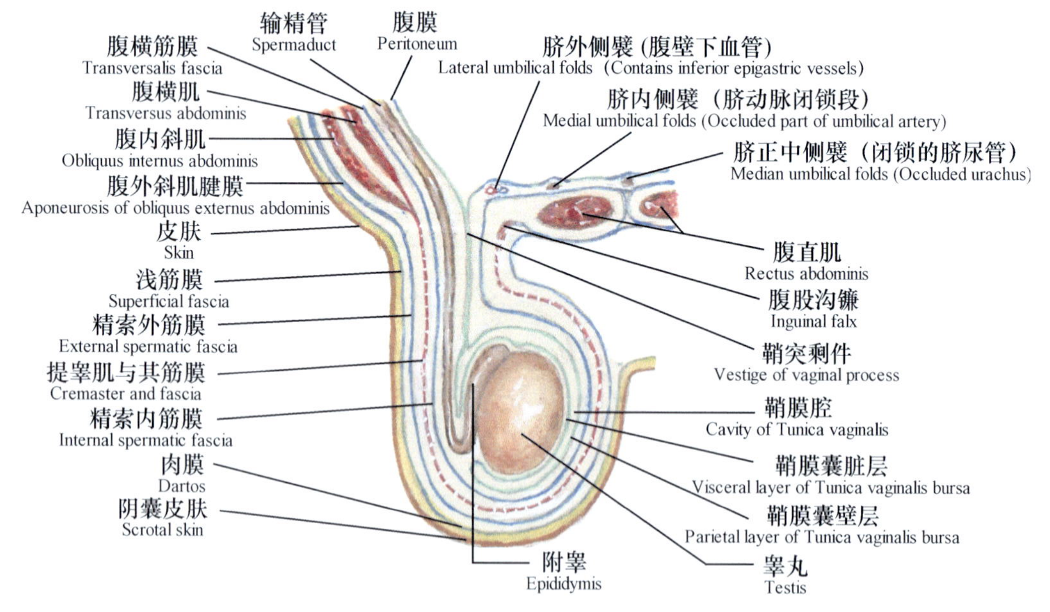

图 2-83 阴囊结构示意图
Sketch of scrotum

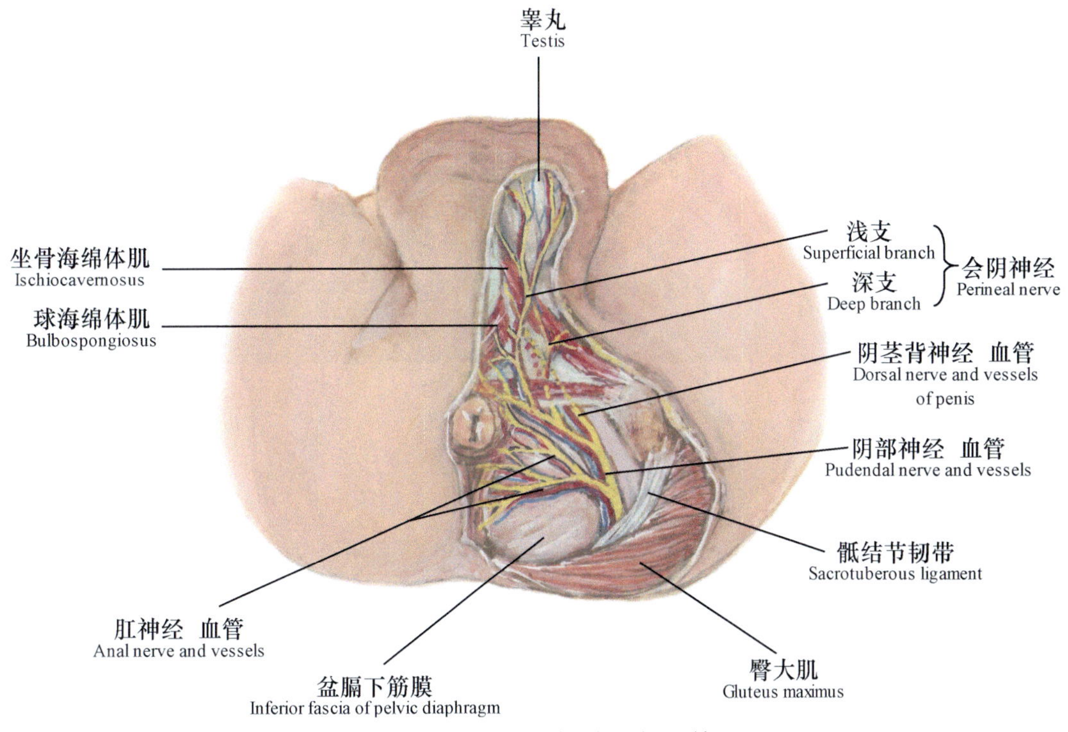

图 2-84 男性阴部神经与血管
Pudendal nerves and blood vessels of male

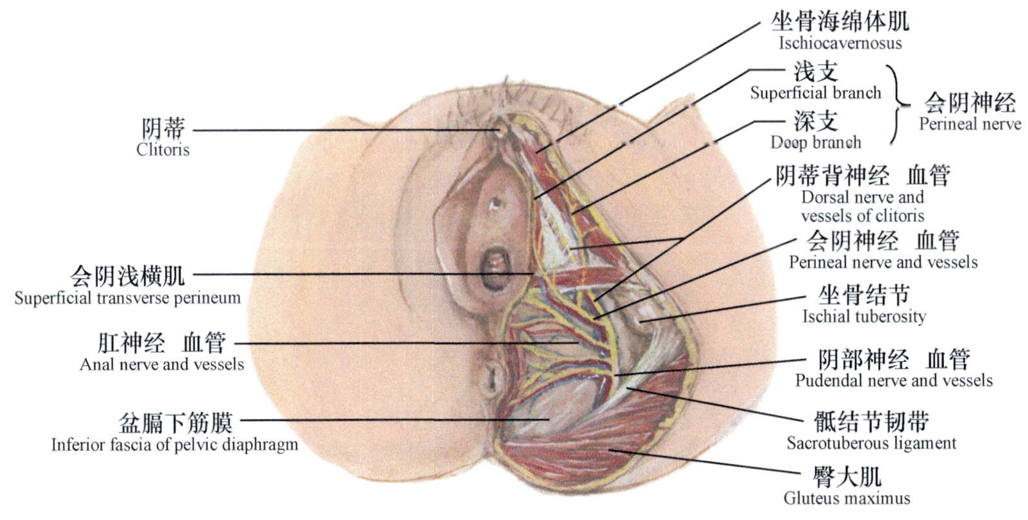

图 2-85 女性阴部神经与血管
Pudendal nerves and vessels of female

第3章

脉管学

ANGIOLOGY

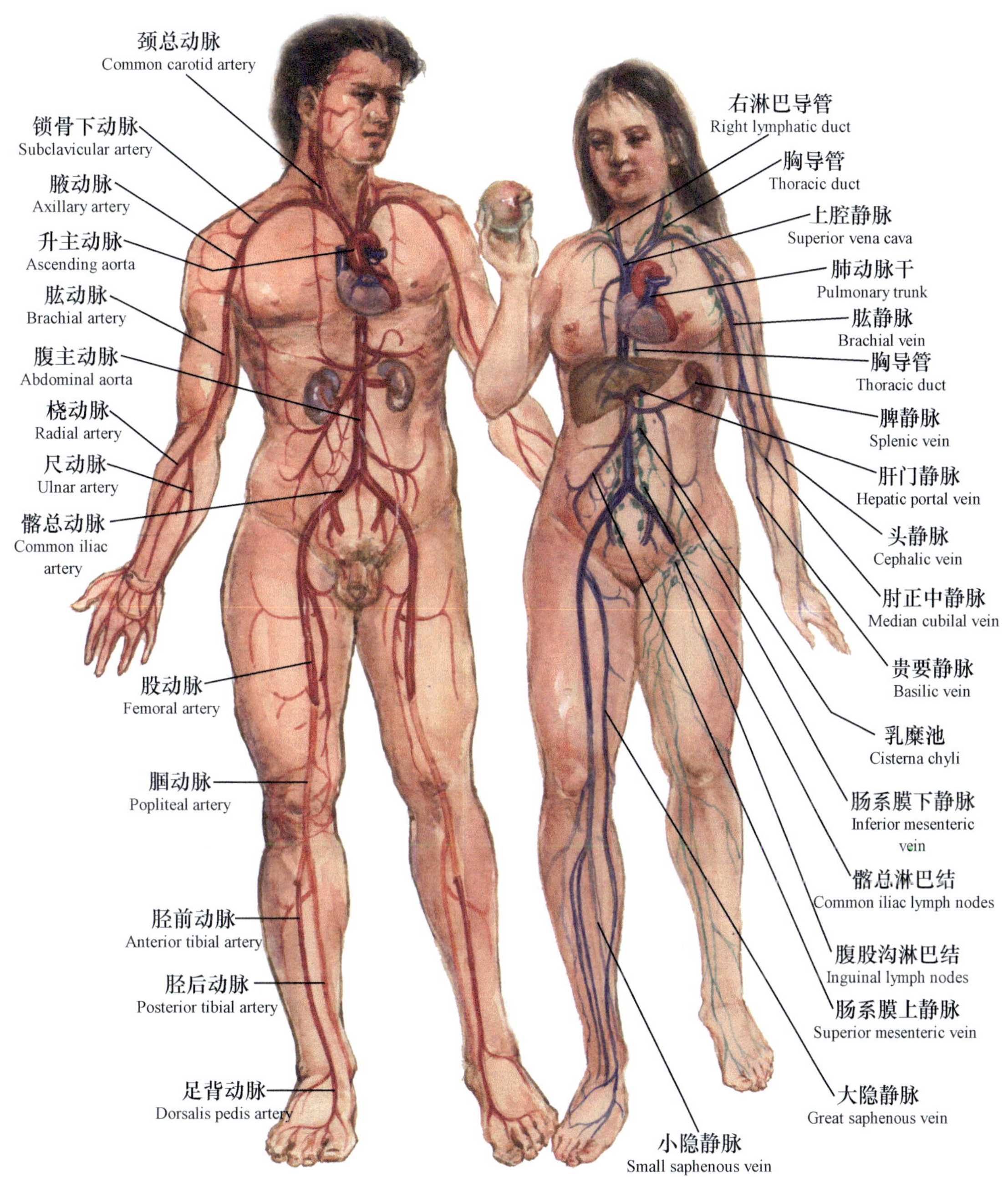

图 3-1 心血管系统和淋巴系统
Cardiovascular and lymphatic system

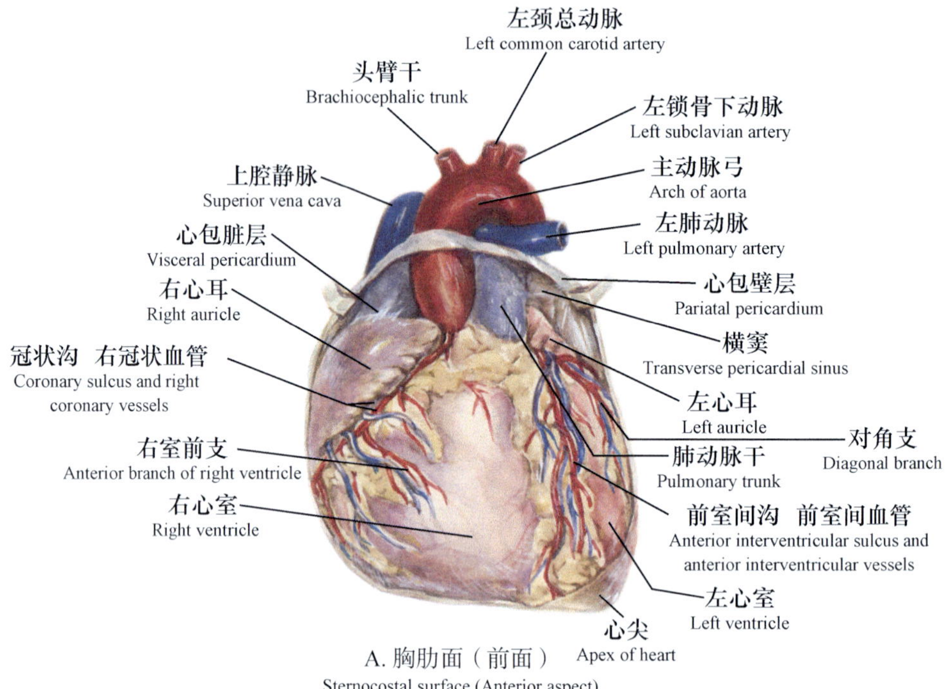

A. 胸肋面（前面）
Sternocostal surface (Anterior aspect)

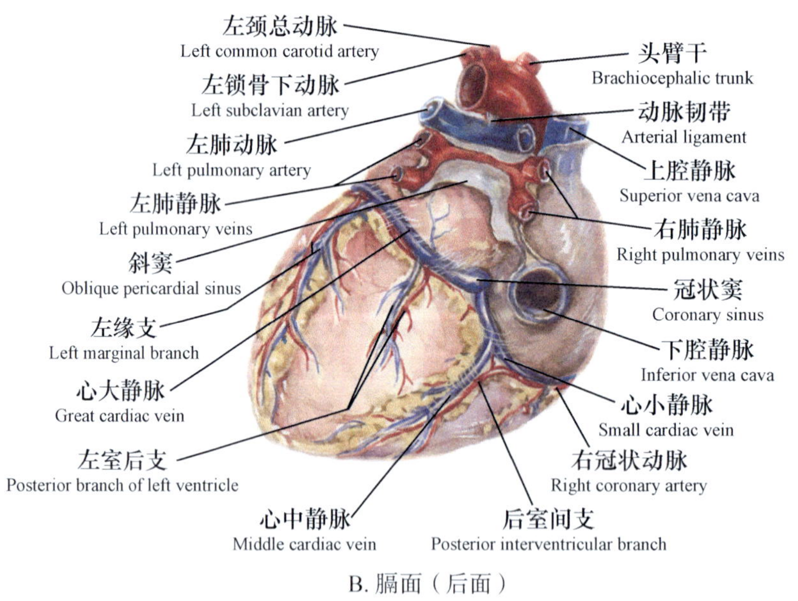

B. 膈面（后面）
Diaphragmatic surface (Posterior aspect)

图 3-2 心外面观
The surface aspect of heart

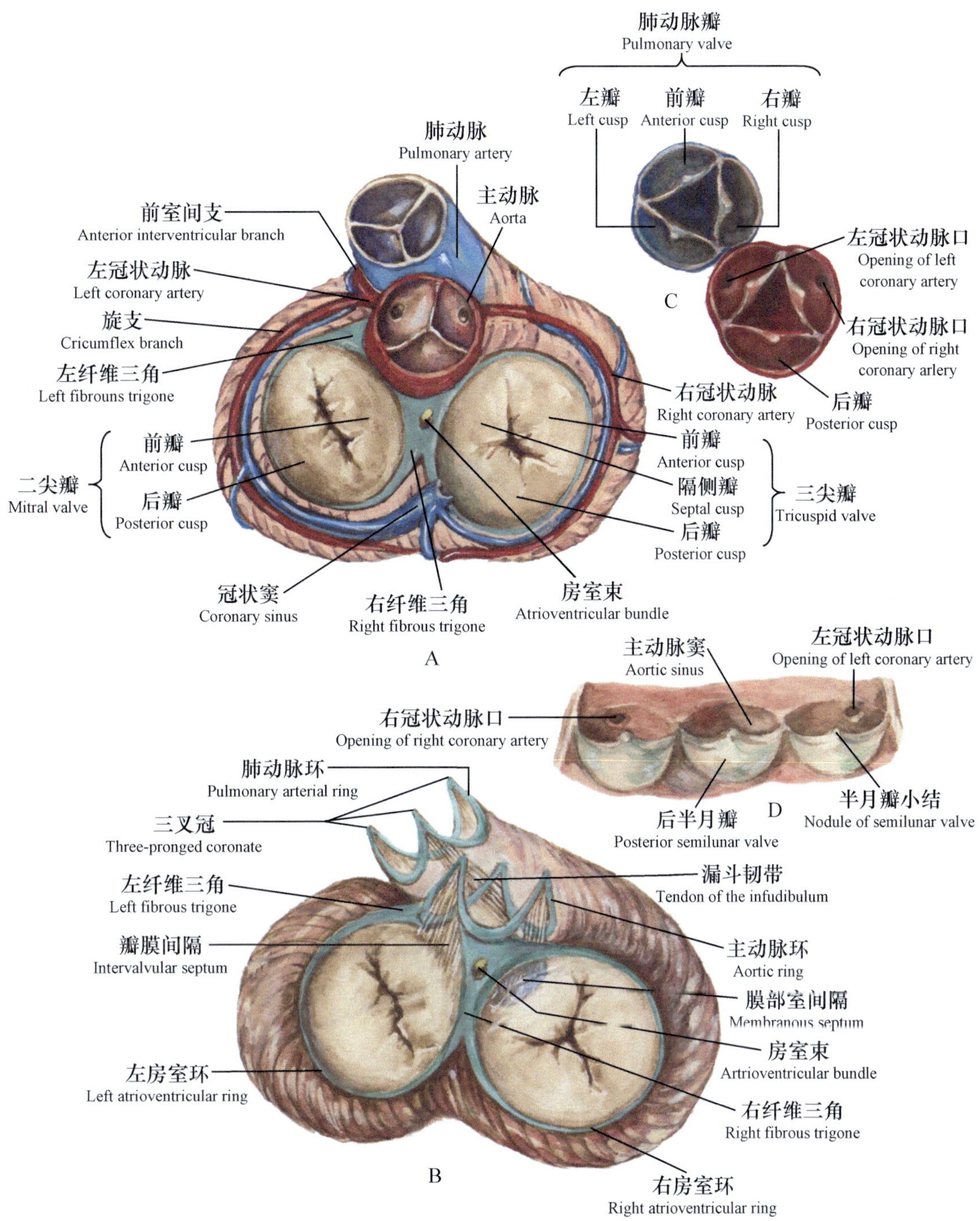

A. 二维结构的纤维环
Two dimensional fibrous ring

C. 心室收缩期的动脉窦膨大，动脉口开放呈三角形
Ventricular in systole the arterial sinus swaling and the opening of artery opened trigonaly

B. 三维结构的纤维环
Three dimensional fibrous ring

D. 主动脉的纵剖面显示三个半月瓣
A longitudinal section of the aorta showing three semilunar valves

注：动脉环的立体结构称三叉冠
The three dimensional structure of arterial ring is could three-pronged coronate

图 3-3 心纤维骨架
Fibrous skeleton of the heart

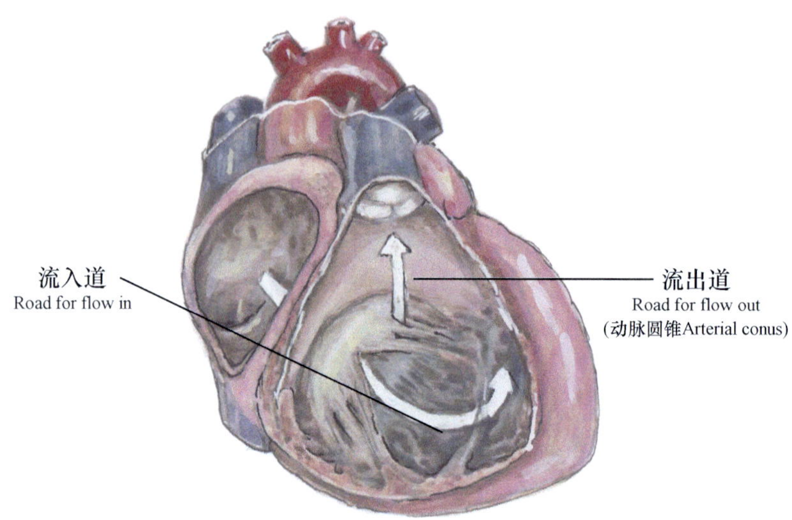

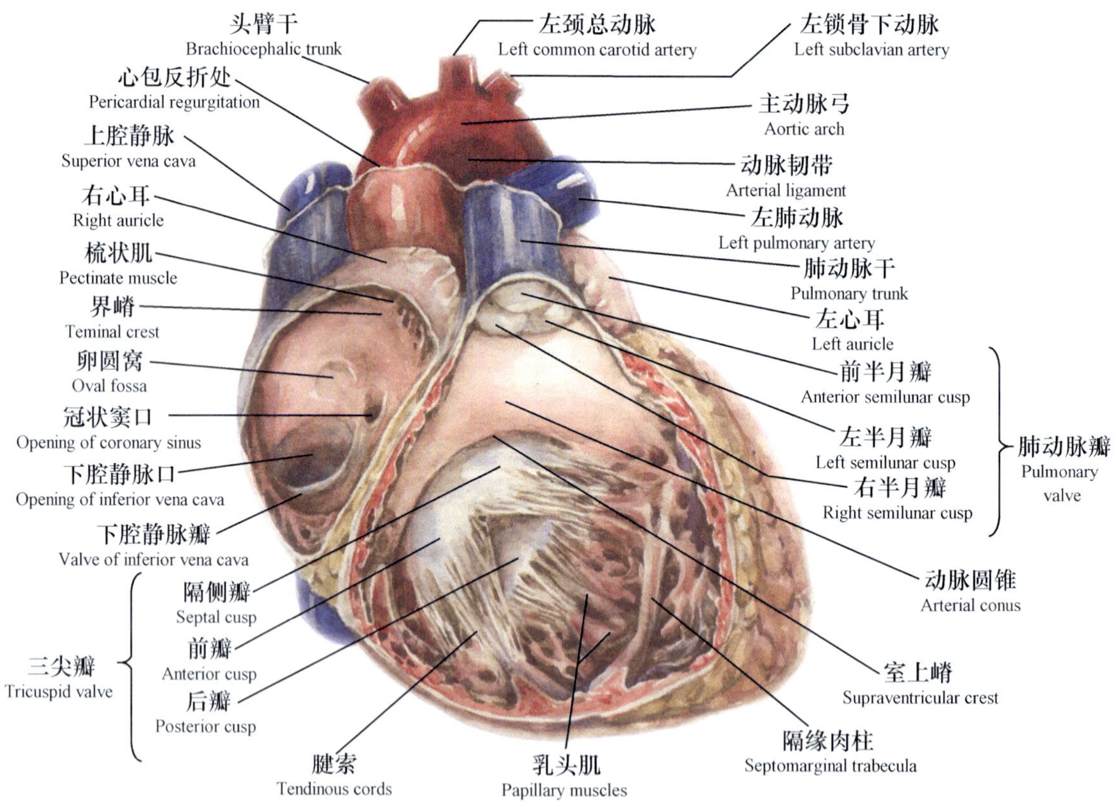

图 3-4 心（前面观）
Heart (Anterior aspect)

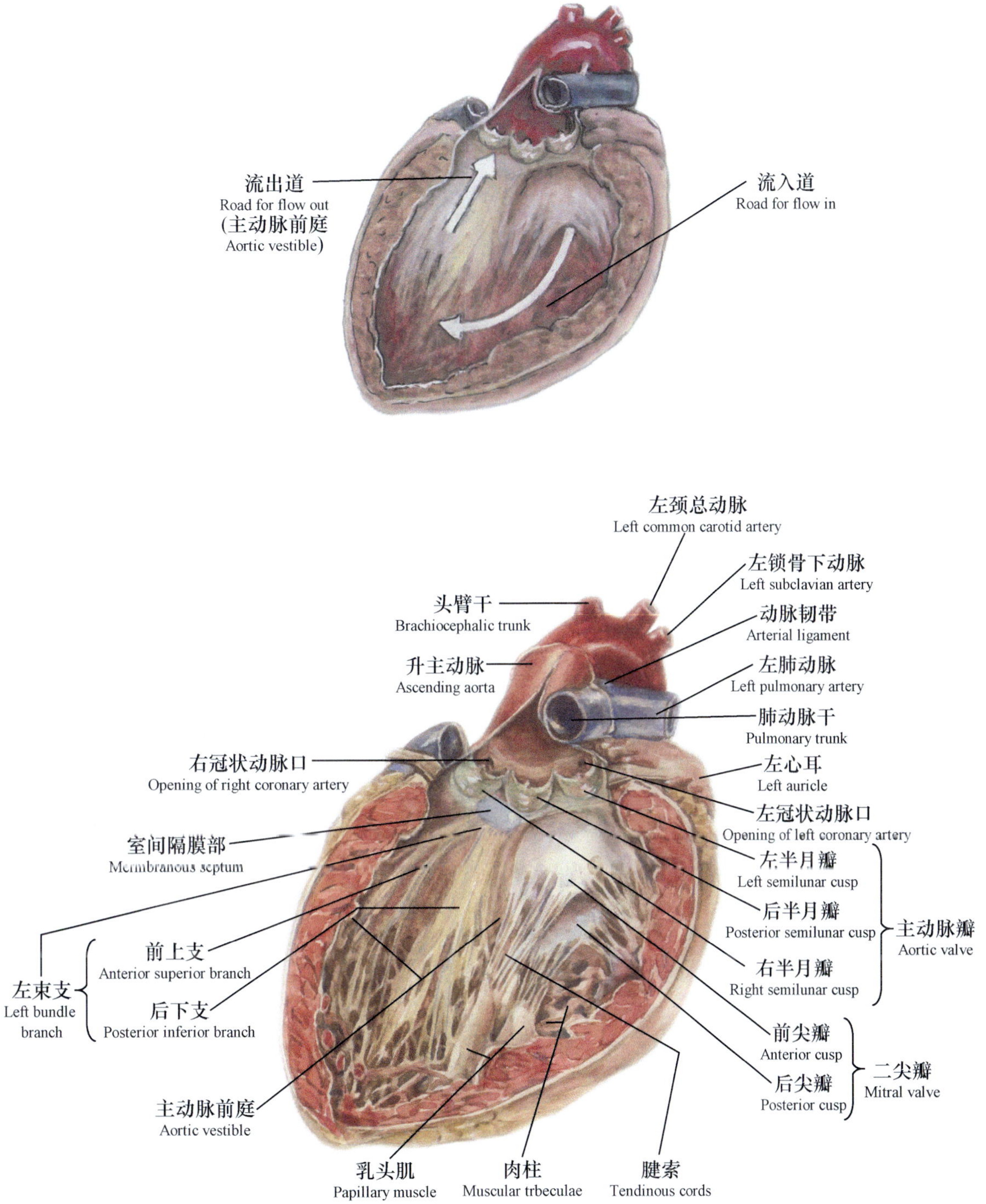

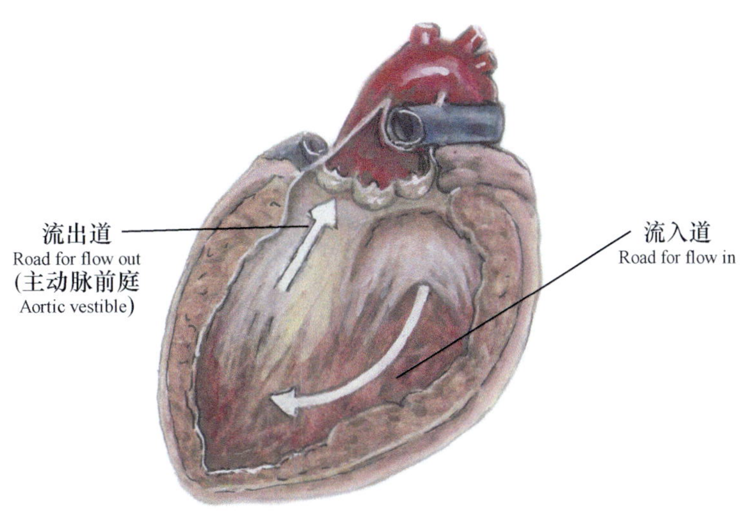

图 3-5　心（左侧面观）
Heart (Left aspect)

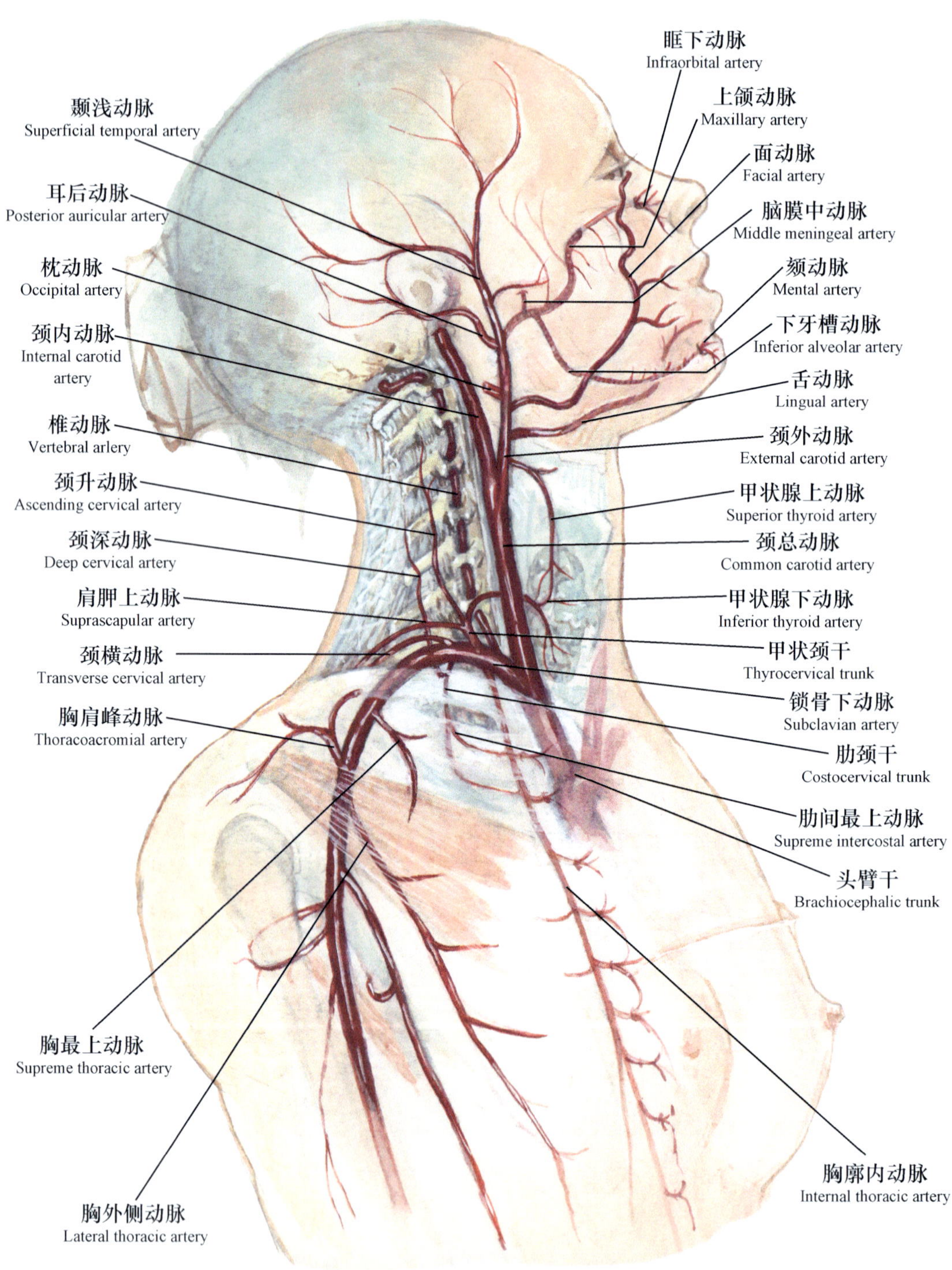

图 3-6 头颈动脉示意图
Diagram of arterial of the head and neck

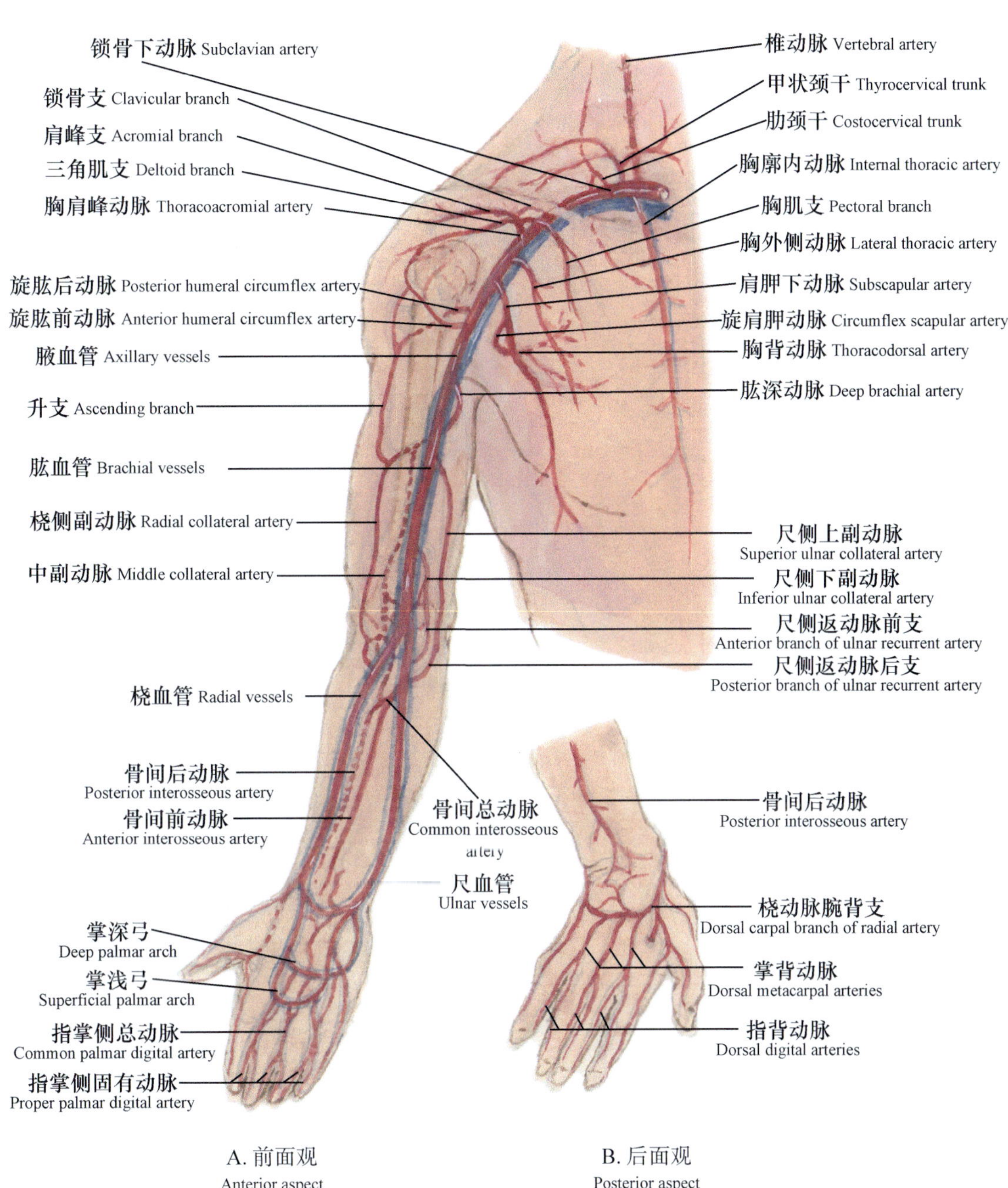

图 3-7 上肢血管
Blood vessels of the upper limb

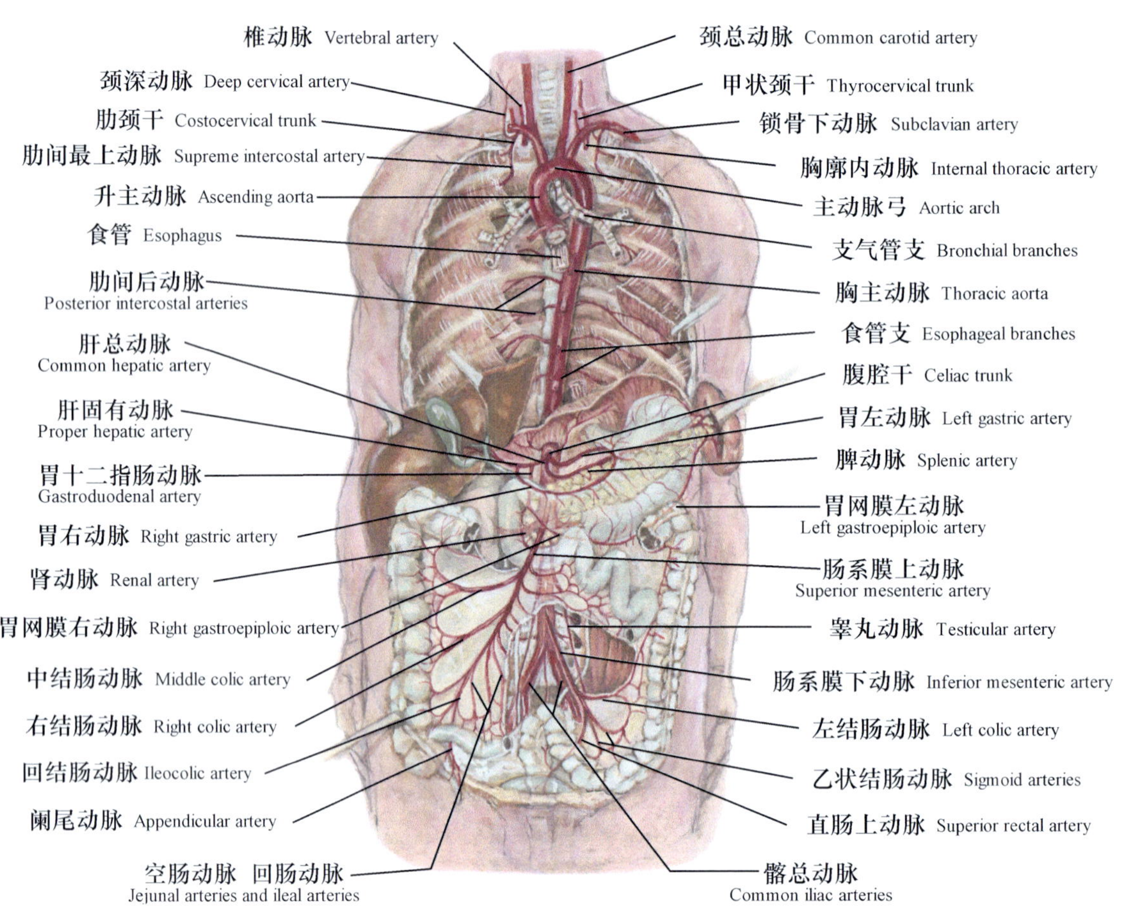

图 3-8 主动脉分支概观
A general view of branches of the aorta

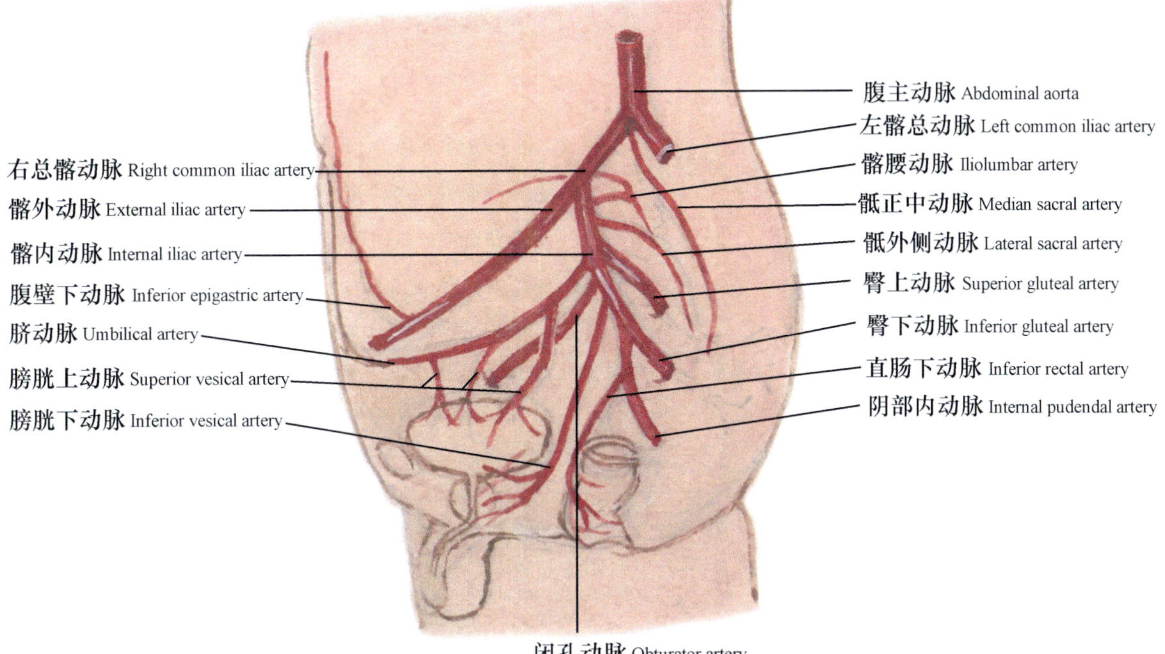

A. 男性
Male

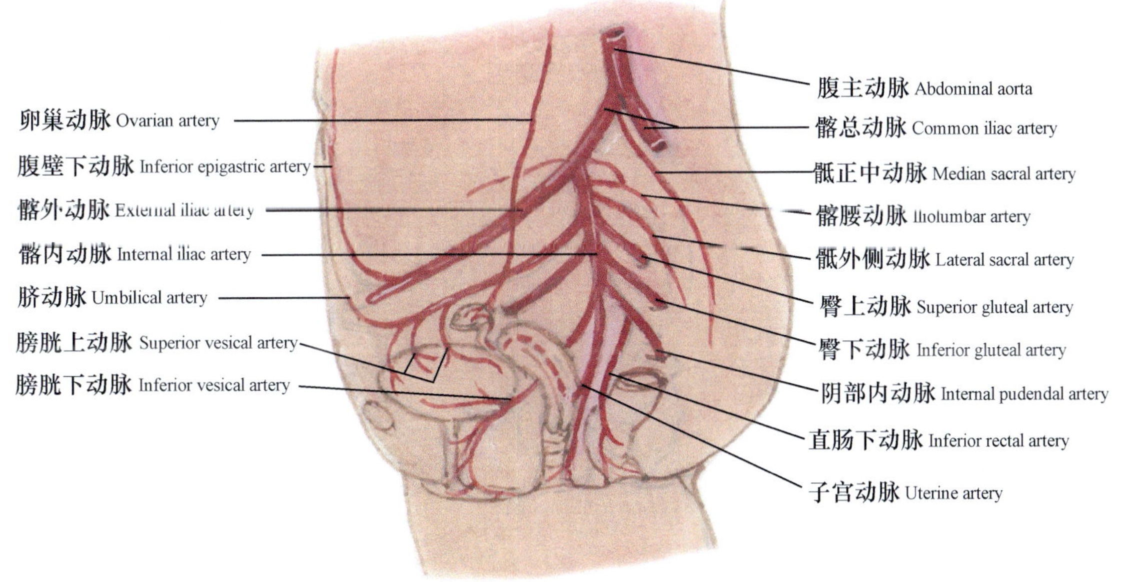

B. 女性
Female

图 3-9 盆腔动脉示意图
A schema of pelvic arteries

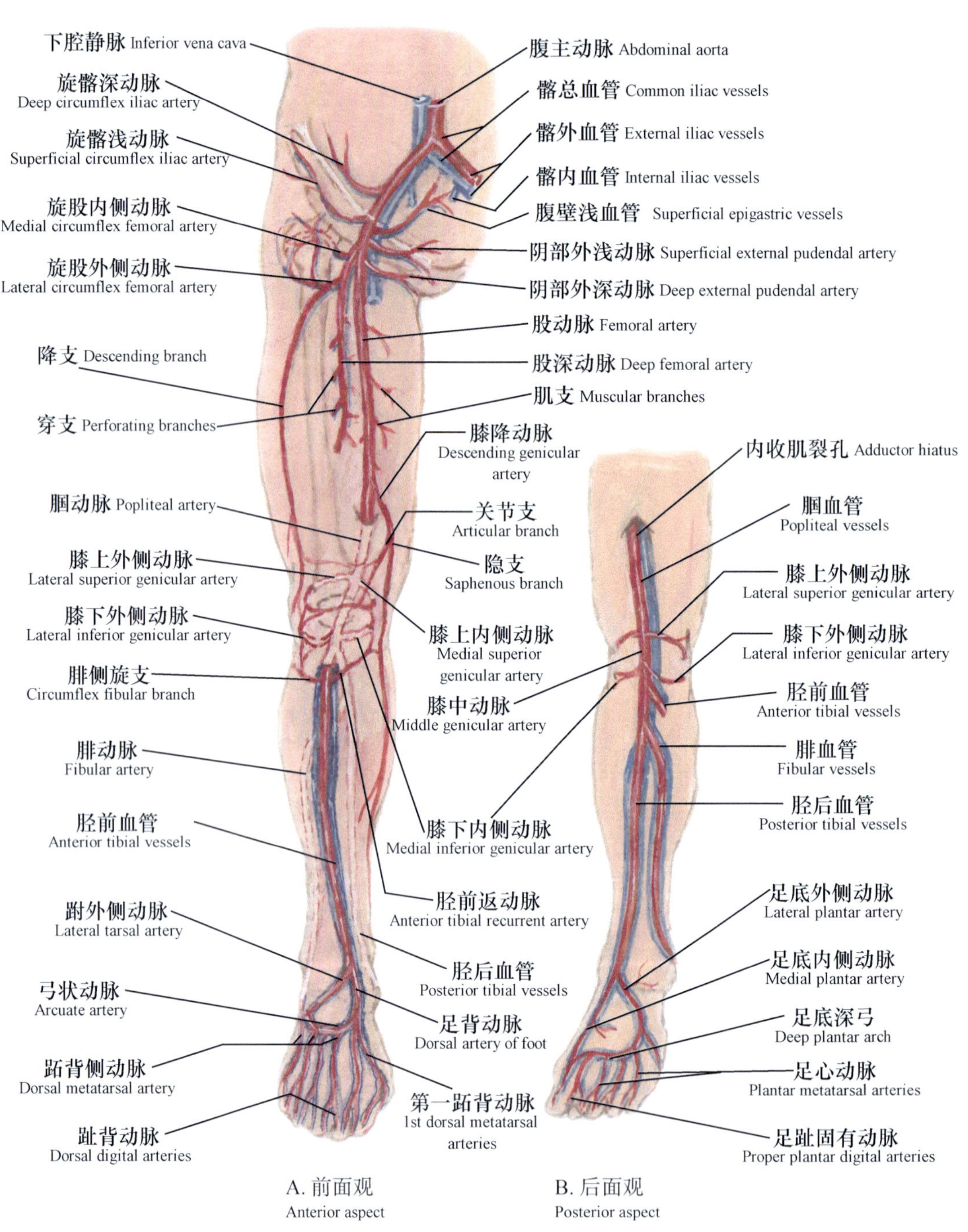

图 3-10 下肢血管
Blood vessels of the lower limb

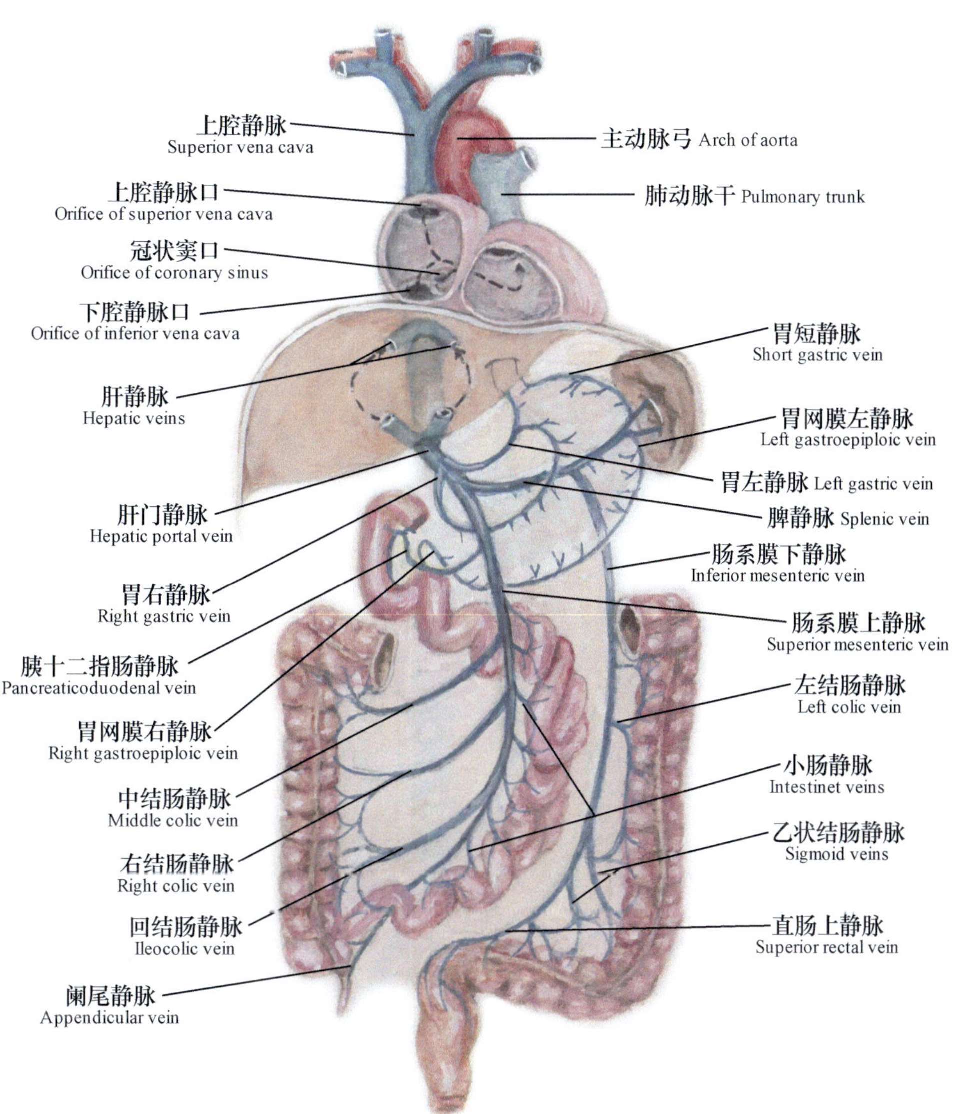

图 3-11 门静脉示意图
A schema of the hepatic portal vein

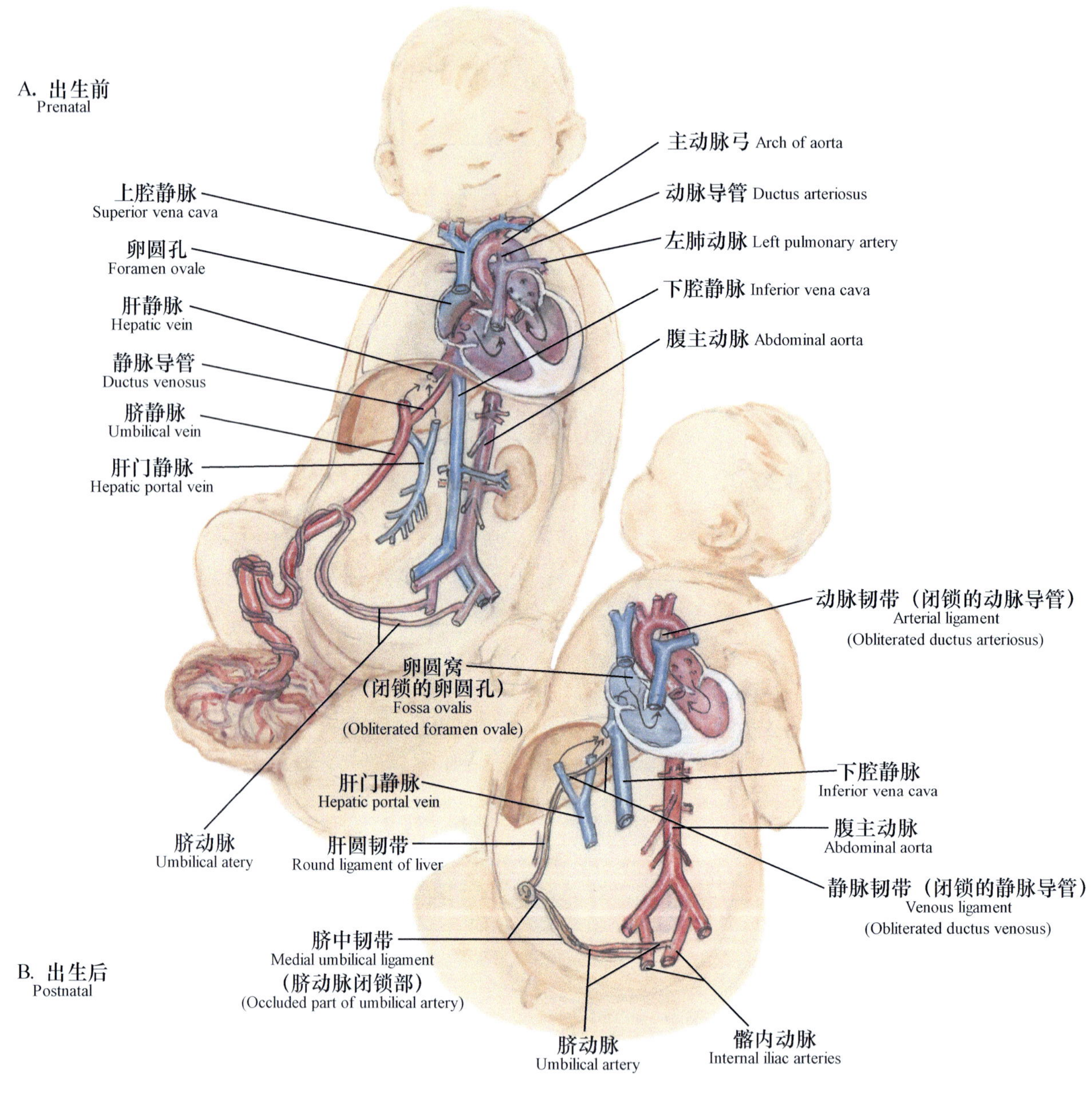

图 3-12 出生前后的血循环
Prenatal and postnatal circulation

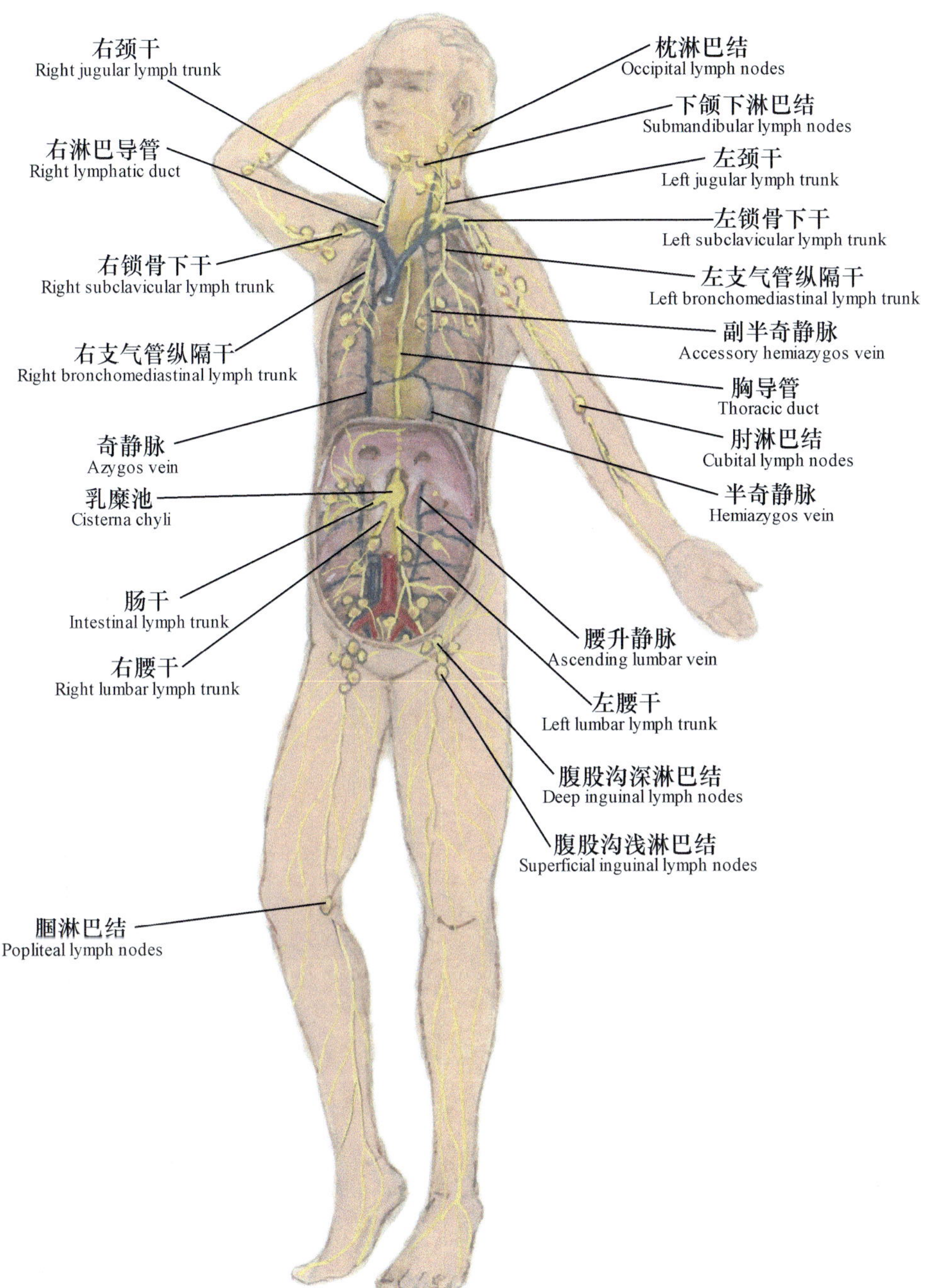

图 3-13 奇静脉与全身淋巴回流示意图

A schema of the azygos vein and the lymphatic drainage the body

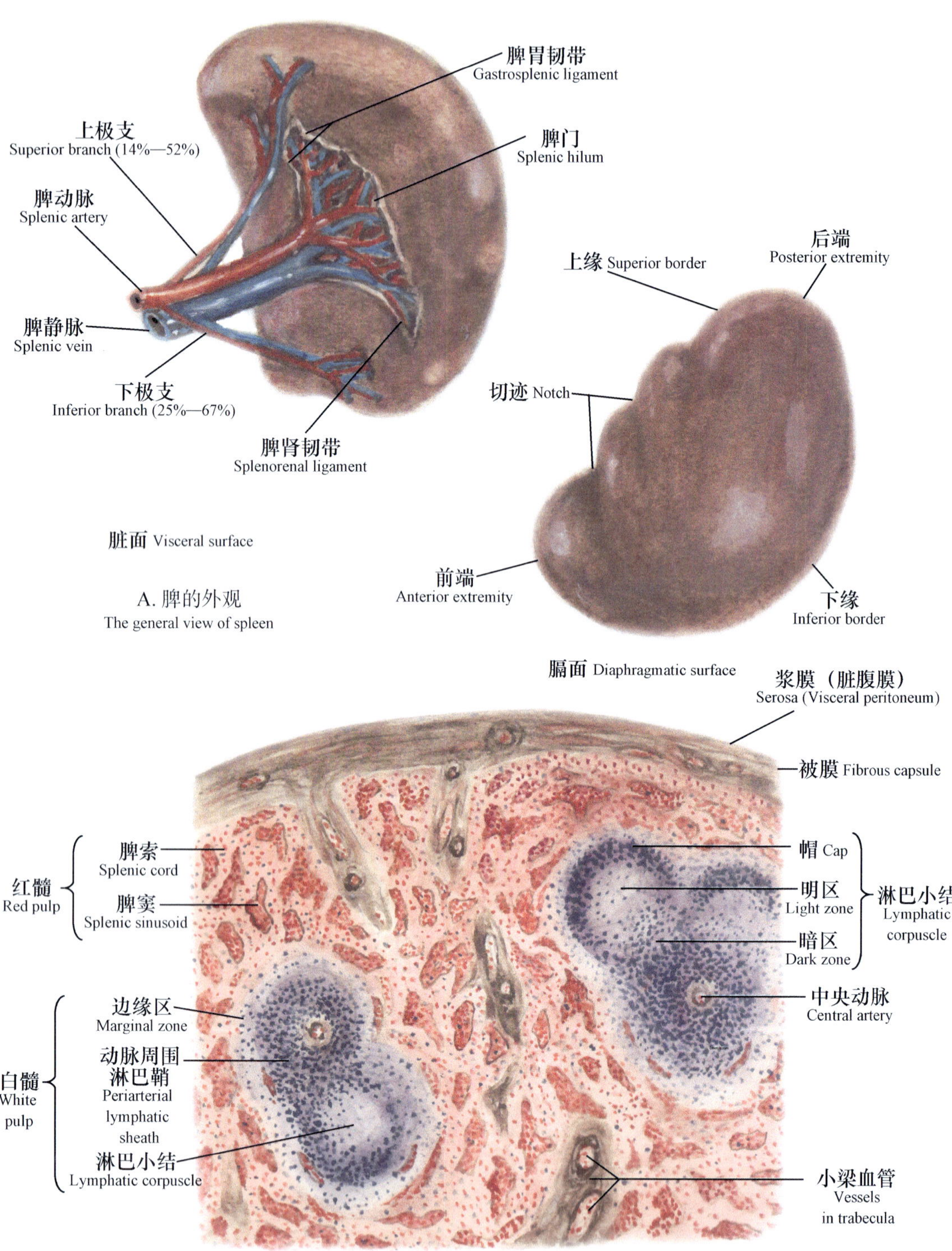

B. 脾微观结构模式图
The diagram of splenic micro structure

图 3-14 脾
Spleen

第4章

神经系统

NERVOUS SYSTEM

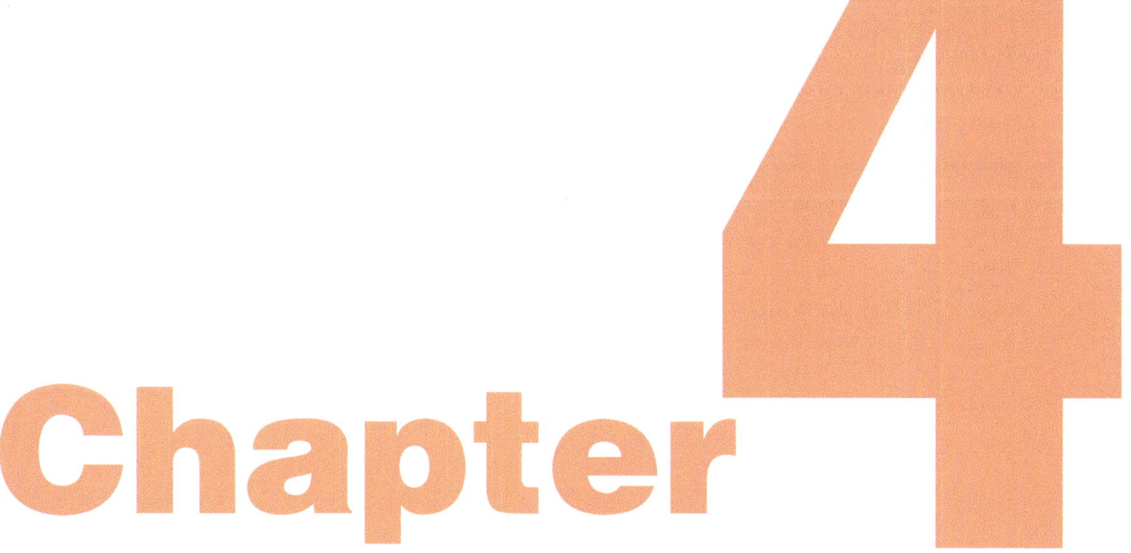

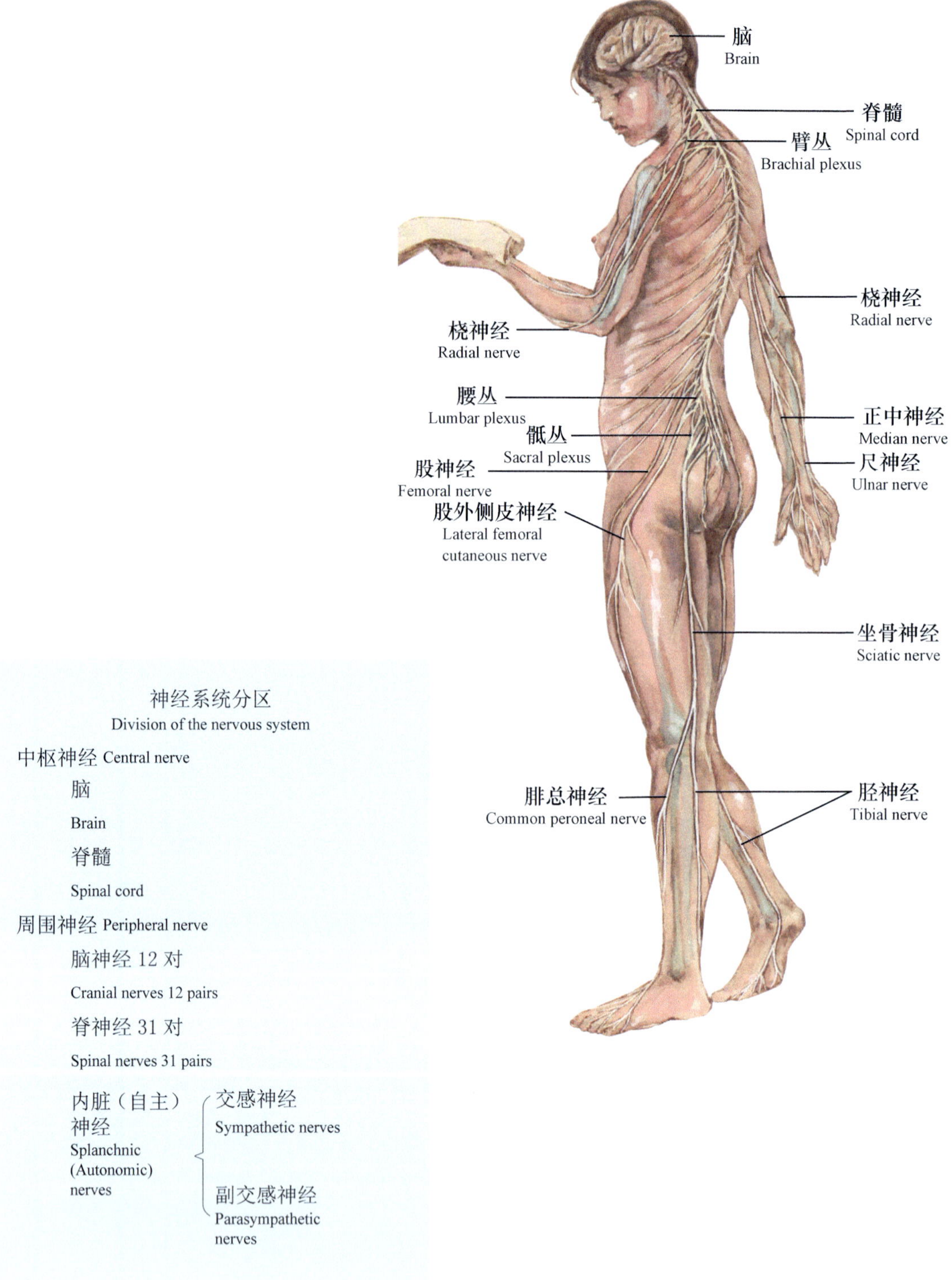

神经系统分区
Division of the nervous system

中枢神经 Central nerve
- 脑
  Brain
- 脊髓
  Spinal cord

周围神经 Peripheral nerve
- 脑神经 12 对
  Cranial nerves 12 pairs
- 脊神经 31 对
  Spinal nerves 31 pairs
- 内脏（自主）神经
  Splanchnic (Autonomic) nerves
  - 交感神经
    Sympathetic nerves
  - 副交感神经
    Parasympathetic nerves

图 4-1 神经系统总观
A general view of the nervous system

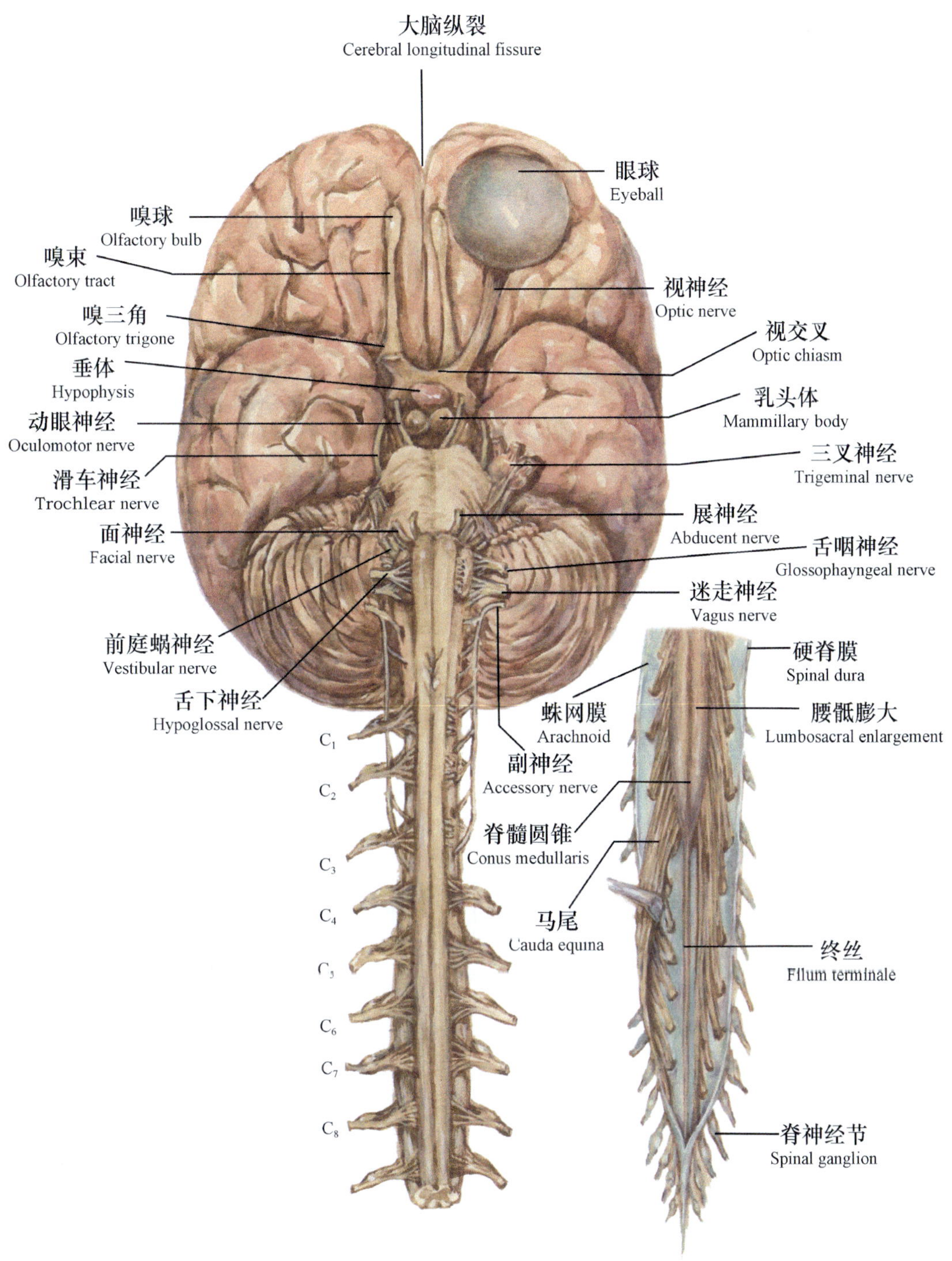

图 4-2 脑脊髓概观
General of cerebrum and spinal cord

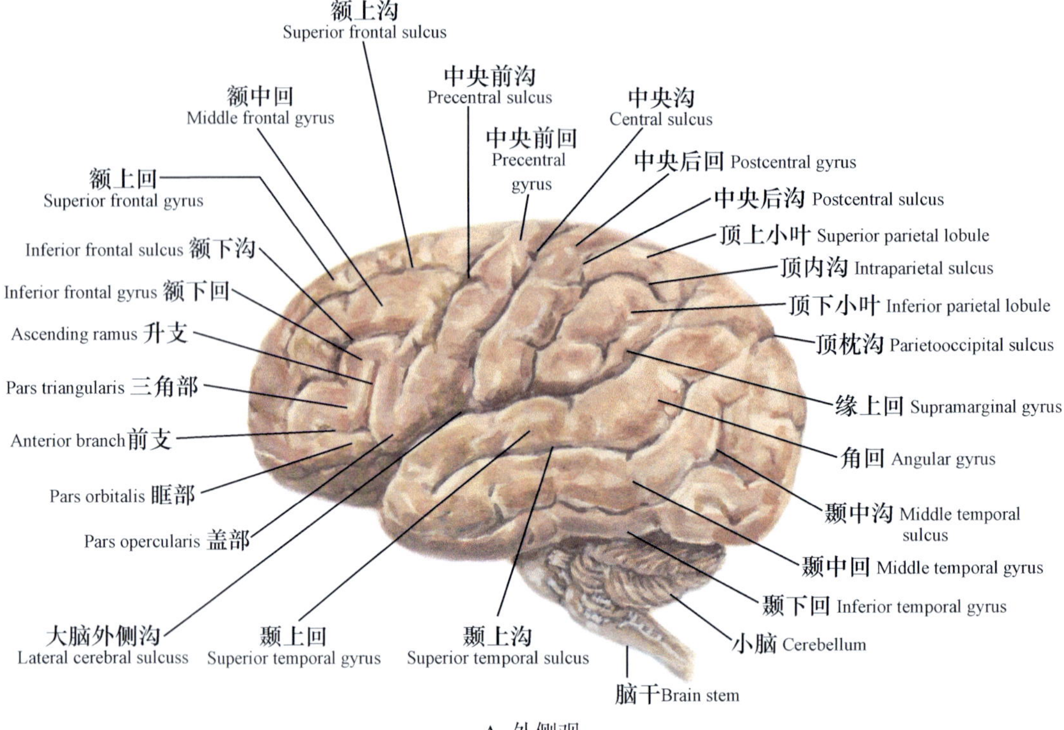

A. 外侧观
Lateral aspect

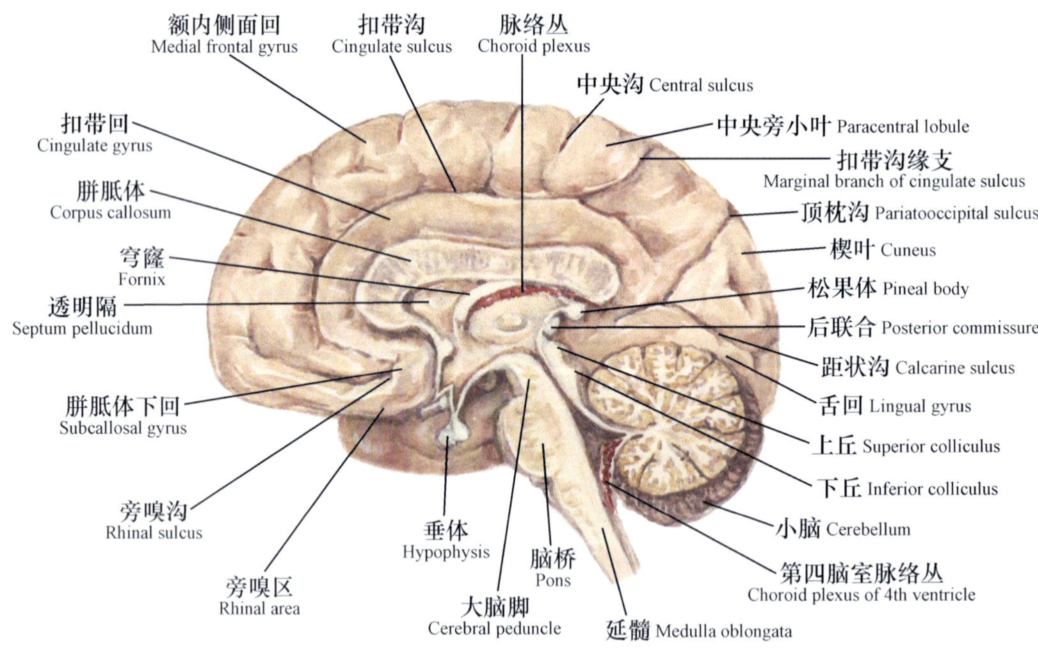

B. 内侧观
Medial aspect

图 4-3 大脑半球外观（1）
The general view of cerebral hemisphere (1)

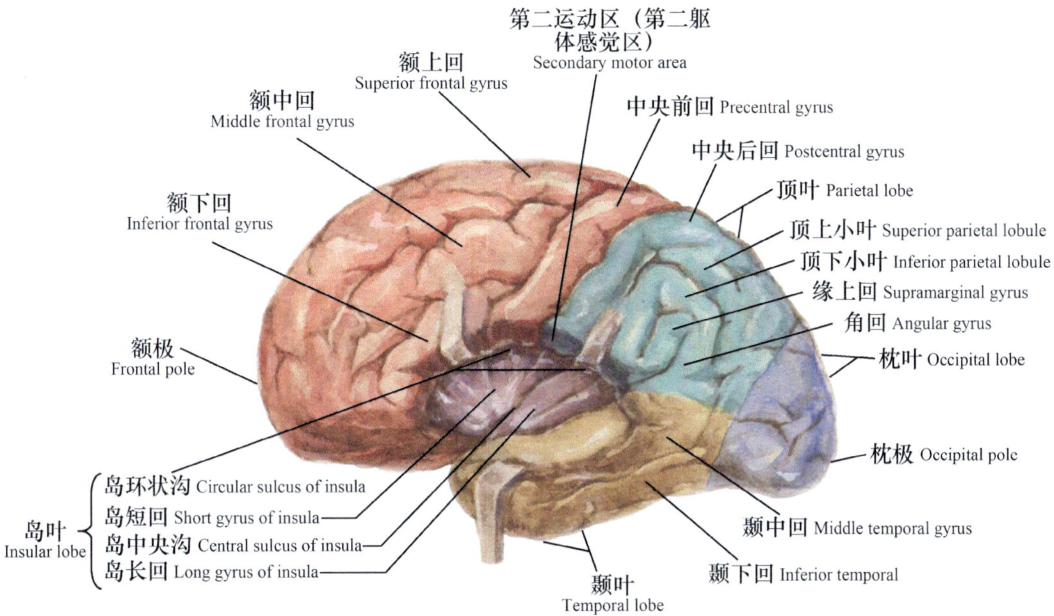

A. 左侧大脑半球外侧观
Lateral aspect of the left cerebral hemisphere

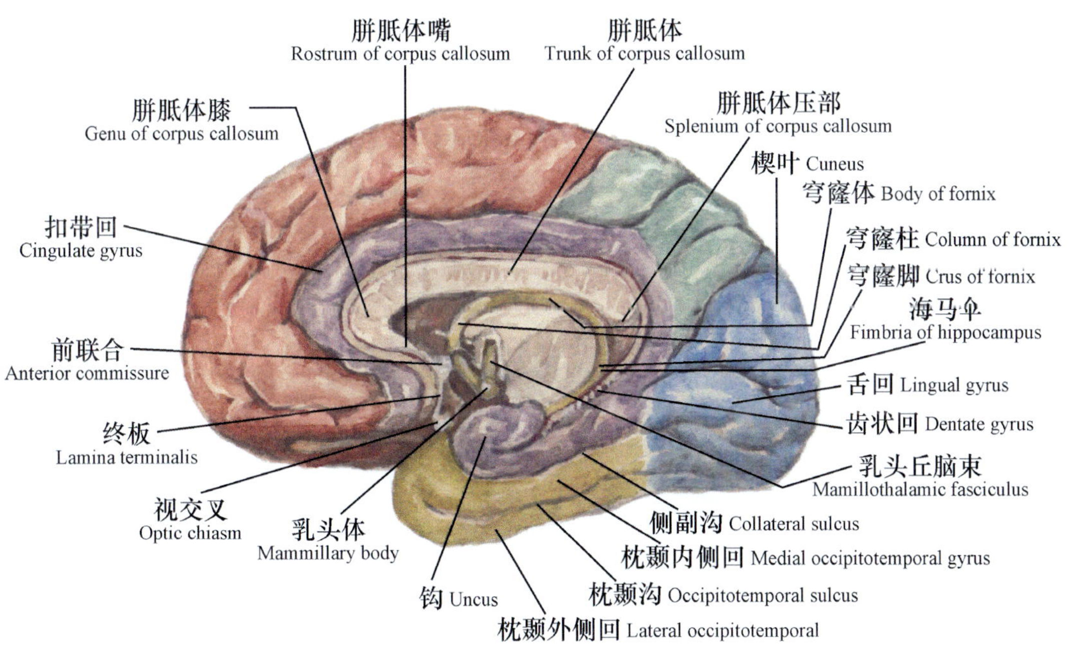

B. 右侧大脑半球内侧面
Medial apesct of the right cerebral hemisphere

图 4-4 大脑半球外观（2）
The general aspect of cerebral hemisphere (2)

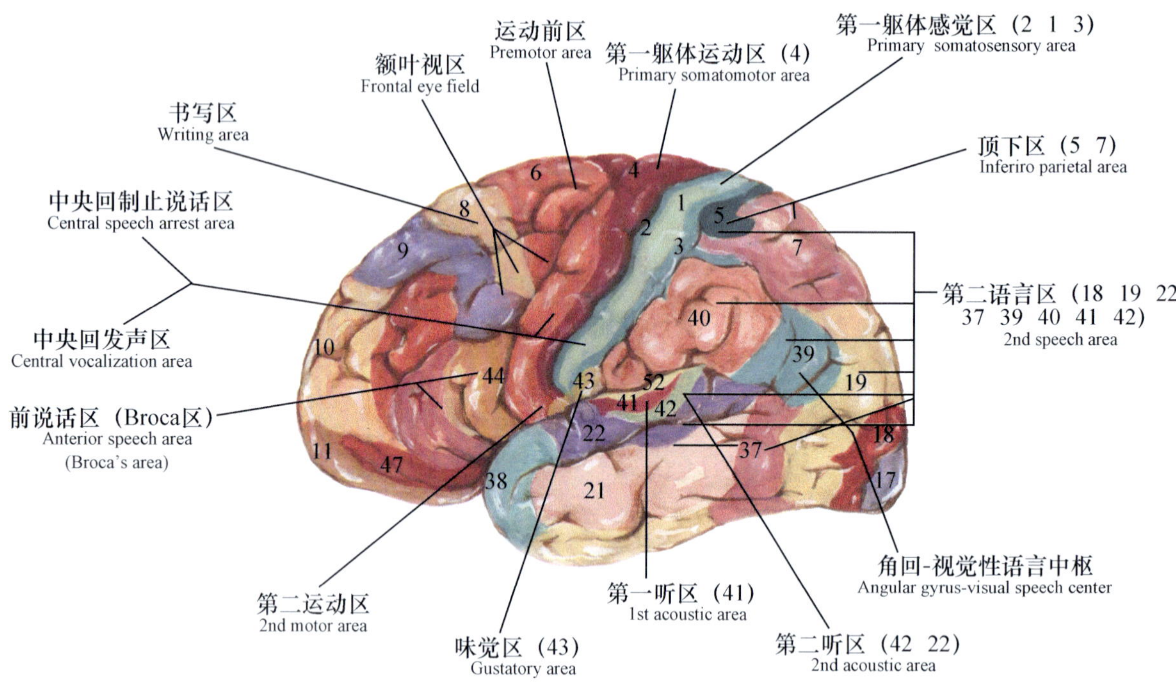

A. 左侧大脑半球外侧观
Lateral aspect of the left cerebral hemisphere

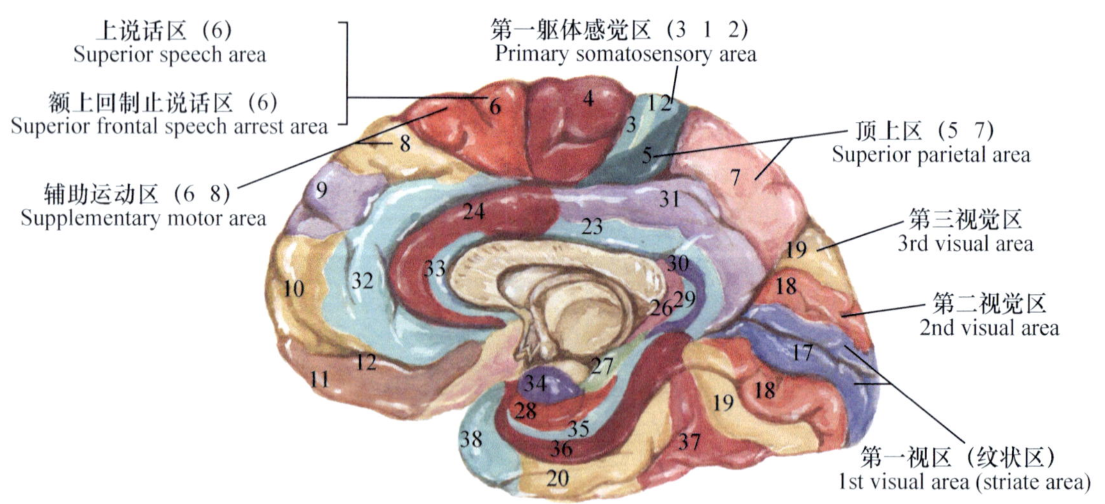

B. 右侧大脑半球内侧观
B. Medial aspect of the right cerebral hemisphere

图 4-5 大脑皮质细胞构筑表面分区及其功能区（Brodmann 分区 1909）
The surface area of the cytoarchitecture and their functions of the human cerebral hemisphere (Brodmann's area 1909)

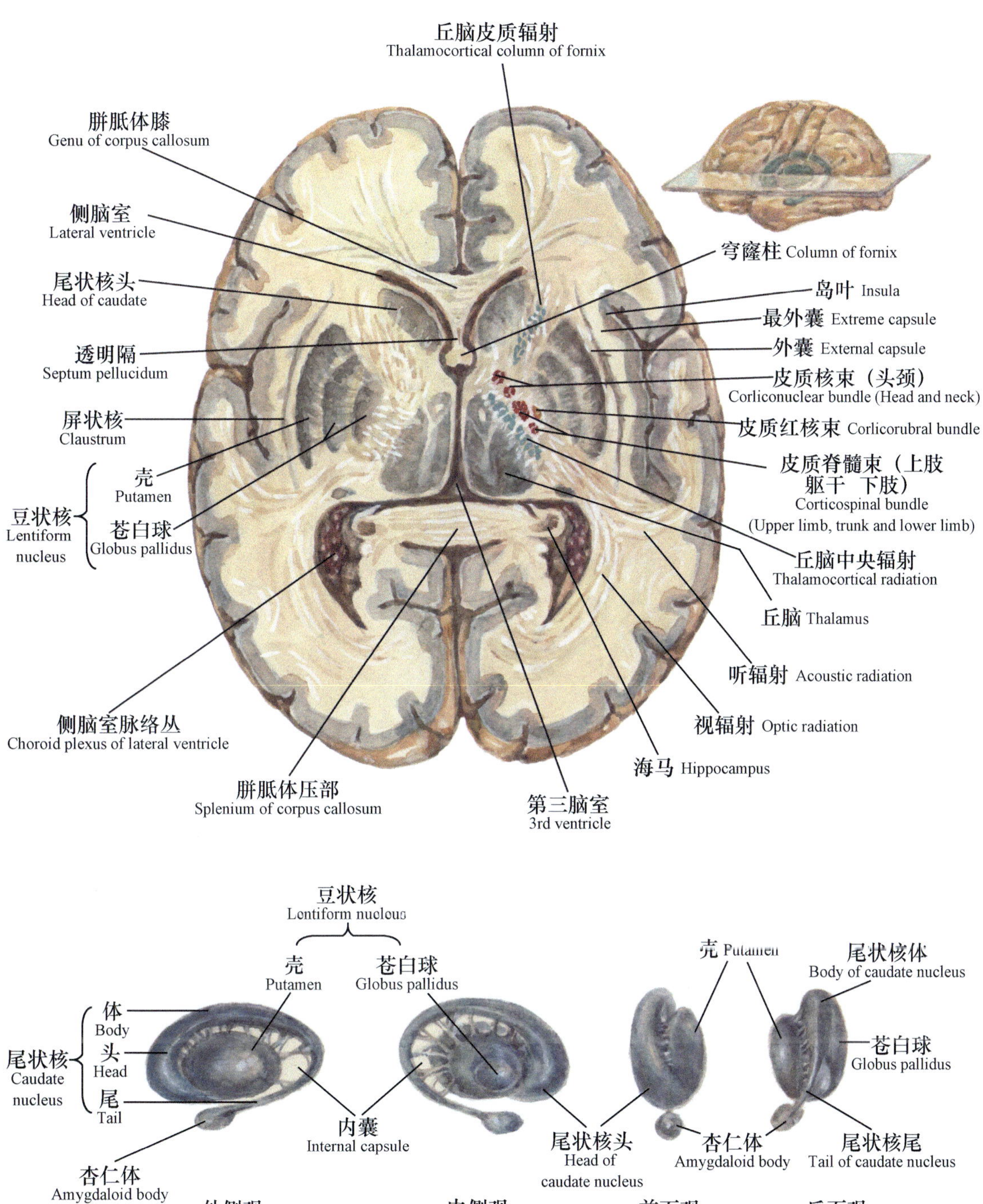

图 4-6　大脑内囊水平切
A horizontal section through the internal capsule of the brain

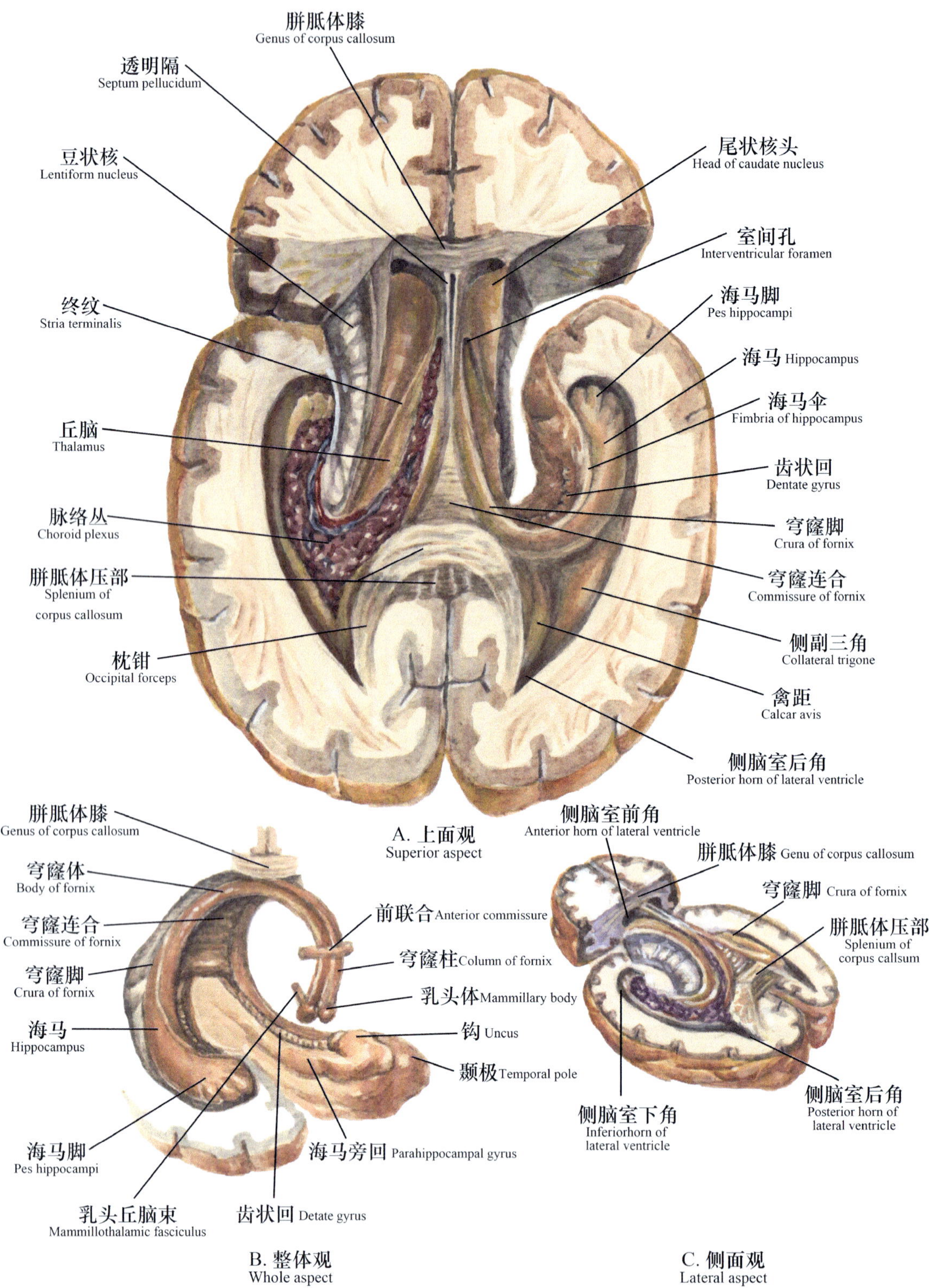

图 4-7 穹窿与海马
Fornix and hippocampus

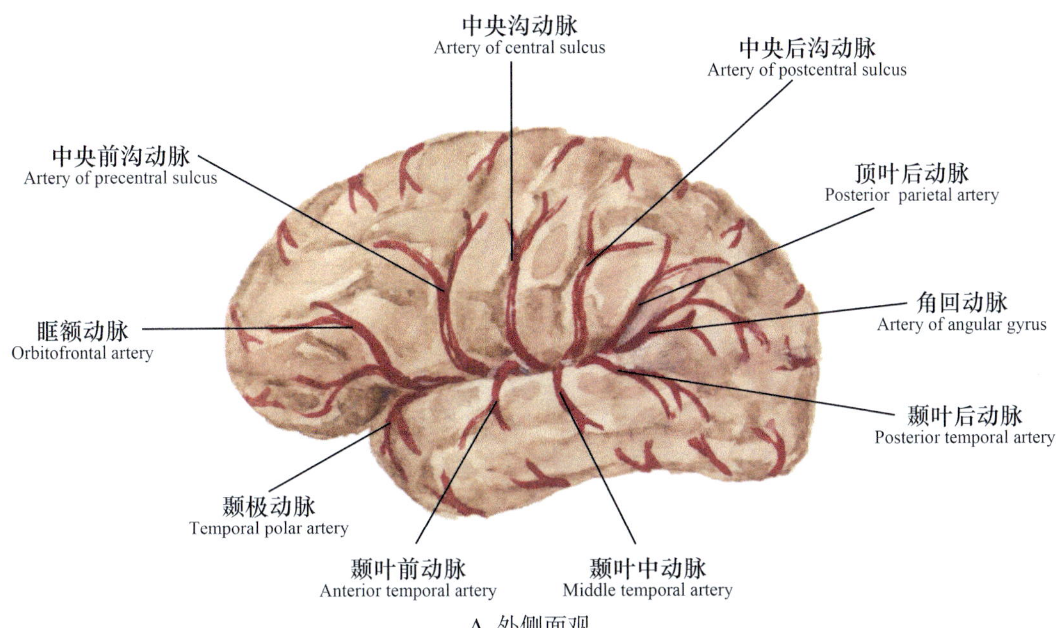

A. 外侧面观
Lateral aspect

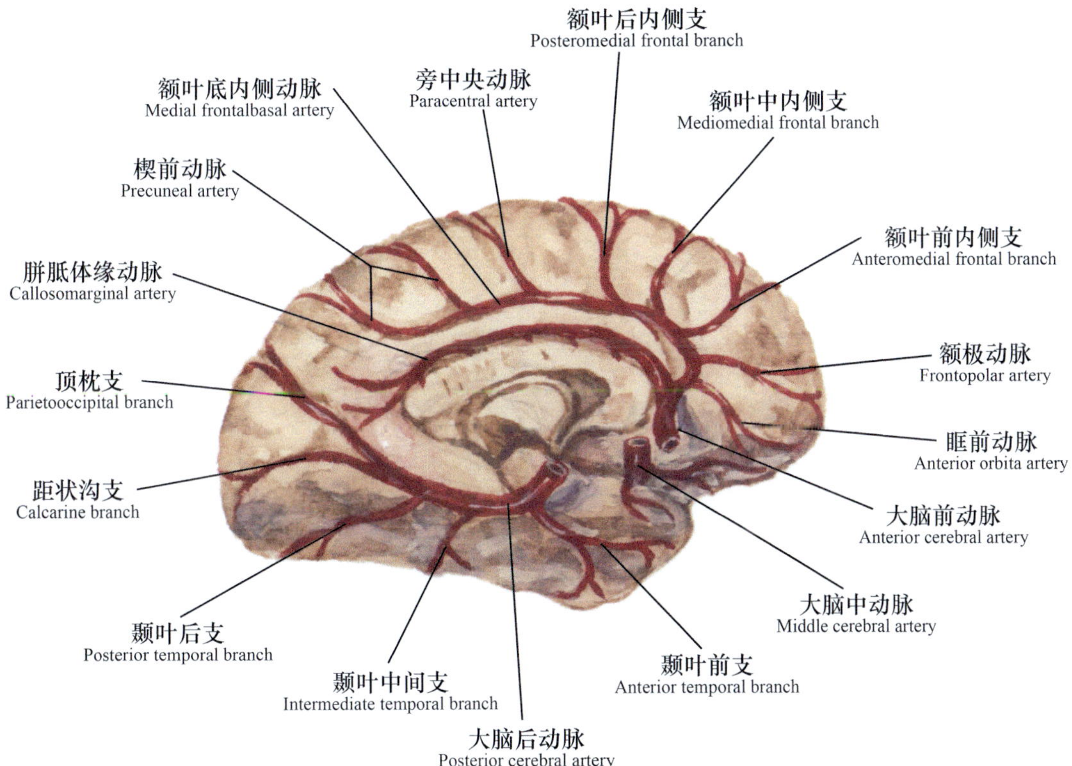

B. 内侧面观
Medical aspect

图 4-8 大脑半球的动脉
Arteries in the cerebral hemisphere

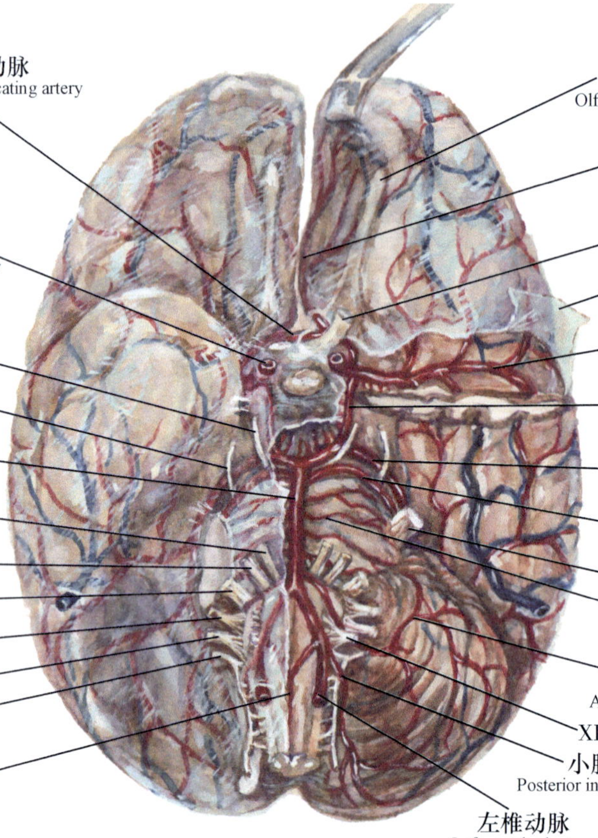

前交通动脉
Anterior communicating artery
嗅球
Olfactory bulb
大脑前动脉
Anterior cerebral artery
Ⅱ
右颈内动脉
Right internal carotid artery
蛛网膜
Arachnoid
大脑中动脉
Middle cerebral artery
Ⅲ
Ⅳ
后交通动脉
Posterior communicating artery
基底动脉
Basilar artery
大脑后动脉
Posterior cerebral artery
Ⅵ
小脑上动脉
Superior cerebellar artery
Ⅶ
Ⅷ
Ⅴ
迷路动脉
Labyrinthine artery
Ⅸ
小脑下前动脉
Anterior inferior cerebellar artery
Ⅹ
XI
XII
脊髓前动脉
Anterior spinal artery
小脑下后动脉
Posterior inferior cerebellar artery
左椎动脉
Left vertebral artery

图 4-9 脑底的动脉
Arteries the base of the brain

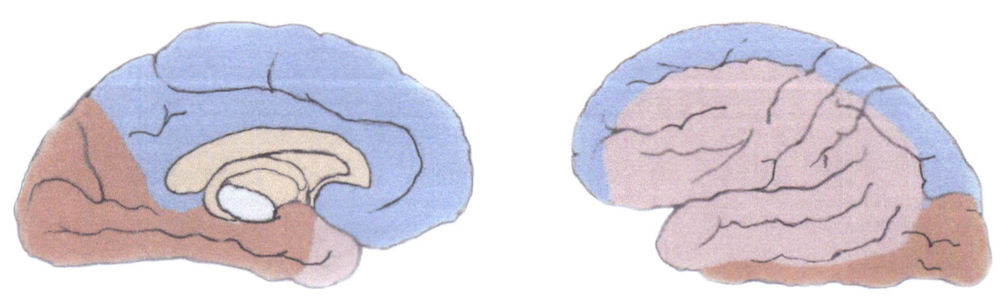

大脑前动脉 - 蓝色区 Blue area by anterior cerebral artery

大脑中动脉 - 粉色区 Pink area by middle cerebral artery

大脑后动脉 - 红色区 Red area by posterior cerebral artery

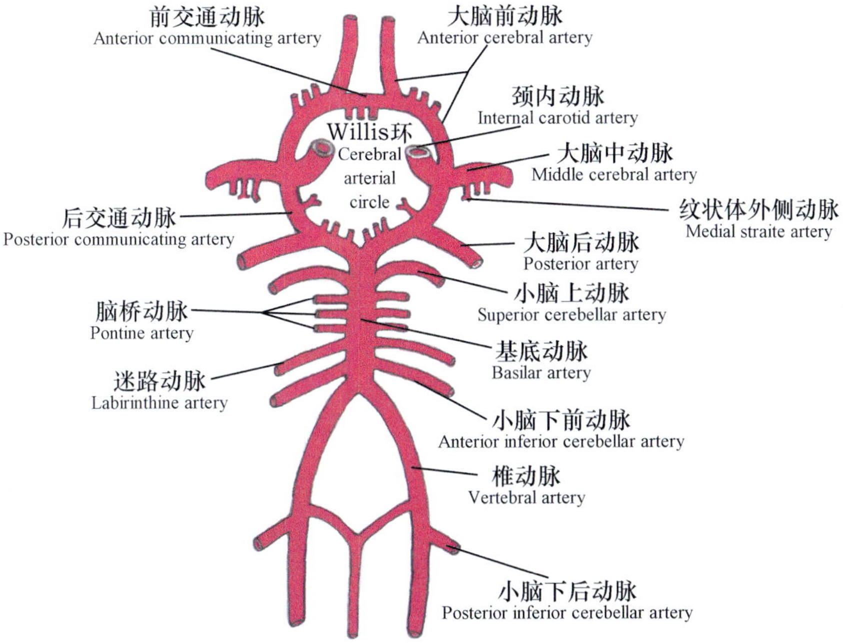

前交通动脉
Anterior communicating artery
大脑前动脉
Anterior cerebral artery
颈内动脉
Internal carotid artery
Willis环
Cerebral
arterial
circle
大脑中动脉
Middle cerebral artery
纹状体外侧动脉
Medial straite artery
后交通动脉
Posterior communicating artery
大脑后动脉
Posterior artery
小脑上动脉
Superior cerebellar artery
脑桥动脉
Pontine artery
基底动脉
Basilar artery
迷路动脉
Labirinthine artery
小脑下前动脉
Anterior inferior cerebellar artery
椎动脉
Vertebral artery
小脑下后动脉
Posterior inferior cerebellar artery

A. 颅底动脉示意图

A diagram of the arteries at the base of the skull

脉络丛前动脉
Anterior choroidal
脉络丛后动脉
Posterior choroidal artery
纹状体外侧动脉
Lateral striate artery
纹状体内侧动脉
Medial striate artery
大脑前动脉
Anterior cerebral artery
丘脑膝状体动脉
Thalamogenicular artery
大脑后动脉
Posterior cerebral artery
颈内动脉
Internal carotid artery
基底动脉
Basilar artery
大脑中动脉
Middle cerebral artery
后交通动脉
Posterior communicating artery
后中央支
Posterior central branch

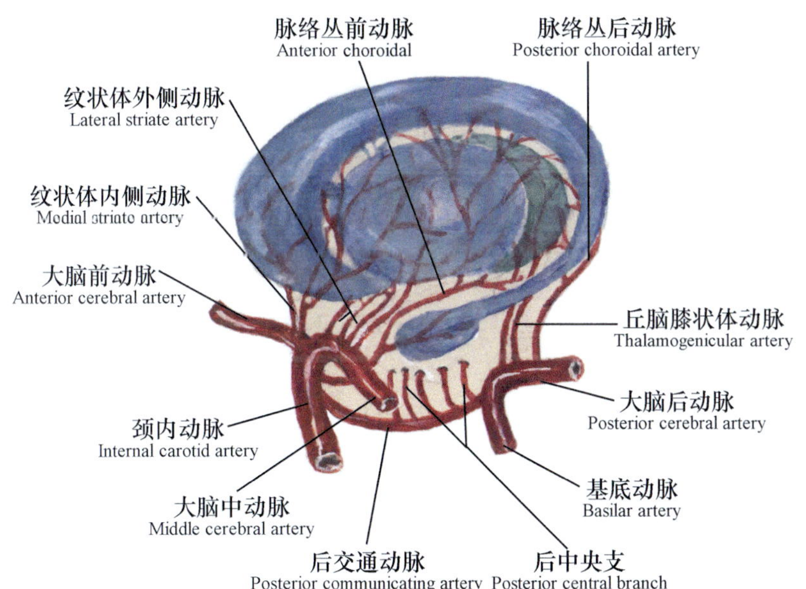

B. 大脑动脉环的中央分支

The central branches of the cerebral arteries circle

图 4-10 大脑动脉环

The central arteries circle

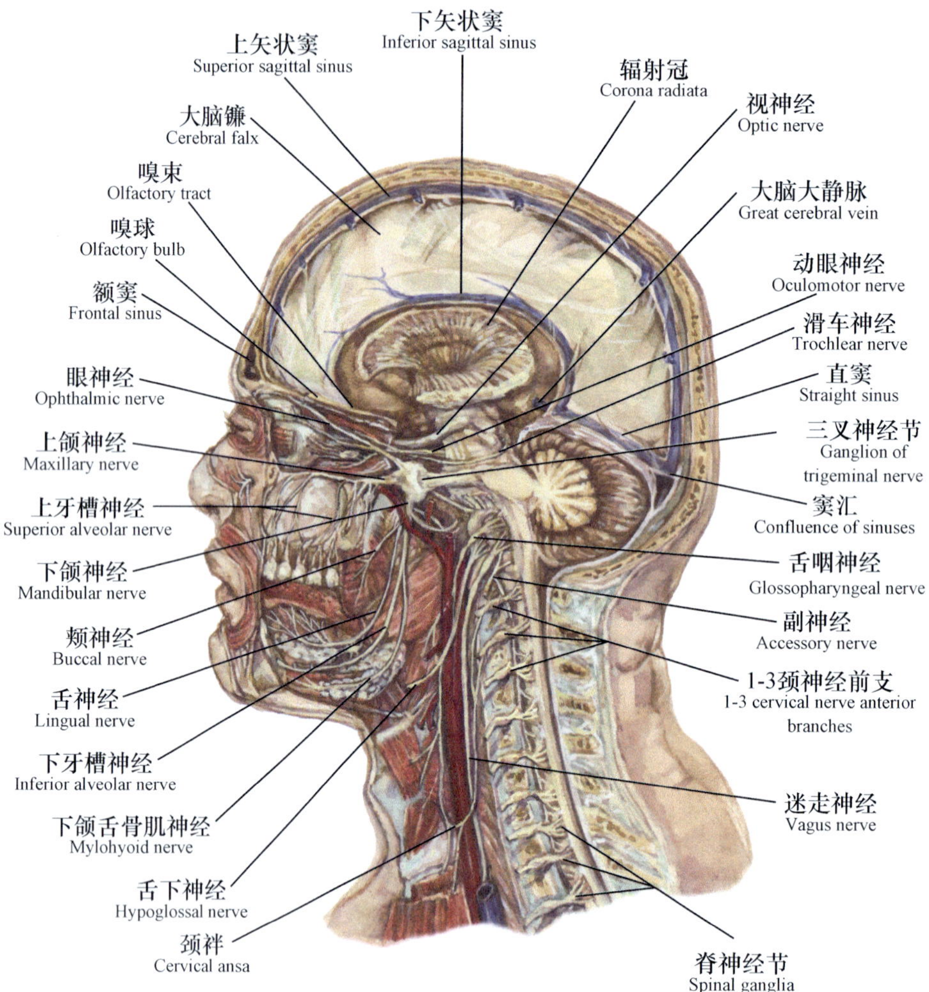

图 4-11 脑神经总观
A general view of the cranial nerves

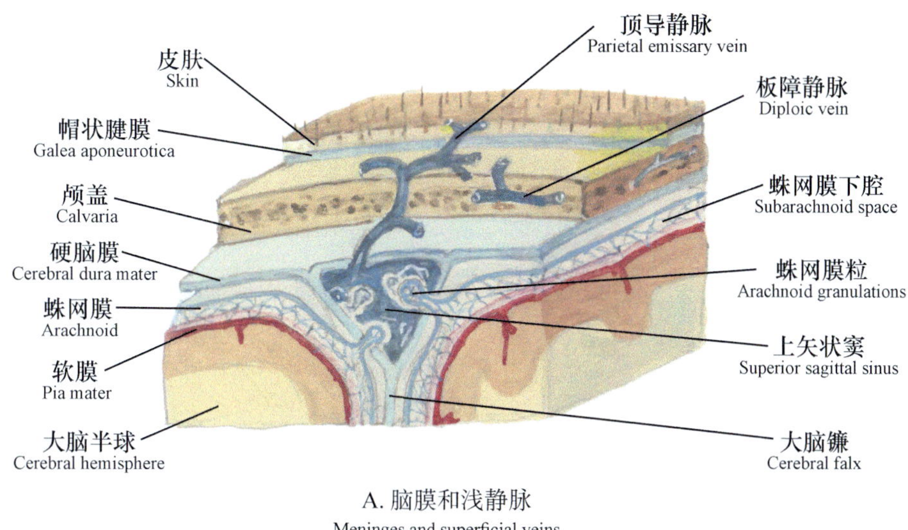

A. 脑膜和浅静脉

Meninges and superficial veins

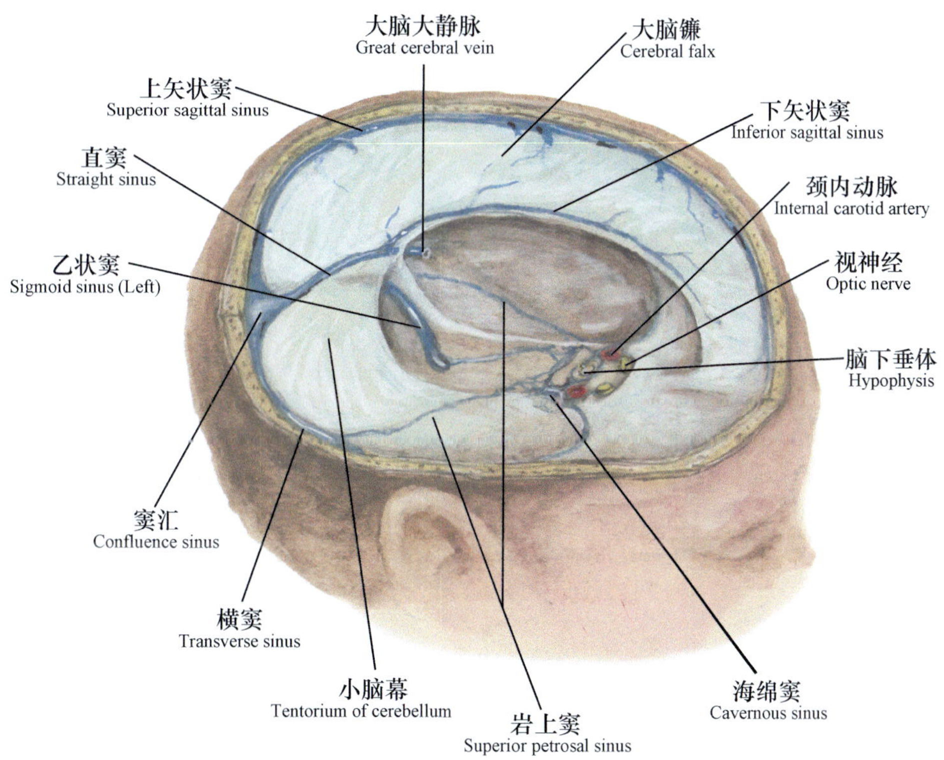

B. 硬膜静脉窦

Dural venous sinuses

图 4-12 脑膜和硬脑膜窦

Meninges and sinuses of dura mater

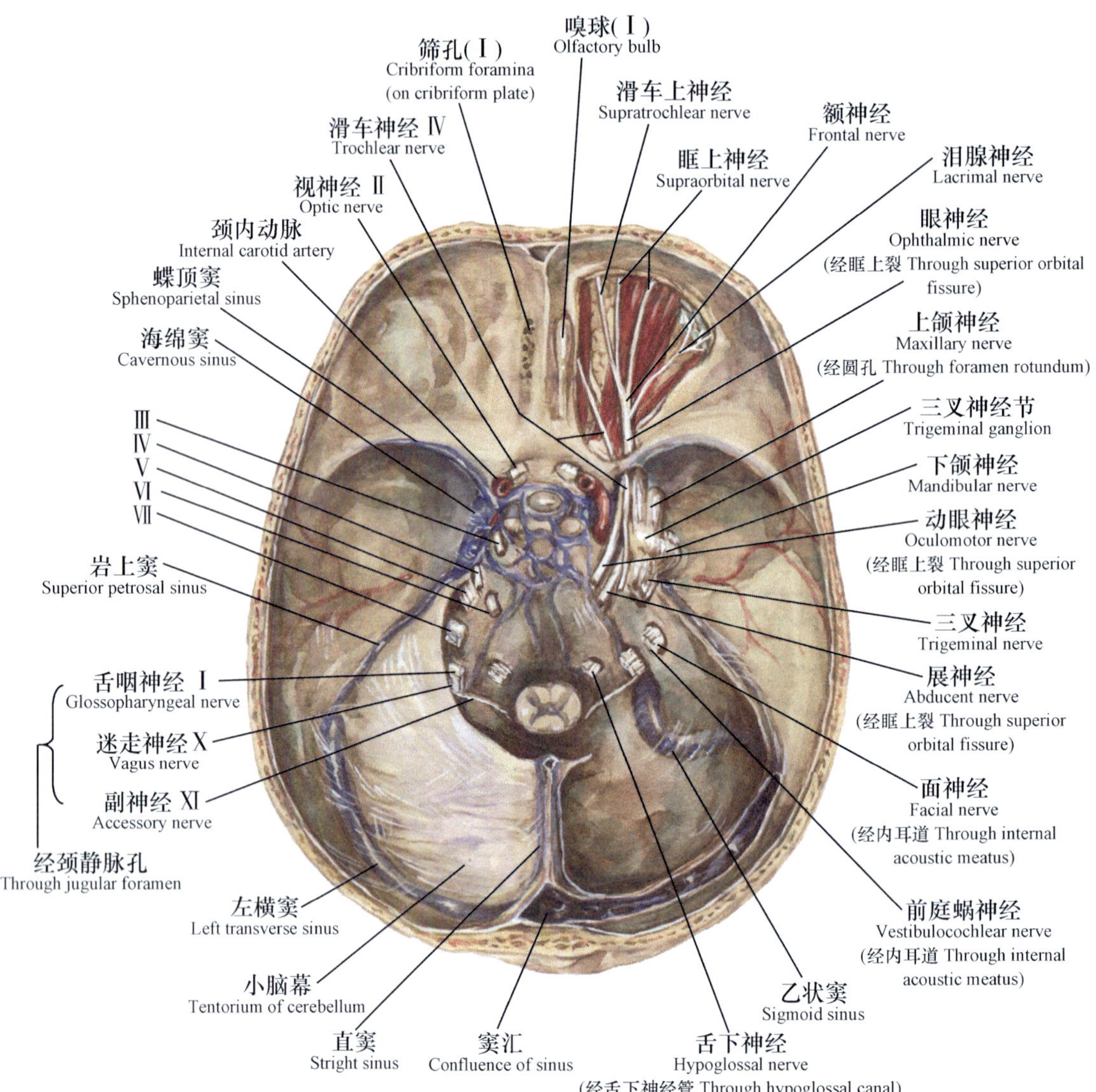

图 4-13 颅底示脑神经出颅位置（孔隙）

Cranial base showing the positions (Foramine) of the cranial nerves

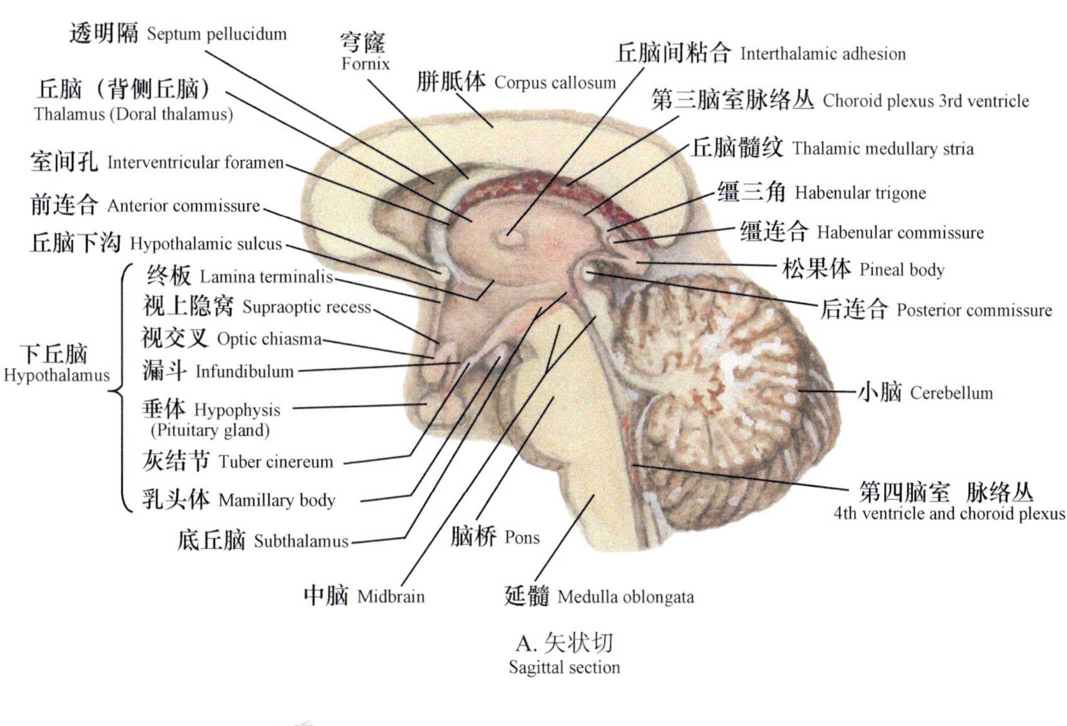

A. 矢状切
Sagittal section

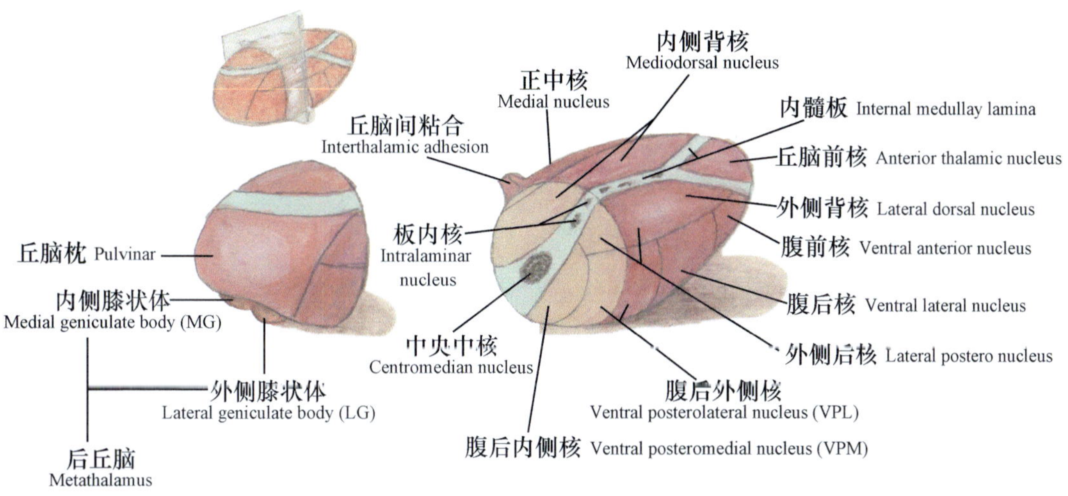

B. 丘脑（背侧丘脑）
Thalamus (Dorsal thalamus)

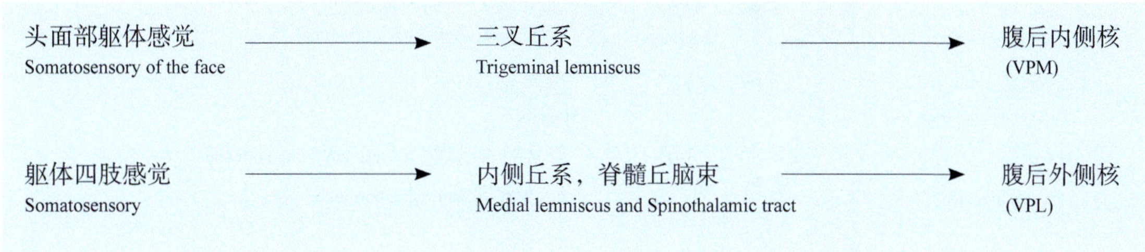

图 4-14 间脑
Diencephalon

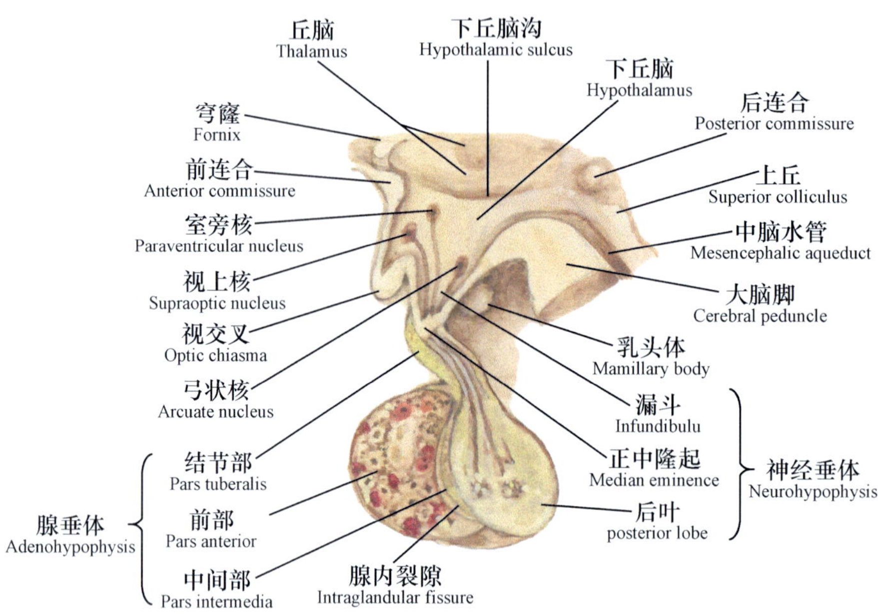

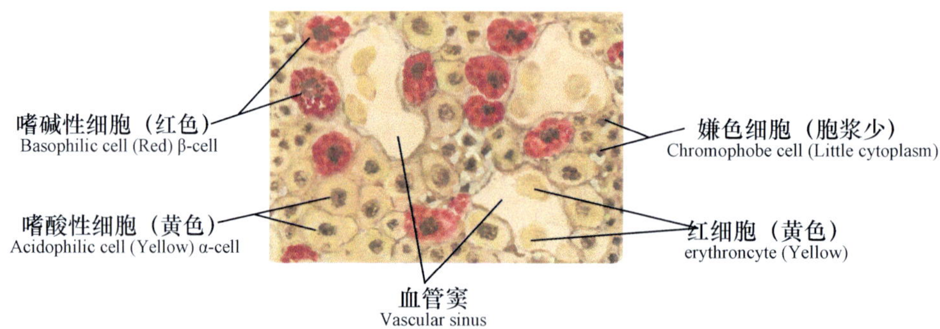

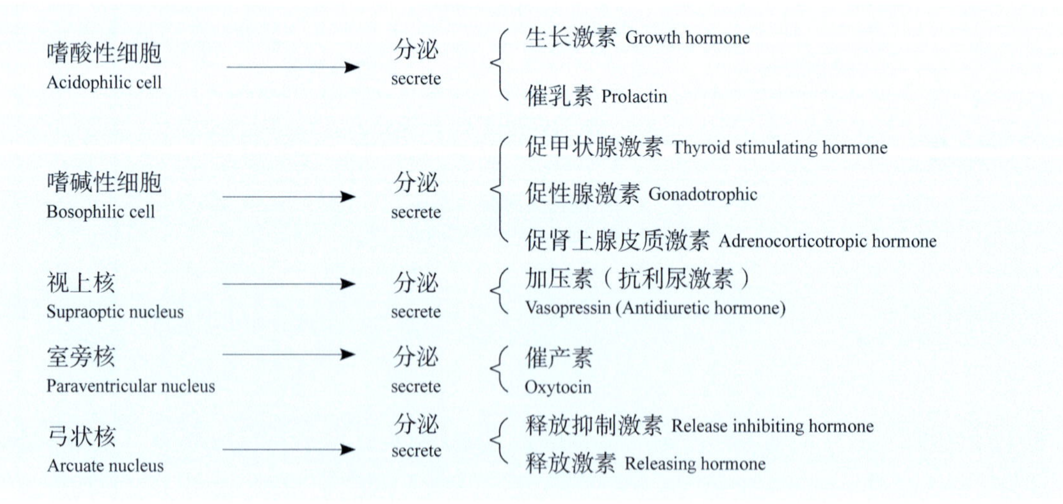

嗜酸性细胞 Acidophilic cell →	分泌 secrete	生长激素 Growth hormone 催乳素 Prolactin
嗜碱性细胞 Bosophilic cell →	分泌 secrete	促甲状腺激素 Thyroid stimulating hormone 促性腺激素 Gonadotrophic 促肾上腺皮质激素 Adrenocorticotropic hormone
视上核 Supraoptic nucleus →	分泌 secrete	加压素（抗利尿激素） Vasopressin (Antidiuretic hormone)
室旁核 Paraventricular nucleus →	分泌 secrete	催产素 Oxytocin
弓状核 Arcuate nucleus →	分泌 secrete	释放抑制激素 Release inhibiting hormone 释放激素 Releasing hormone

图 4-15 垂体
Hypophysis

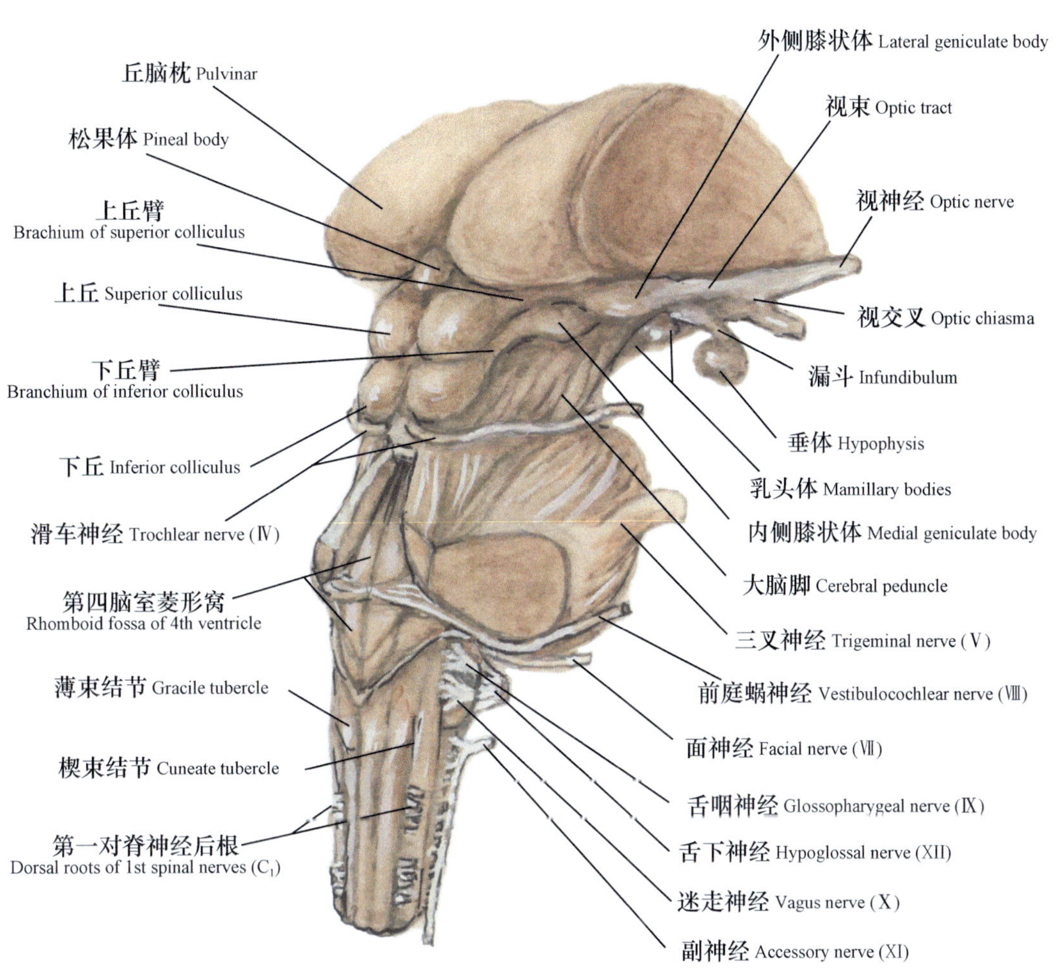

图 4-16 脑干外形
The shape of brain stem

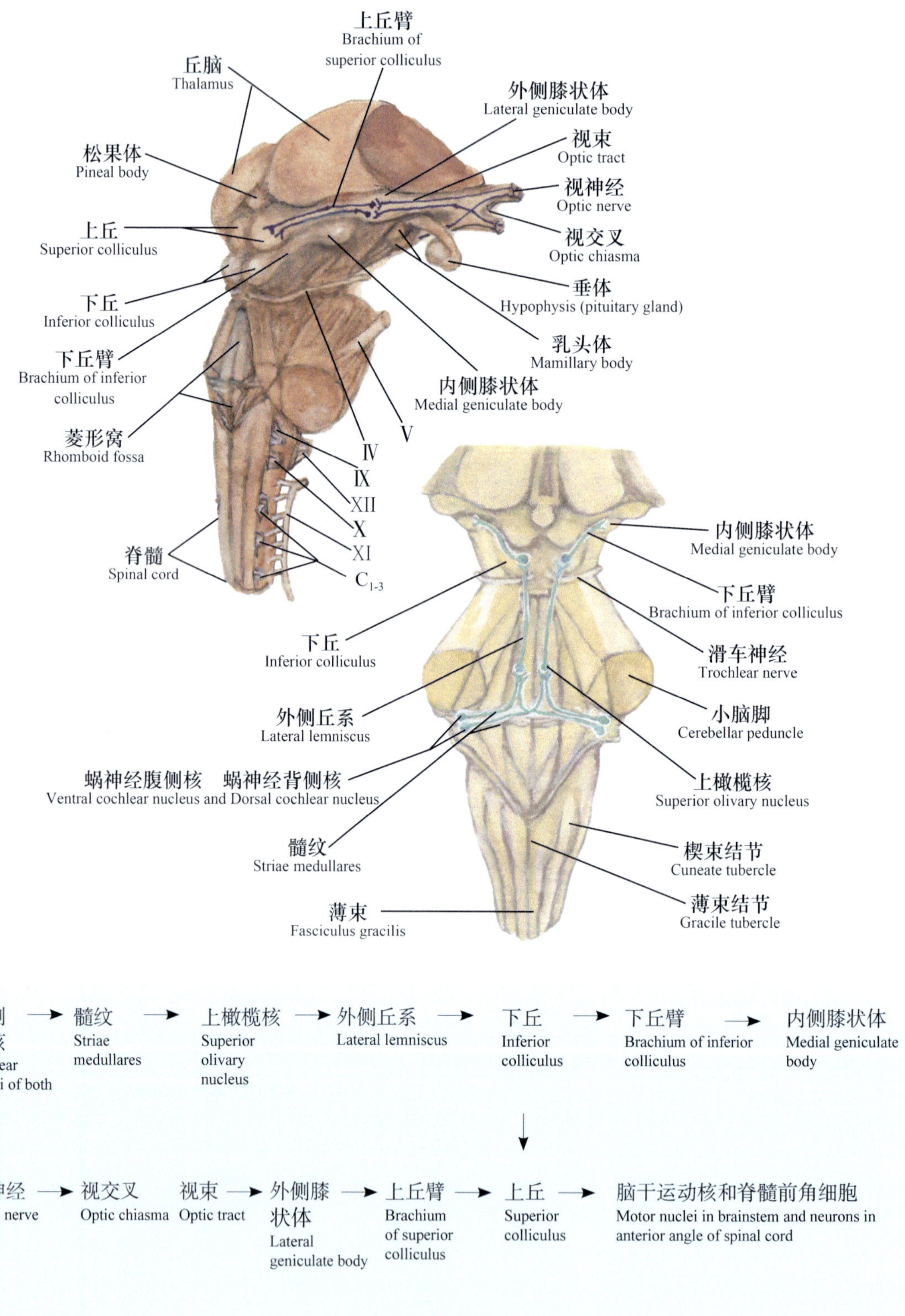

双侧蜗核 Cochear nuclei of both sides → 髓纹 Striae medullares → 上橄榄核 Superior olivary nucleus → 外侧丘系 Lateral lemniscus → 下丘 Inferior colliculus → 下丘臂 Brachium of inferior colliculus → 内侧膝状体 Medial geniculate body

↓

视神经 Optic nerve → 视交叉 Optic chiasma 视束 Optic tract → 外侧膝状体 Lateral geniculate body → 上丘臂 Brachium of superior colliculus → 上丘 Superior colliculus → 脑干运动核和脊髓前角细胞 Motor nuclei in brainstem and neurons in anterior angle of spinal cord

图 4-17 脑干部视听传导
The visual and auditory conduction of brain stem

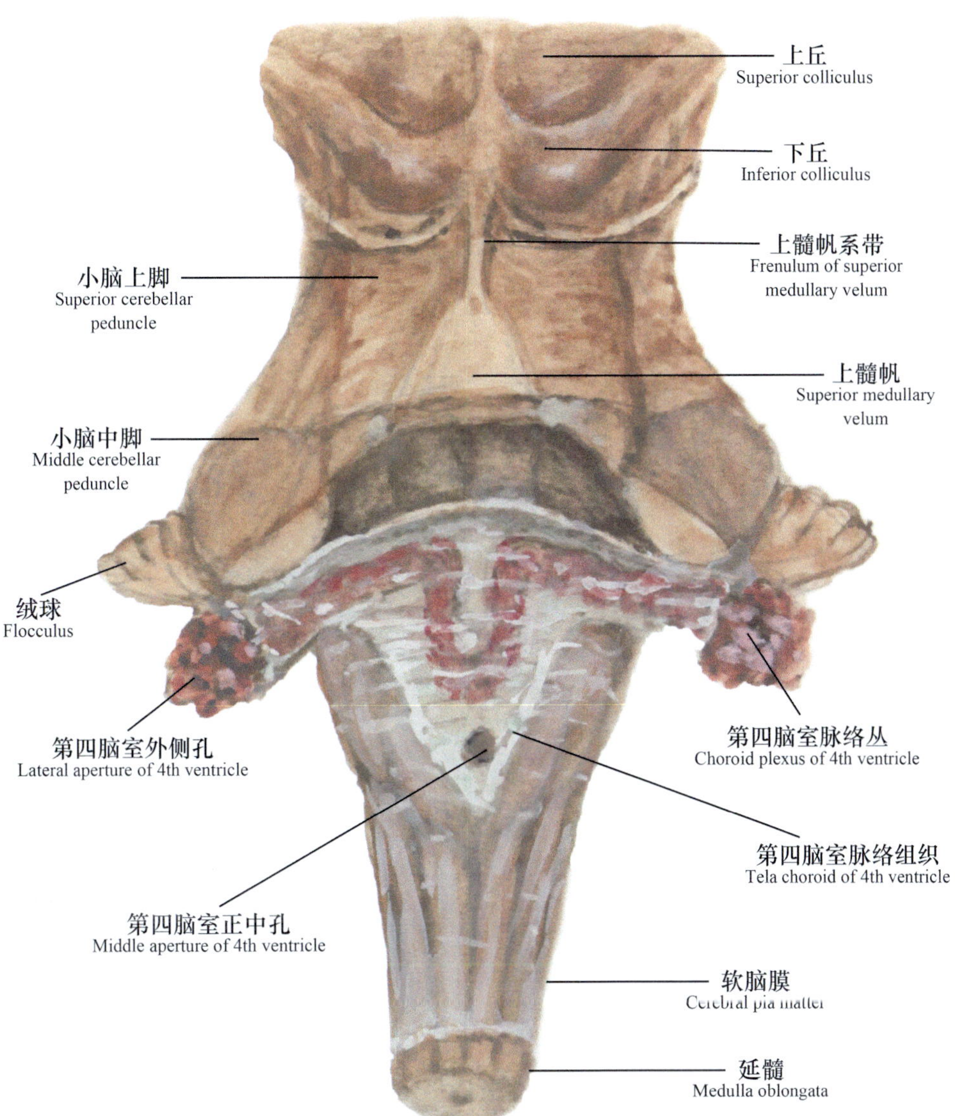

图 4-18 第四脑室脉络组织
Tela choroidea of fourth ventricle

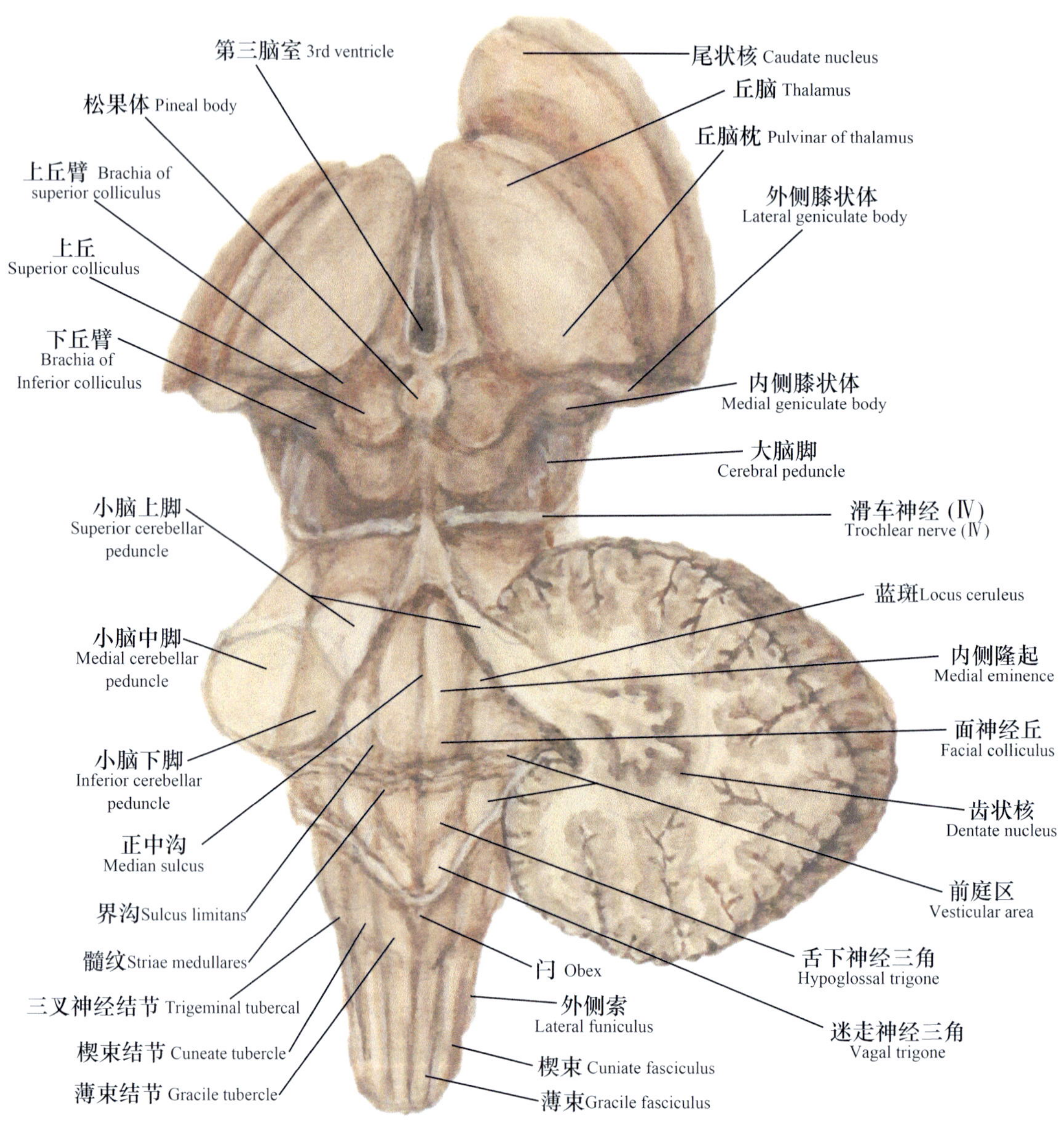

图 4-19 脑干背侧观
Dorsal aspect of the brain stem

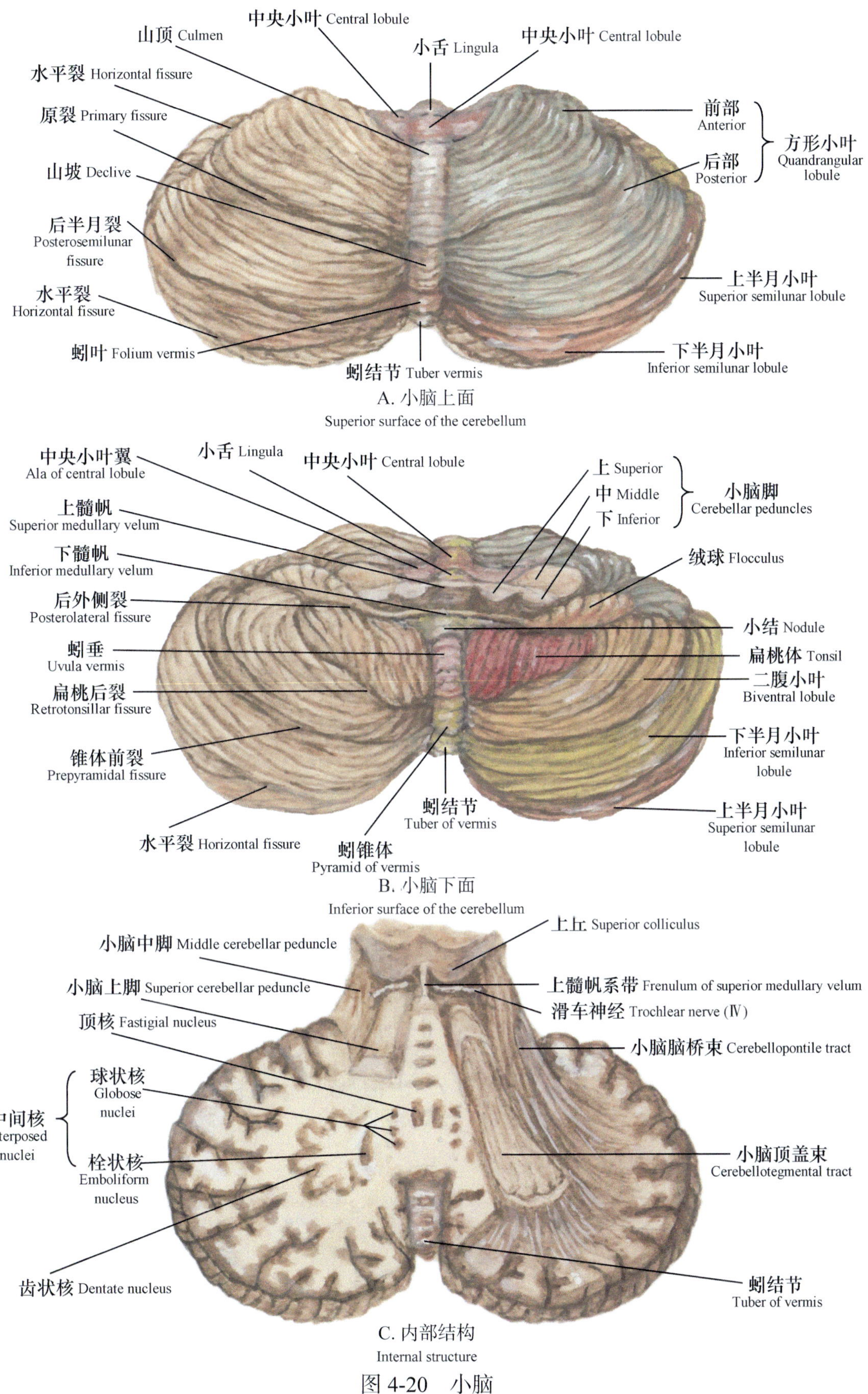

图 4-20 小脑
The cerebellum

小脑分叶表
A table showing the morphological subdivision of the cerebellum

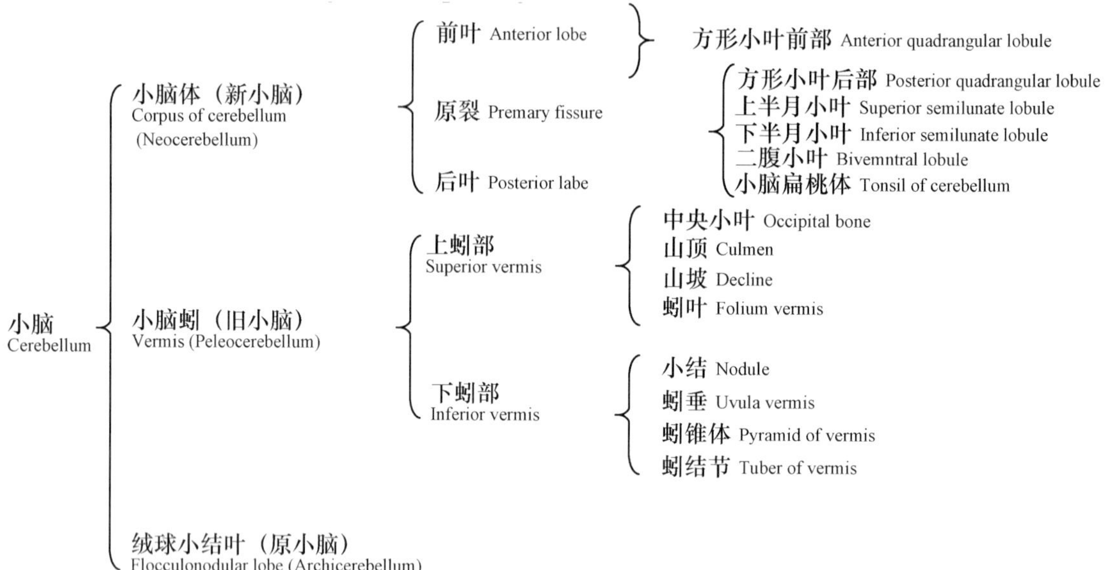

小脑出入纤维表
A table show the output and input connexion of fiber of the cerebellum

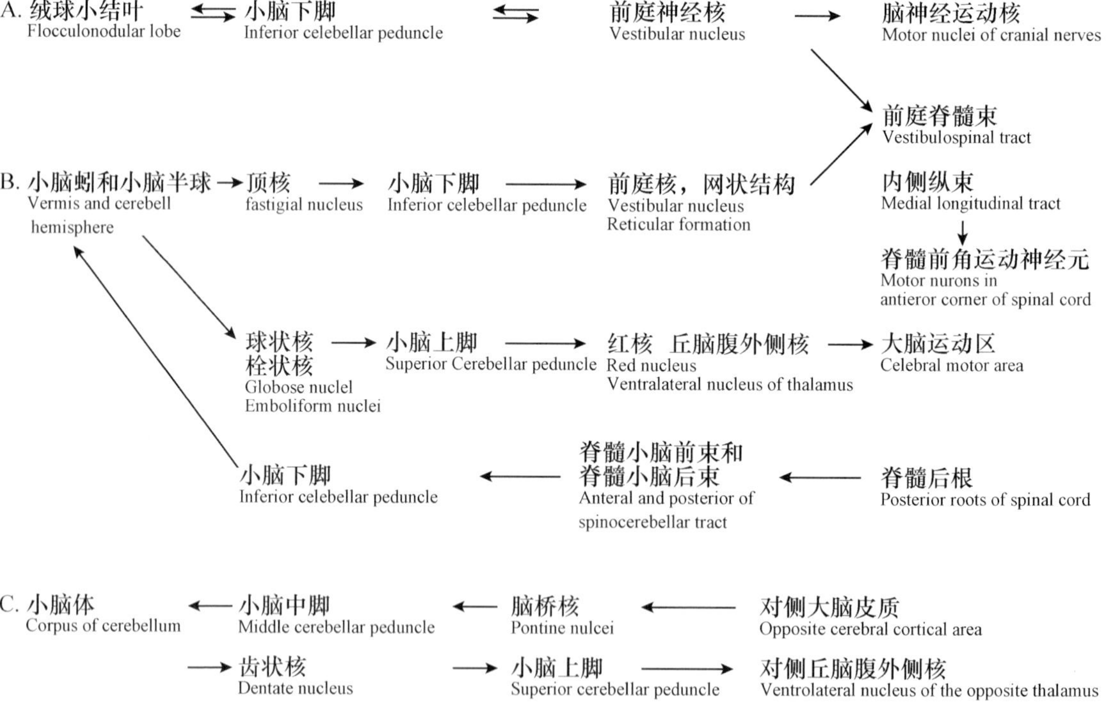

图 4-21 小脑内部结构
Internal structure of the cerebellum

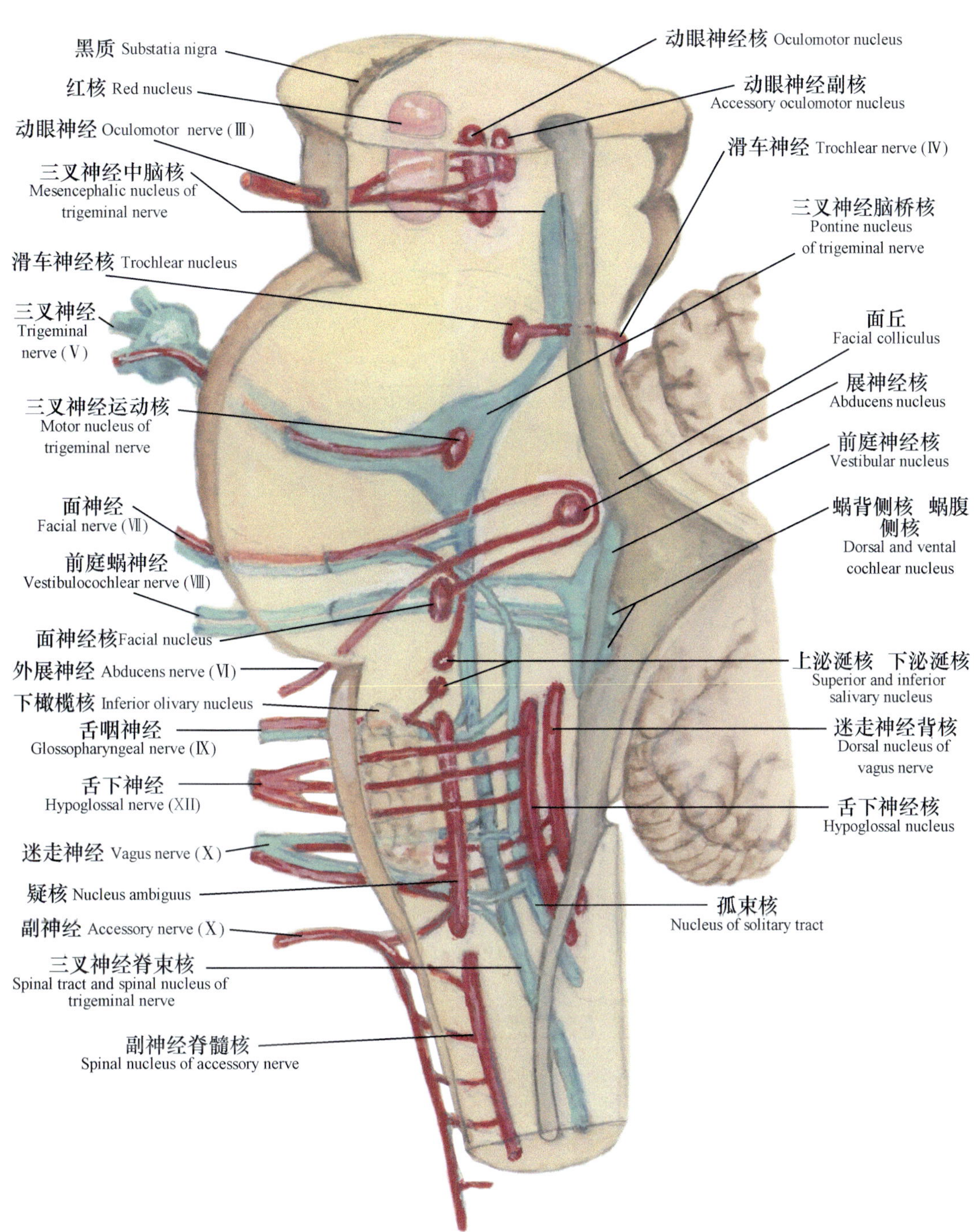

图 4-22 脑干神经核（1）
Nucleus of brain stem (1)

A. 副交感神经核 Parasympathetic nuclei

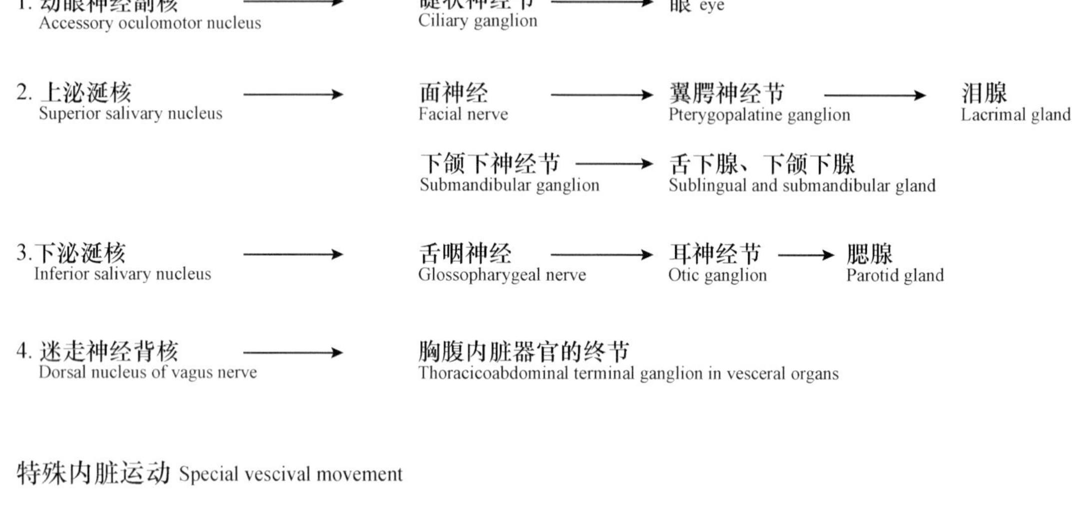

B. 特殊内脏运动 Special vescival movement

C. 味觉传导 Gustatory(taste)transmission

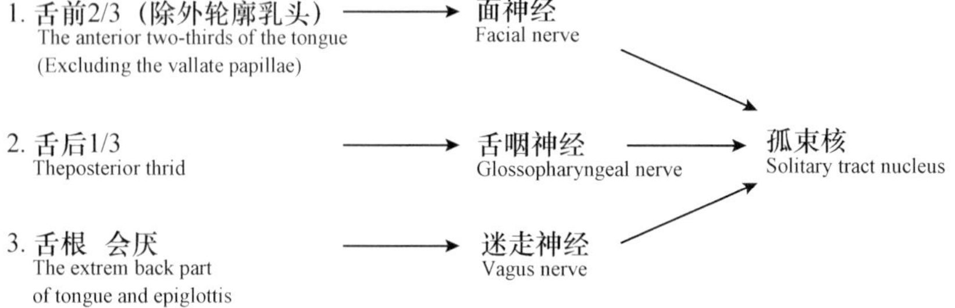

图 4-23 脑干神经核（2）
Nucleus of brain stem (2)

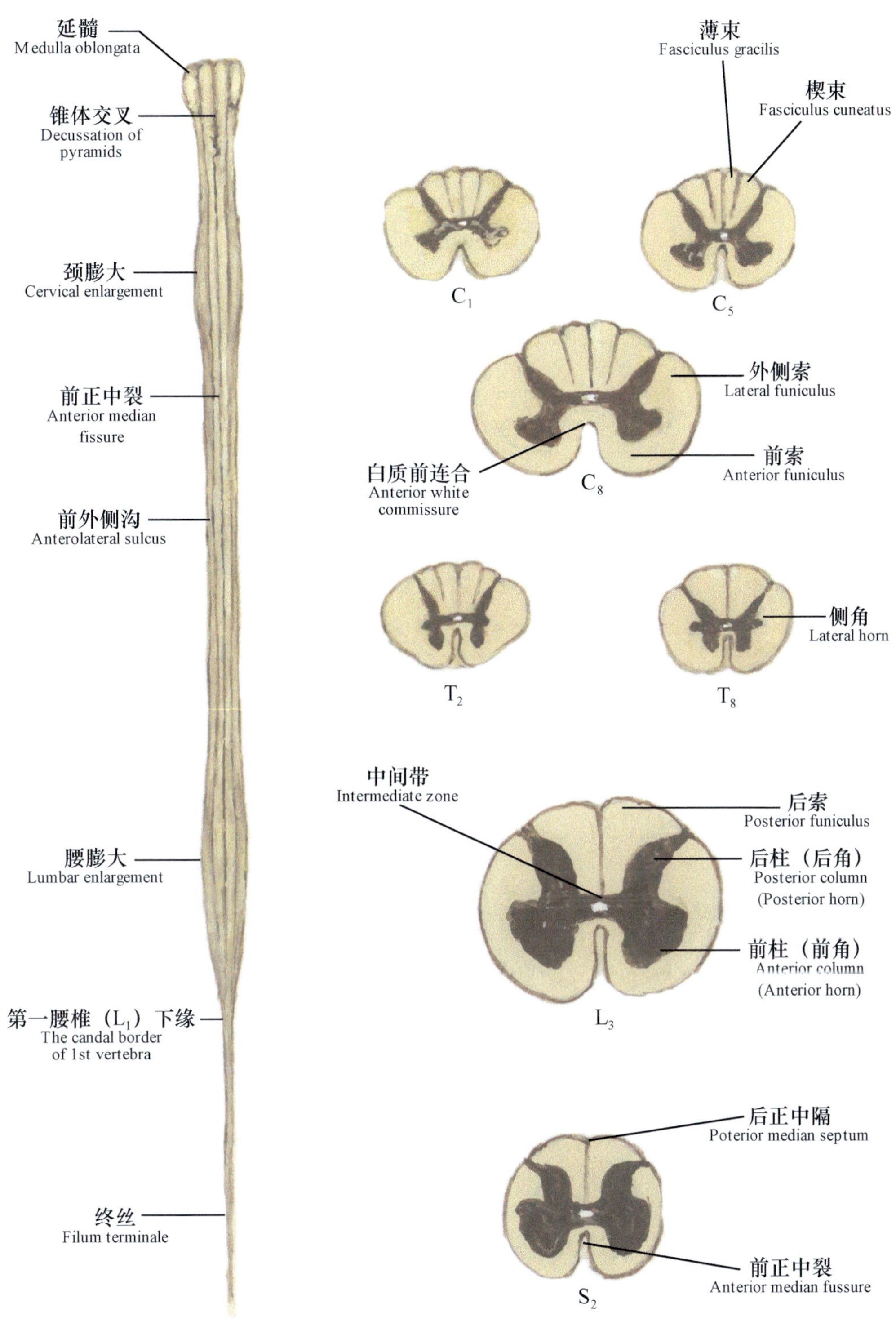

图 4-24 脊髓各段断面示意图

Diagrams of transverse sections through the spinal cord at representative levels

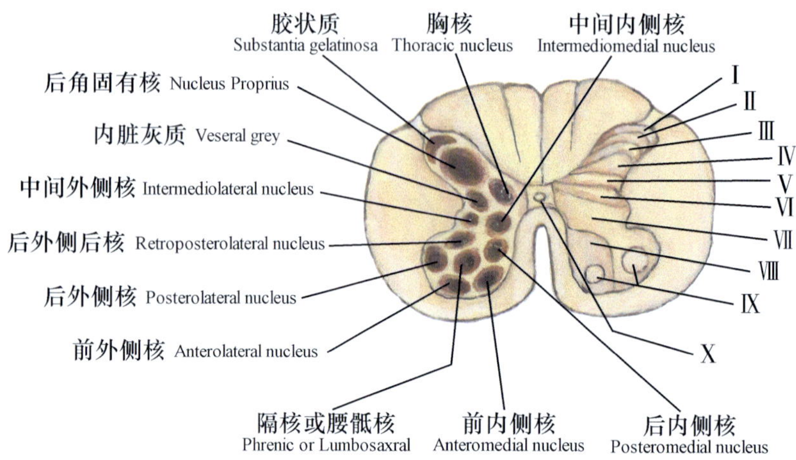

A. 脊髓灰质主要核团和 Rexed 分层模式图

The main nuclei of gray matter in spinal cord and the laminar ideograph according to rexed

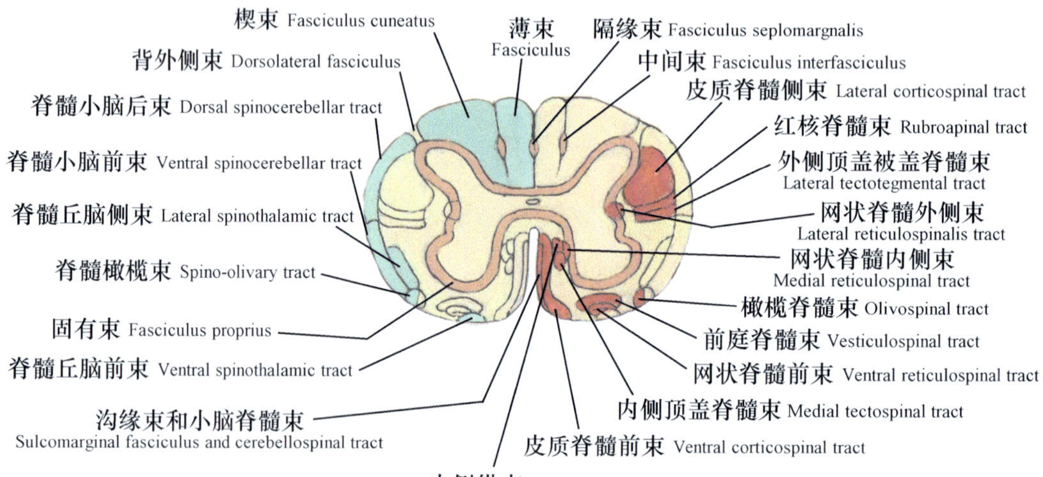

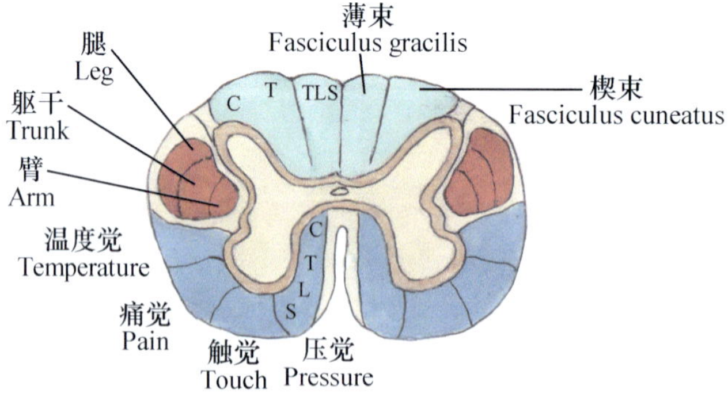

B. 脊髓白质神经纤维束

Neura fasciculus of white matter in spinal cord

图 4-25 脊髓

The spinal cord

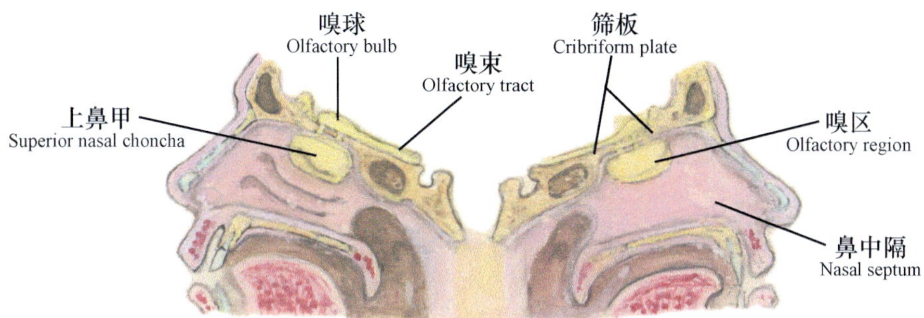

A. 右侧鼻腔的嗅区
The olfactory area in the right nasal cavity

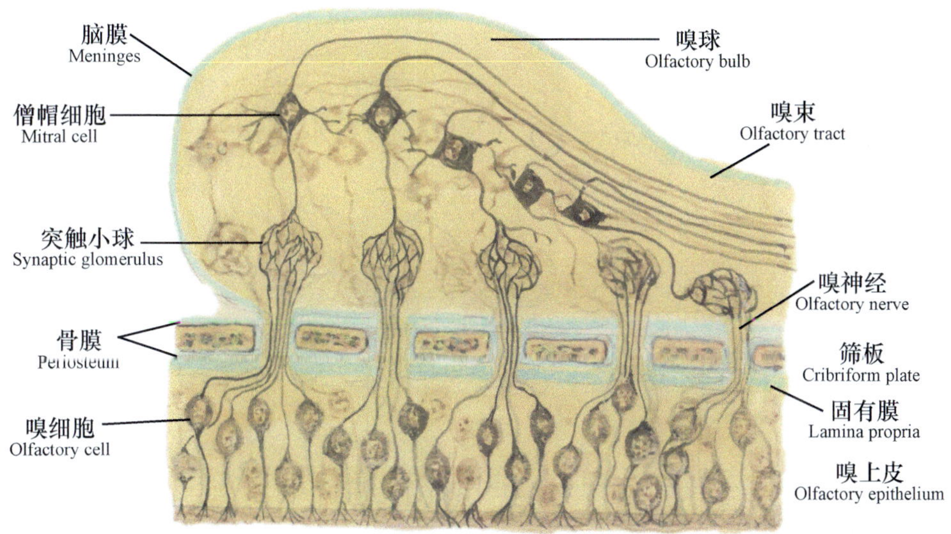

B. 嗅神经与嗅球的传导
Transmiting between the olfactory nerves and the olfactory bulb

图 4-26 嗅觉的传导
Olfactory transmission

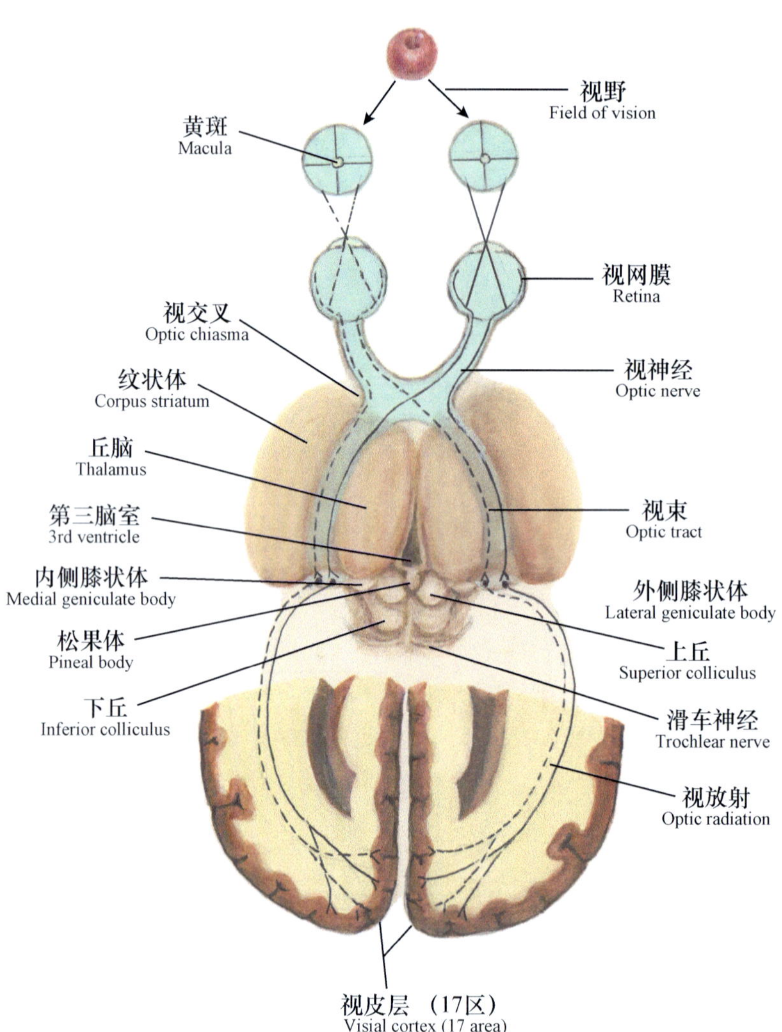

图 4-27 视神经示意图（传导图）
Schema for the optic nerve (Visual pathway)

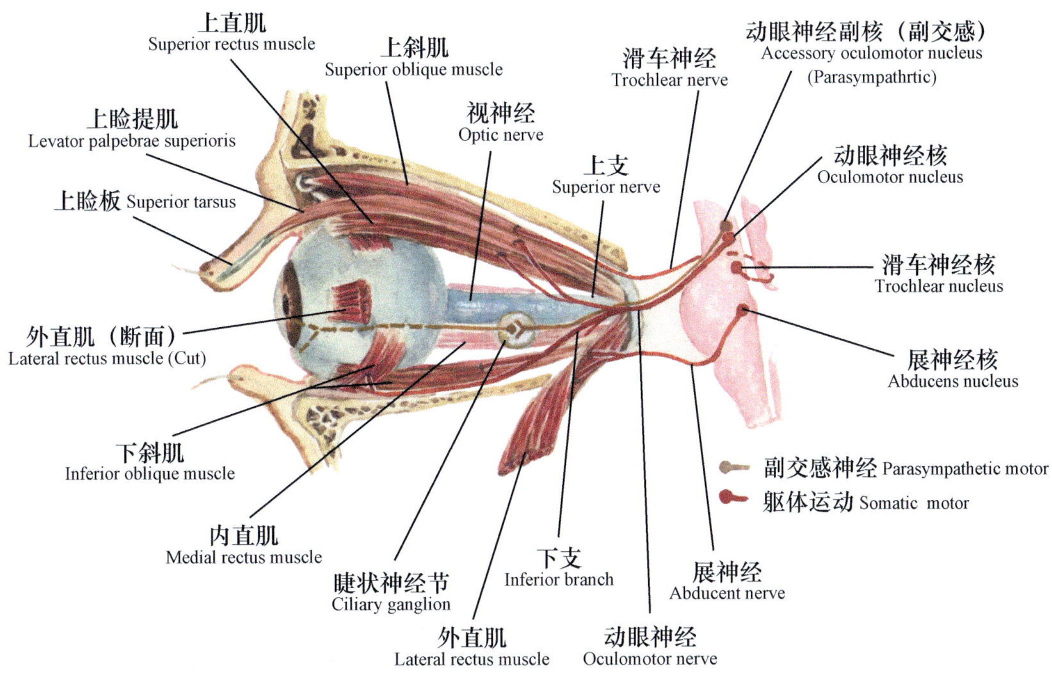

A. Ⅱ Ⅲ Ⅳ Ⅵ脑神经示意图
A diagram showing the Ⅱ, Ⅲ, Ⅳ, Ⅵ cranial nerves

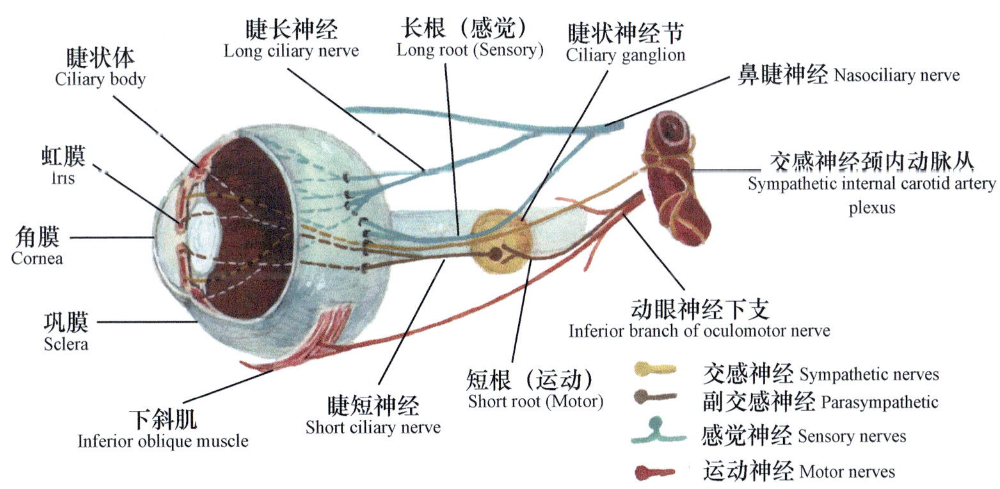

B. 睫状神经节示意图
A diagram showing the ciliary ganglion

图 4-28 眶内神经分布
The distribution of nerve in orbit

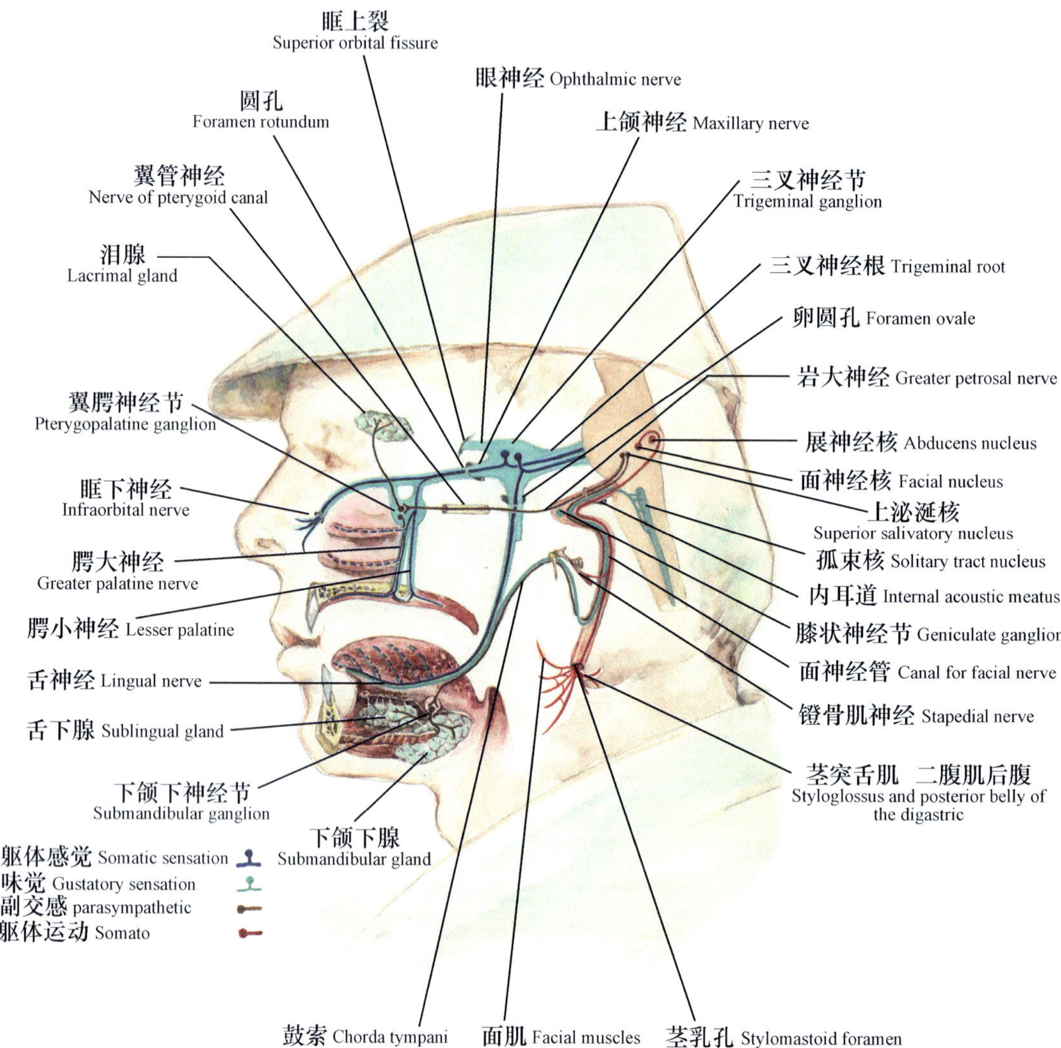

图 4-29 面神经及三叉神经分支分布示意图

A diagram showing the branches displayed of the facial nerve and trigeminal nerve

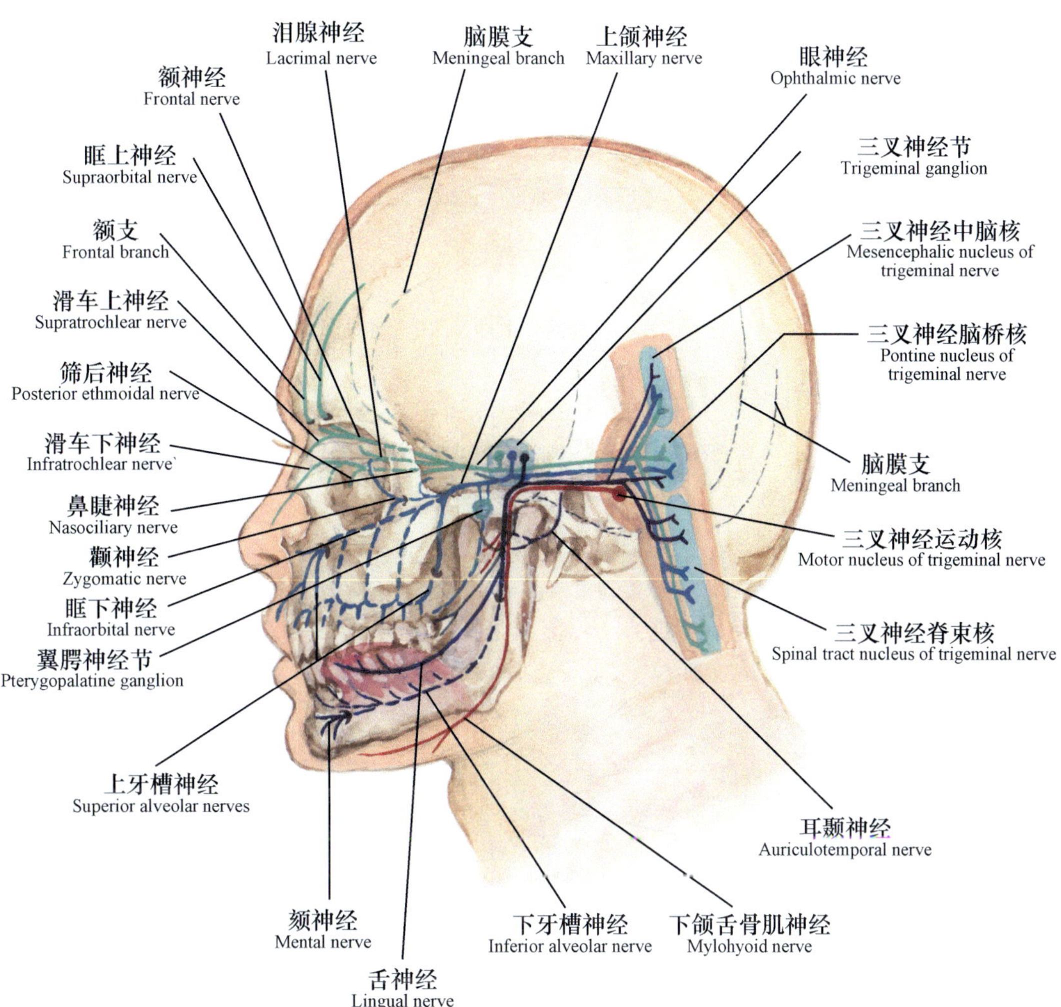

图 4-30 三叉神经运动根分布示意图
A diagram showing the supply of the motor root of the trigeminal nerve

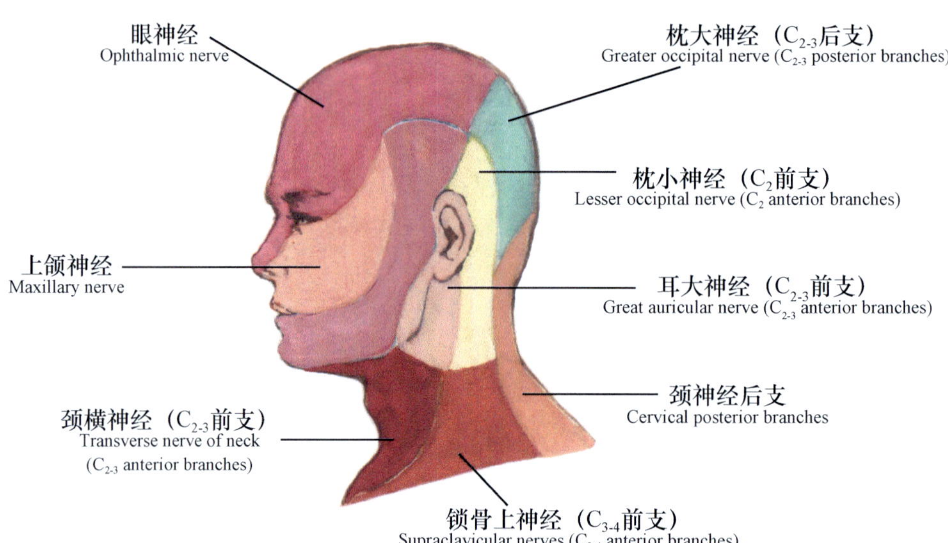

A. 头颈皮神经分布示意图

A diagram showing the cutanous nerve supply of face and neck

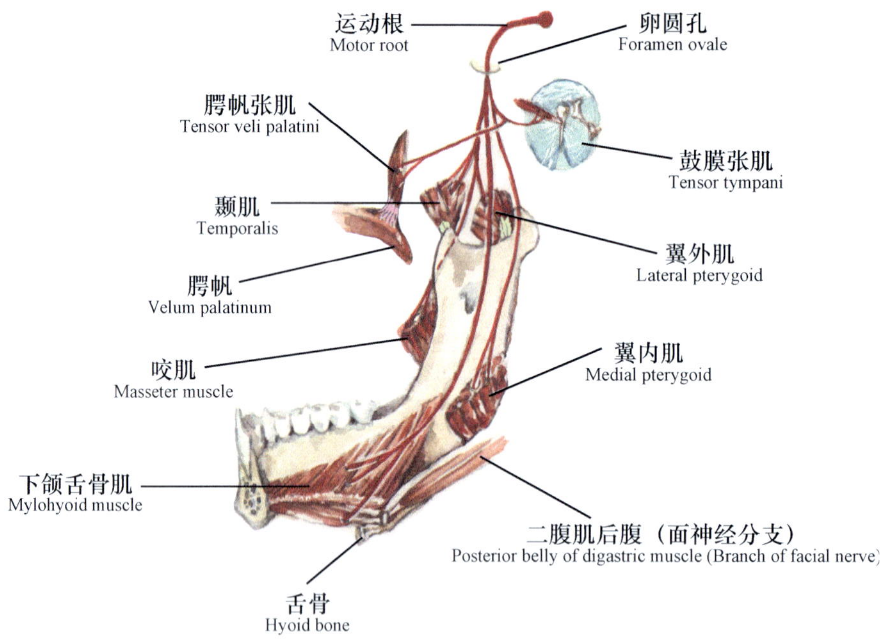

B. 三叉神经分布示意图

A diagram showing the supply of the trigeminal nerve

图 4-31 三叉神经的皮支和肌支

Cutaneous and muscularis branches of trigeminal nerve

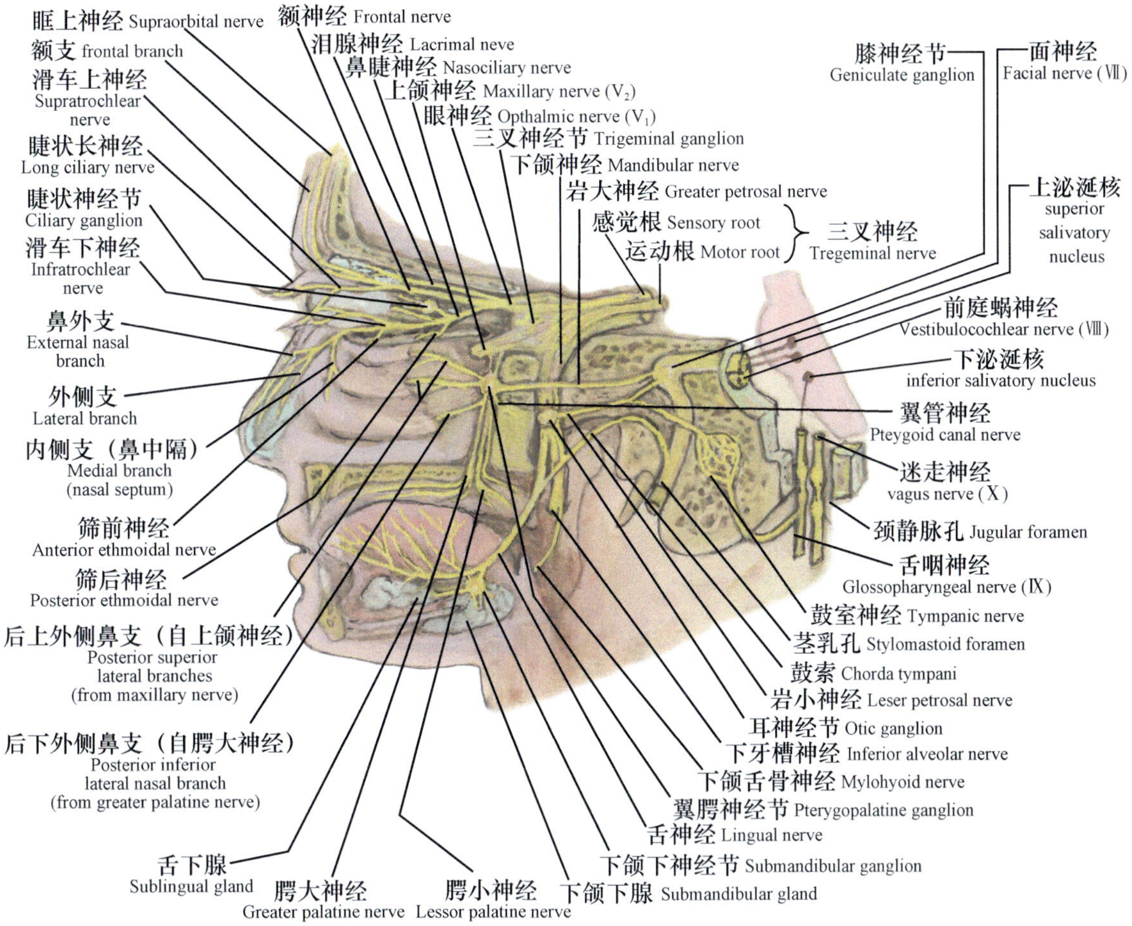

眶上神经 Supraorbital nerve
额支 frontal branch
滑车上神经 Supratrochlear nerve
睫状长神经 Long ciliary nerve
睫状神经节 Ciliary ganglion
滑车下神经 Infratrochlear nerve
鼻外支 External nasal branch
外侧支 Lateral branch
内侧支（鼻中隔） Medial branch (nasal septum)
筛前神经 Anterior ethmoidal nerve
筛后神经 Posterior ethmoidal nerve
后上外侧鼻支（自上颌神经） Posterior superior lateral branches (from maxillary nerve)
后下外侧鼻支（自腭大神经） Posterior inferior lateral nasal branch (from greater palatine nerve)
舌下腺 Sublingual gland
腭大神经 Greater palatine nerve
腭小神经 Lessor palatine nerve
额神经 Frontal nerve
泪腺神经 Lacrimal neve
鼻睫神经 Nasociliary nerve
上颌神经 Maxillary nerve (V_2)
眼神经 Opthalmic nerve (V_1)
三叉神经节 Trigeminal ganglion
下颌神经 Mandibular nerve
岩大神经 Greater petrosal nerve
感觉根 Sensory root
运动根 Motor root
三叉神经 Tregeminal nerve
膝神经节 Geniculate ganglion
面神经 Facial nerve (Ⅶ)
上泌涎核 superior salivatory nucleus
前庭蜗神经 Vestibulocochlear nerve (Ⅷ)
下泌涎核 inferior salivatory nucleus
翼管神经 Pteygoid canal nerve
迷走神经 vagus nerve (Ⅹ)
颈静脉孔 Jugular foramen
舌咽神经 Glossopharyngeal nerve (Ⅸ)
鼓室神经 Tympanic nerve
茎乳孔 Stylomastoid foramen
鼓索 Chorda tympani
岩小神经 Leser petrosal nerve
耳神经节 Otic ganglion
下牙槽神经 Inferior alveolar nerve
下颌舌骨神经 Mylohyoid nerve
翼腭神经节 Pterygopalatine ganglion
舌神经 Lingual nerve
下颌下神经节 Submandibular ganglion
下颌下腺 Submandibular gland

A. 三叉神经相关的神经节模式图
Schema for ganglions connected with the trigeminal nerve

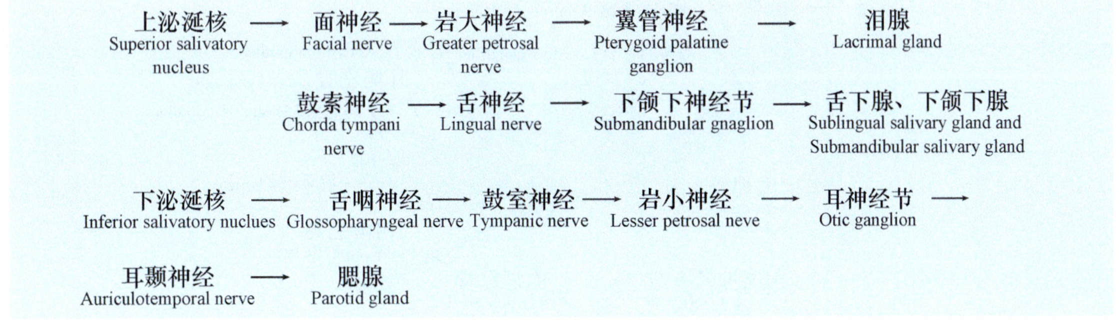

B. 三叉神经副交感神经节的行程表
A diagram showing the connection of parasymathetic ganglions of the trigeminal nerve

图 4-32 三叉神经
The trigeminal nerve

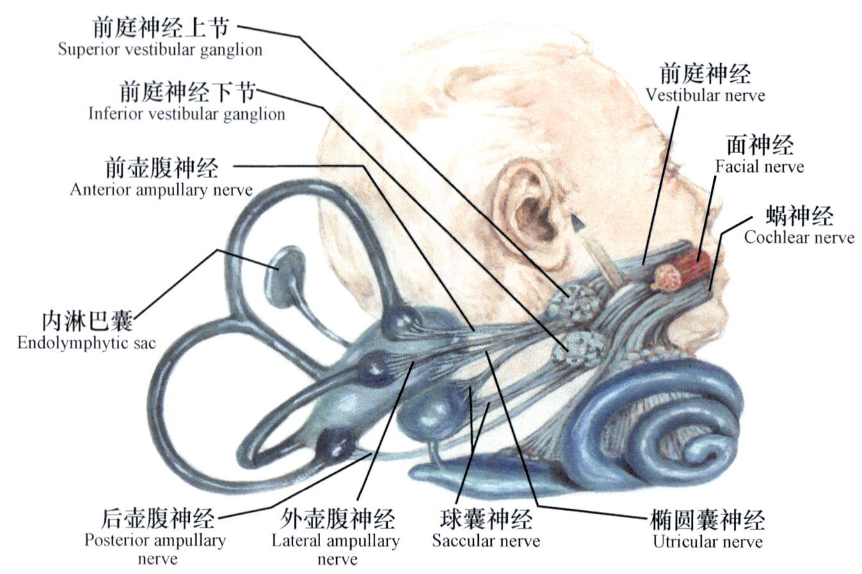

A. 外侧观
Lateral aspect

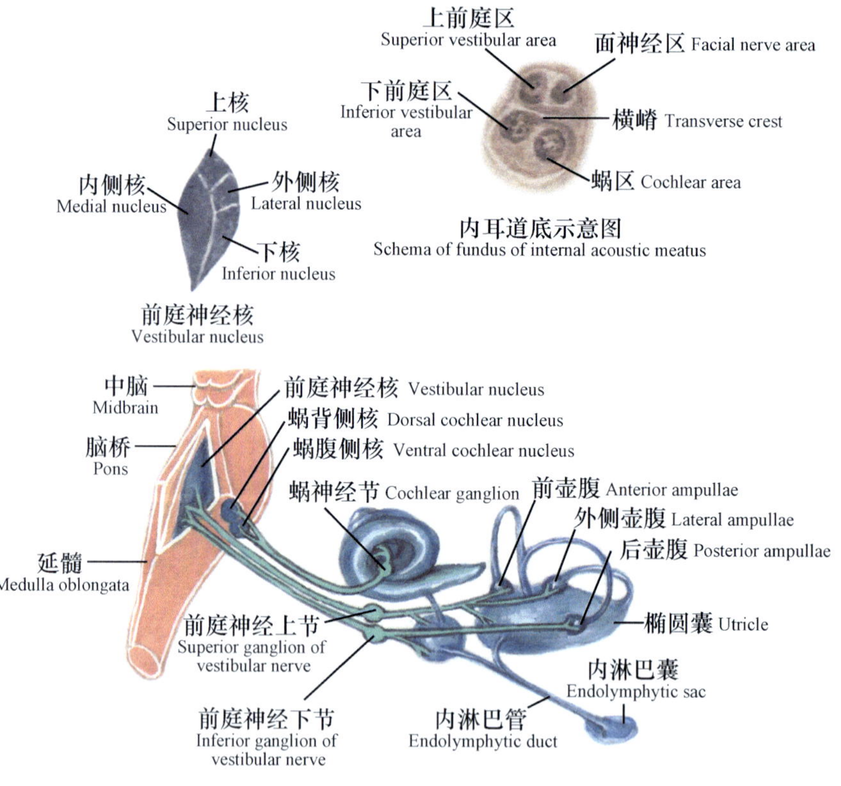

B. 内侧观
Medial aspect

图 4-33 前庭蜗神经示意图
A Scheme of the vestibulocochlear nerve

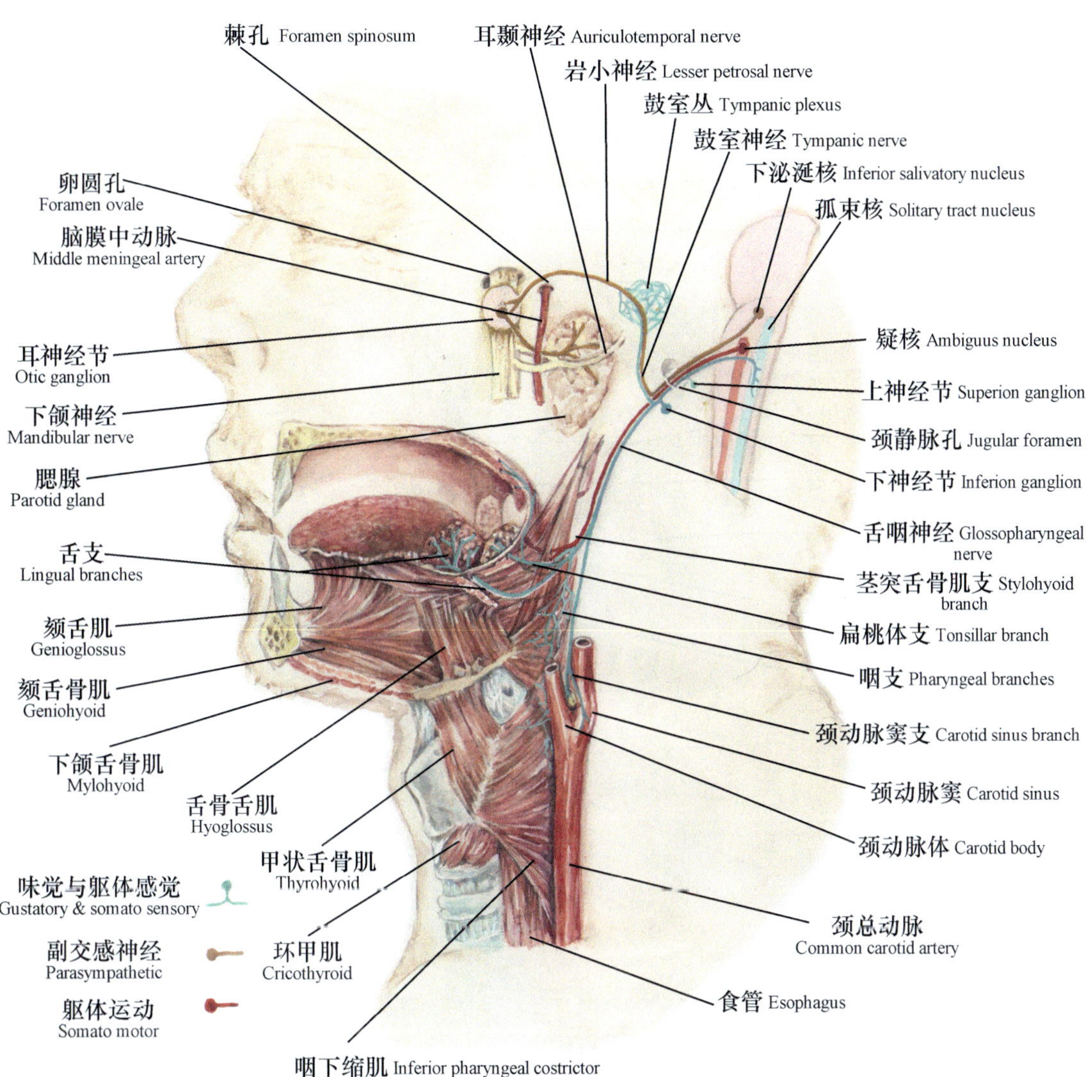

图 4-34 舌咽神经示意图

A diagram showing the glossopharyngeal nerve

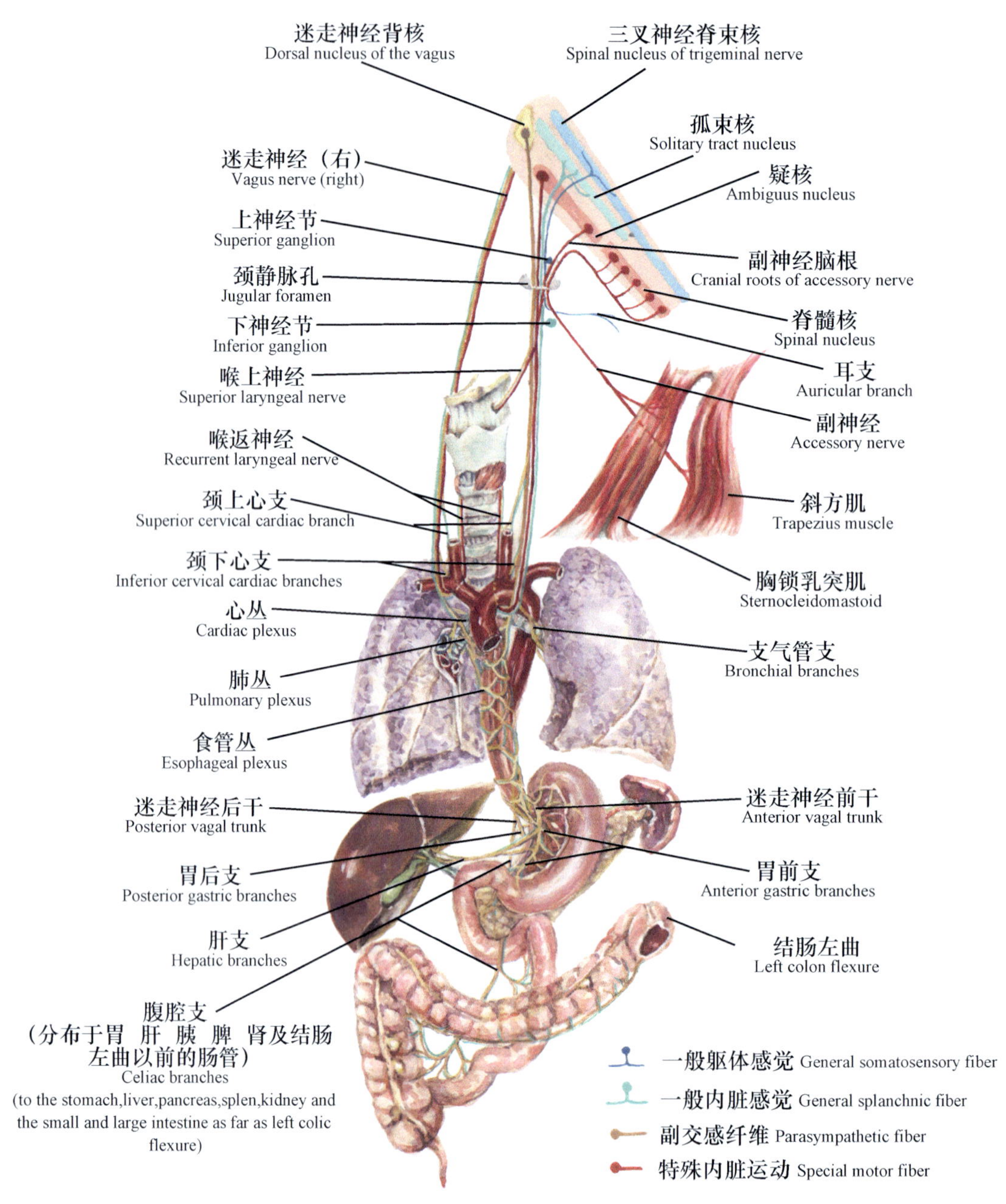

图 4-35 迷走神经和副神经示意图
A diagram of vagus and accessory nerves

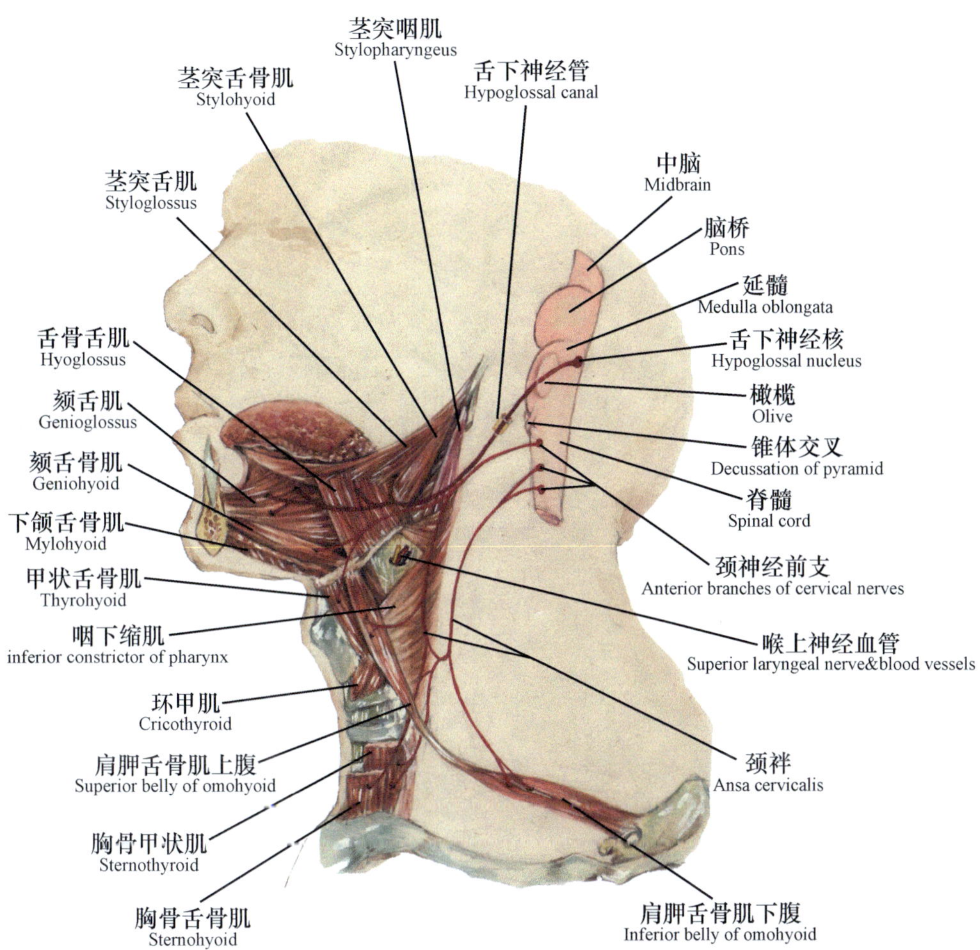

图 4-36　舌下神经示意图
A diagram of hypoglossal nerve

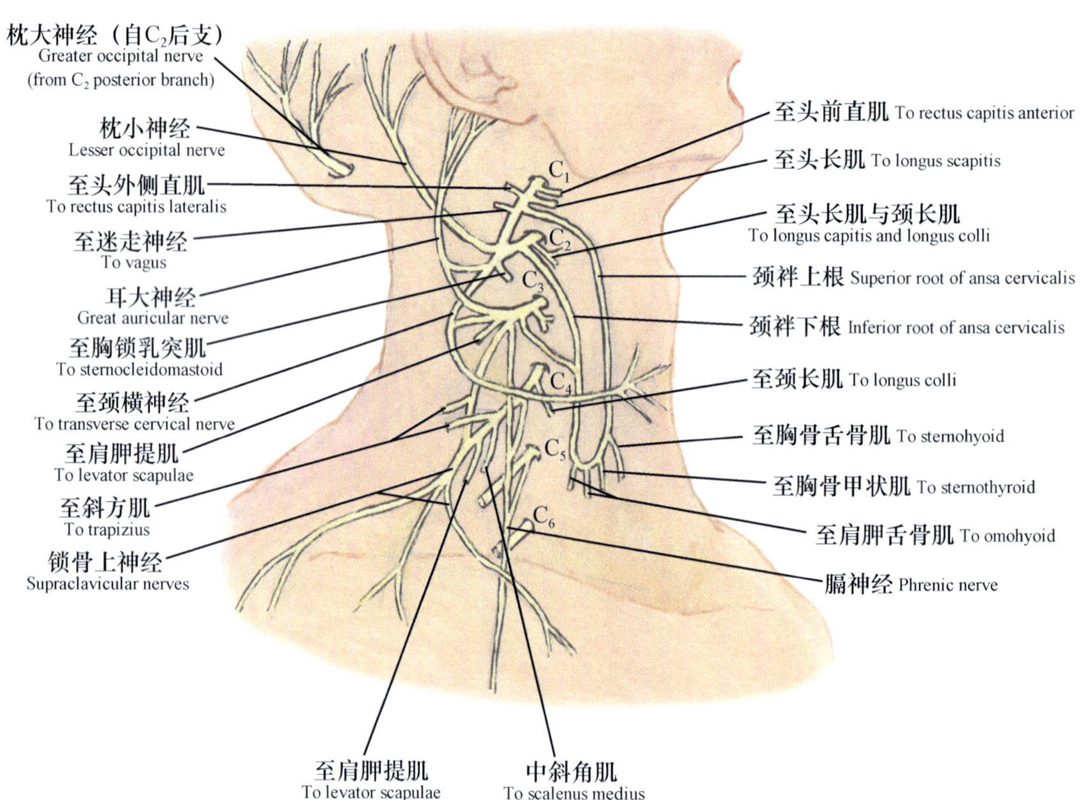

图 4-37　颈丛
The cervical plexus

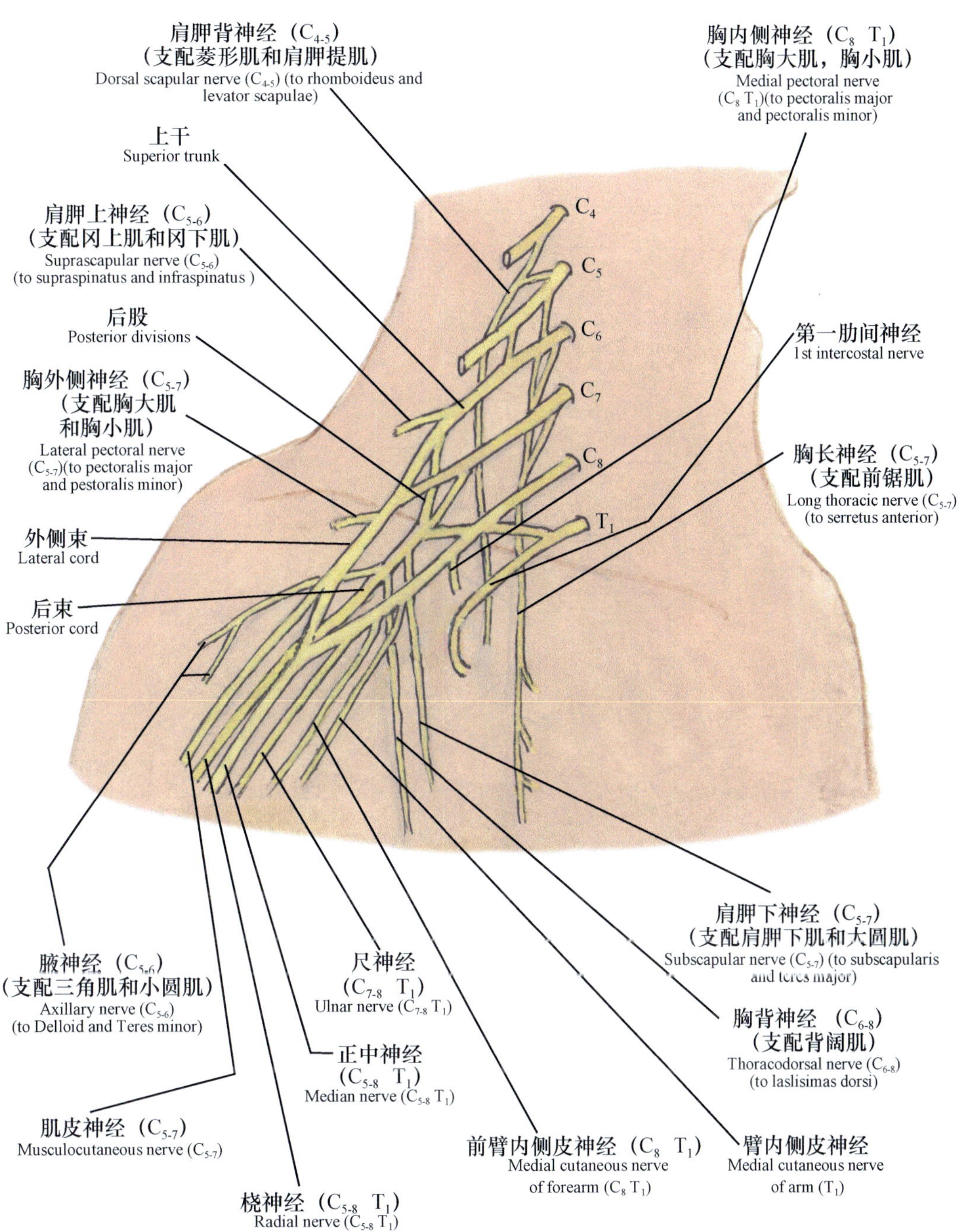

图 4-38 臂丛示意图

A schema showing the brachial plexus

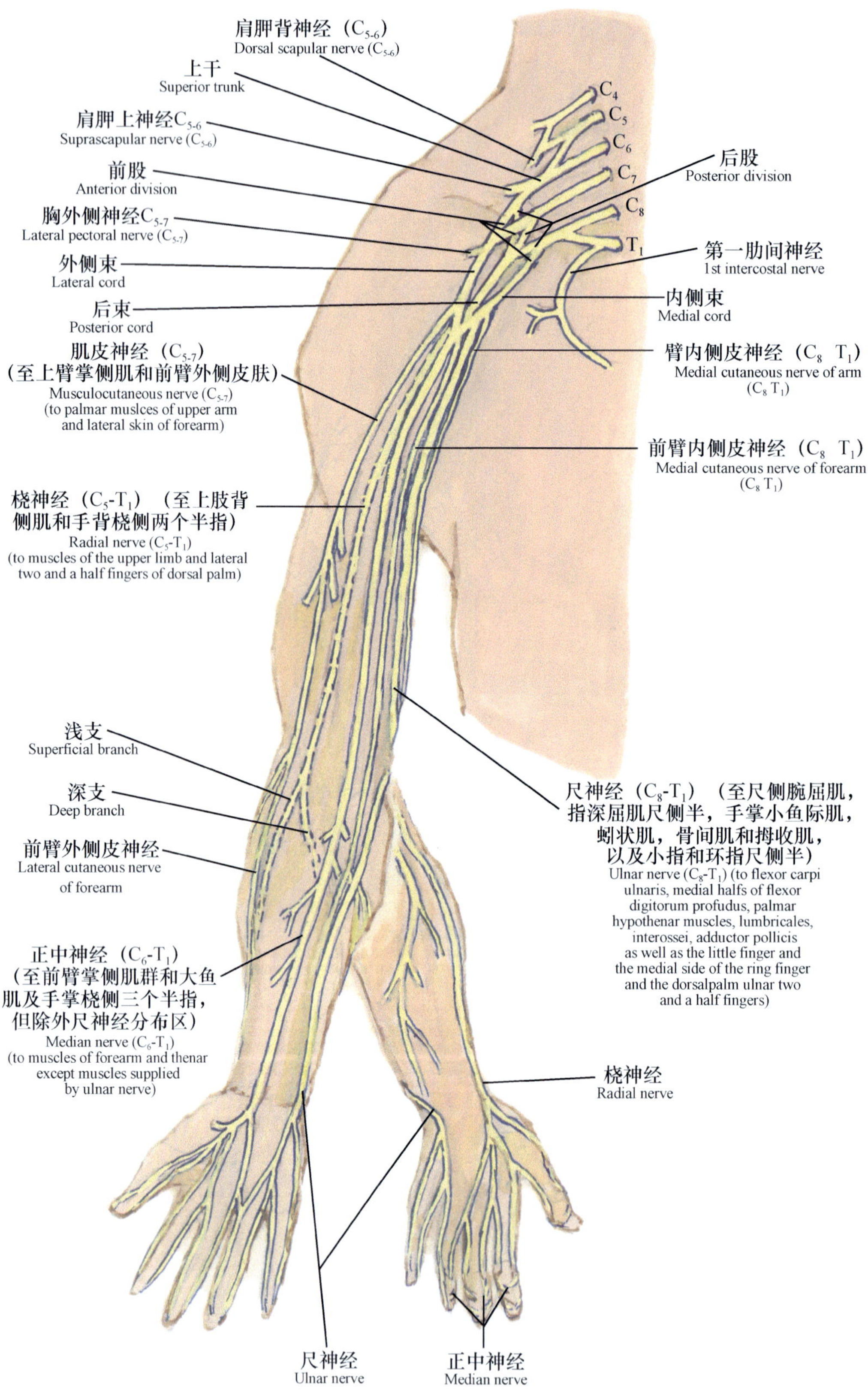

图 4-39 上肢神经示意图

A scheme showing the nerves of upper limb

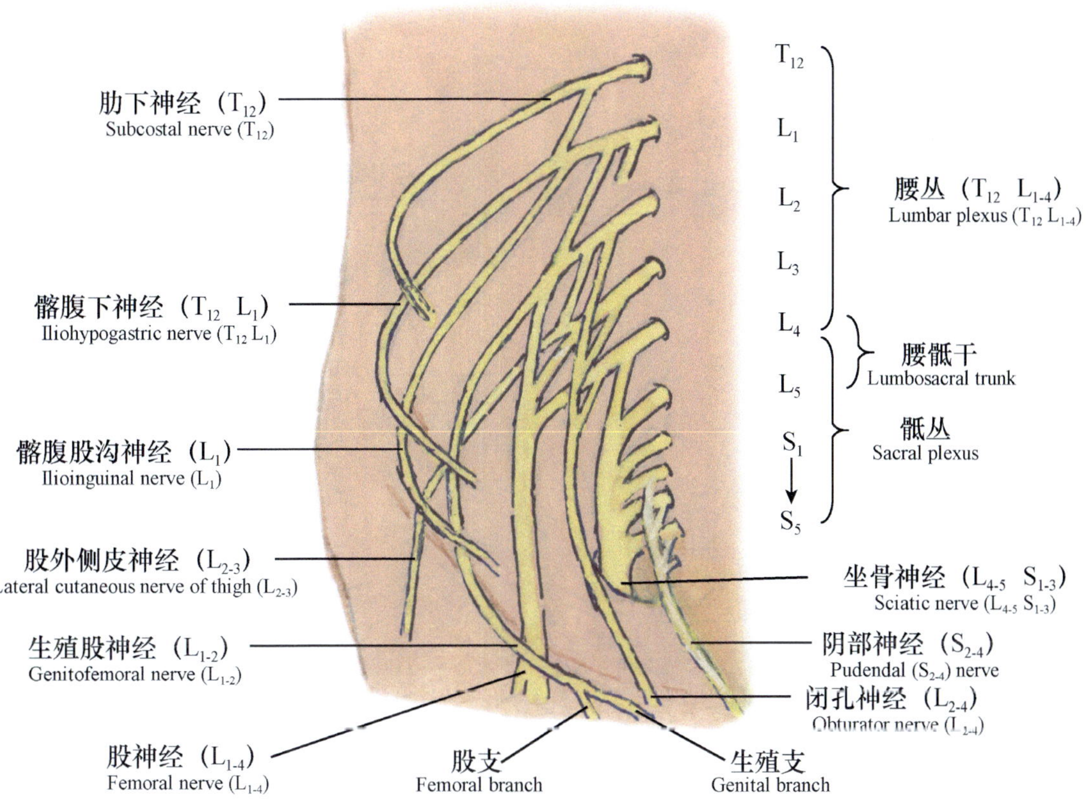

图 4-40 腰丛和骶丛示意图
A schema showing the lumbar and sacral plexus

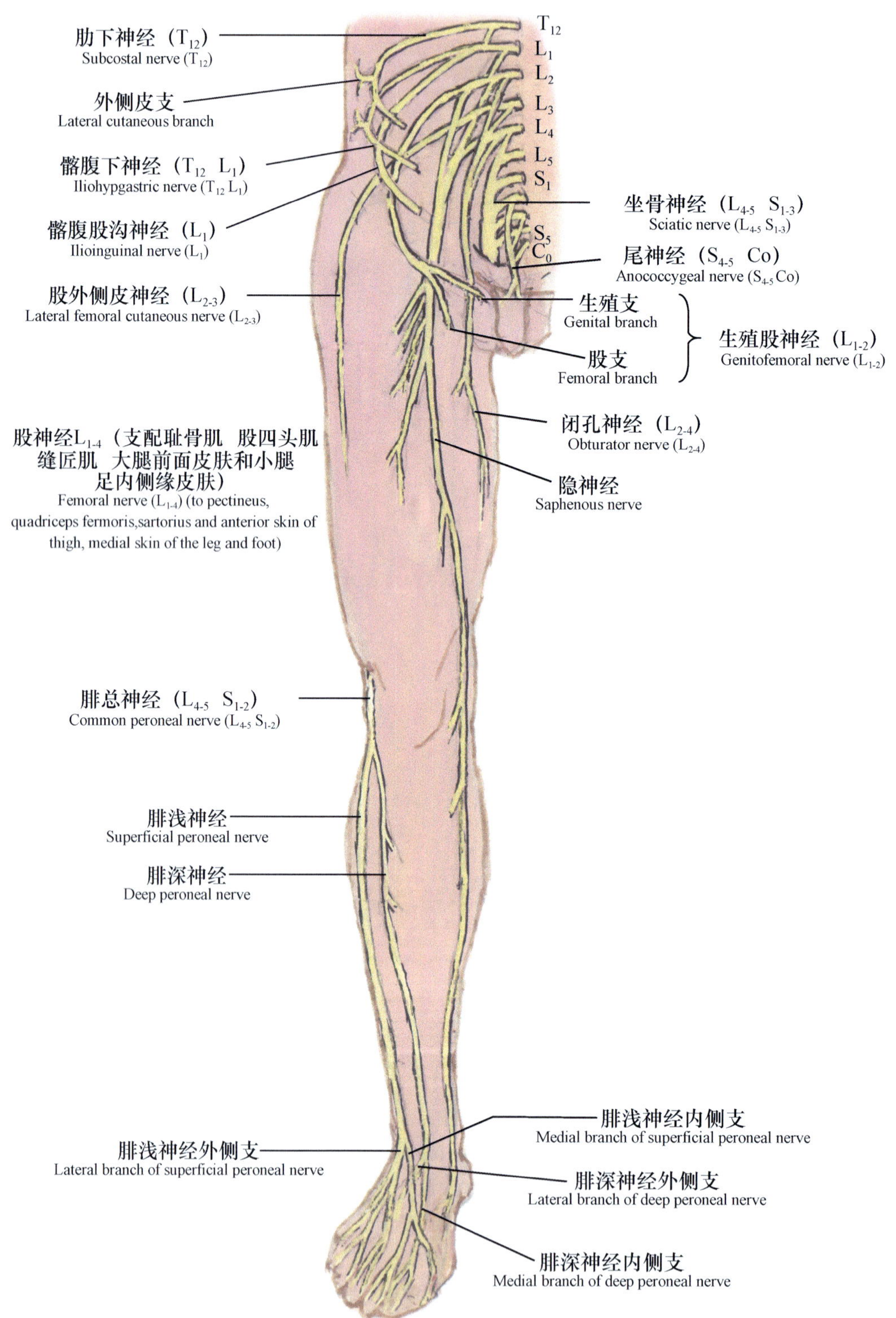

图 4-41 右下肢前面神经分布示意图

A scheme showing the anterior aspect of the nervous distribution of the right lower limb

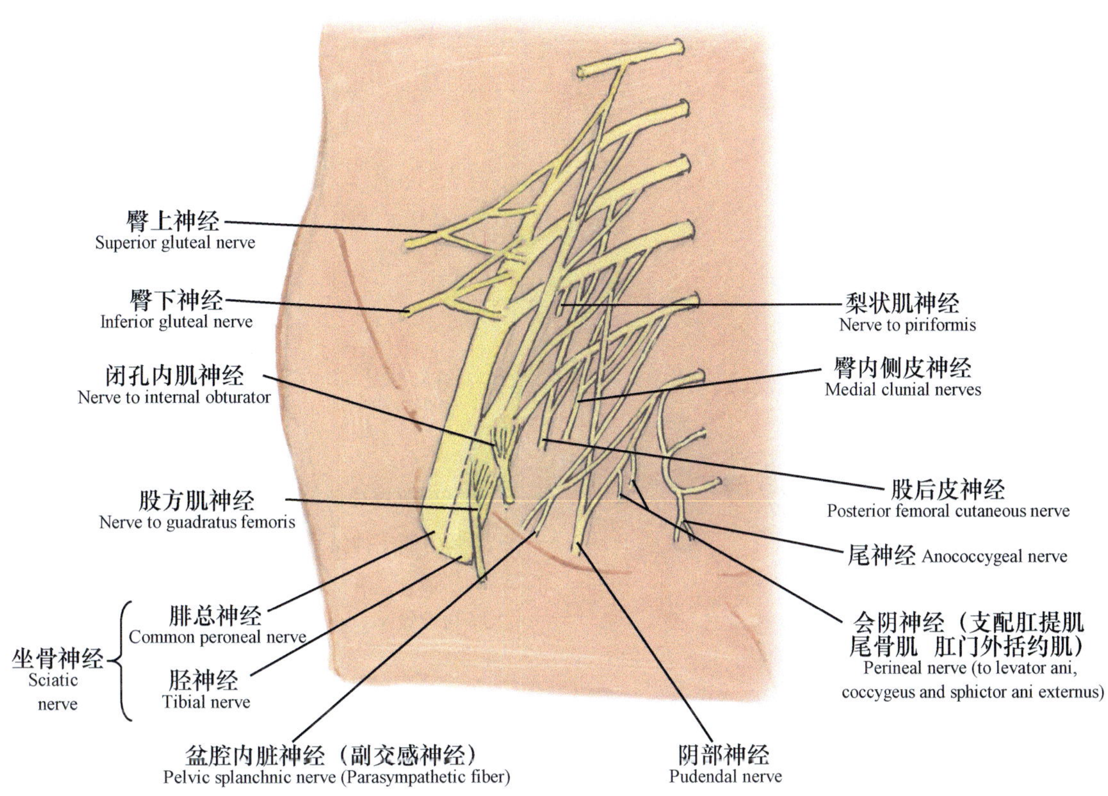

图 4-42 骶丛组成及分支示意图
A scheme showing composition and branches of the sacral plexus

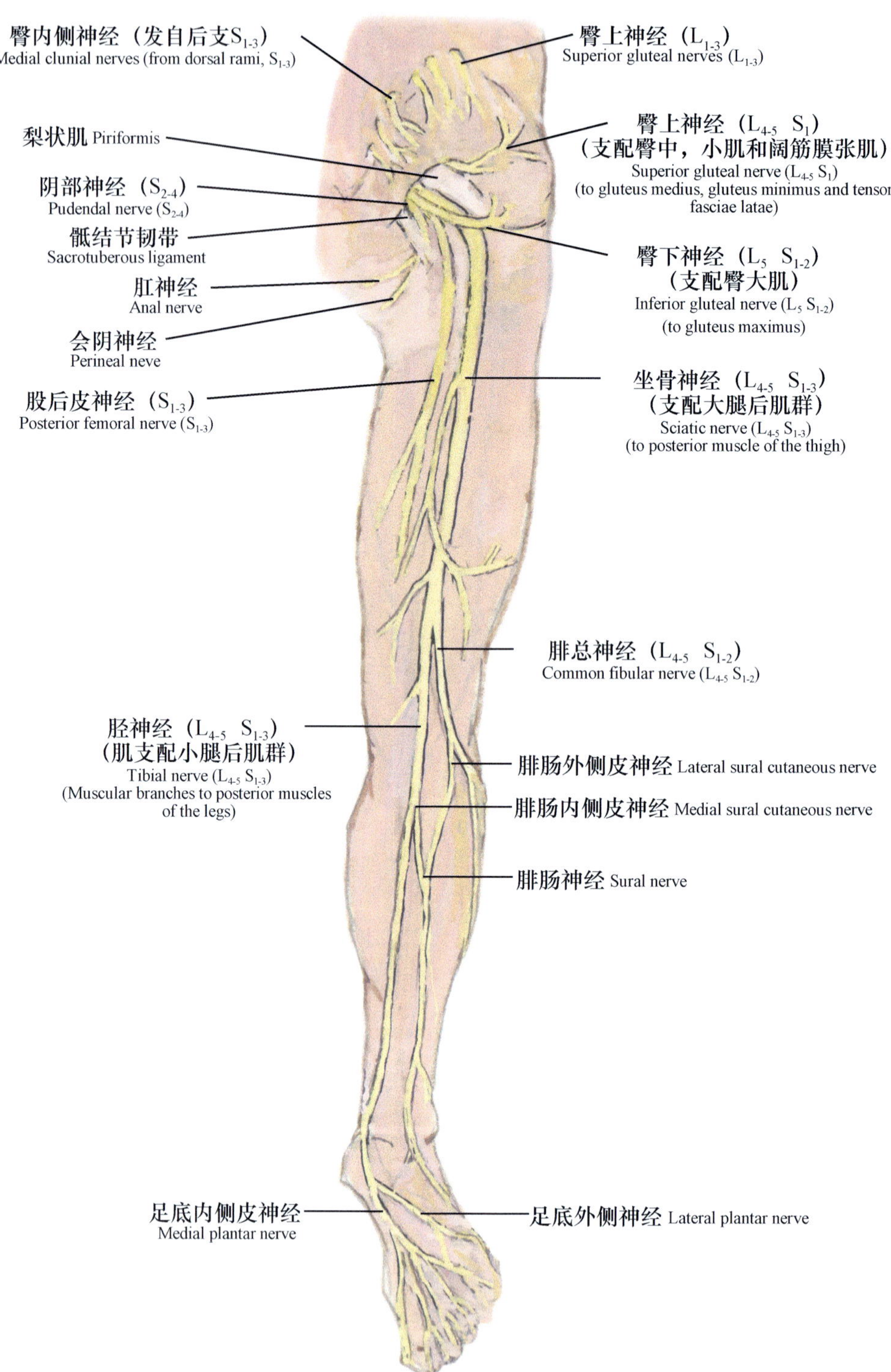

图 4-43　下肢背侧神经分布示意图

A scheme showing the nervous distribution of the dorsal aspect of the right lower limb

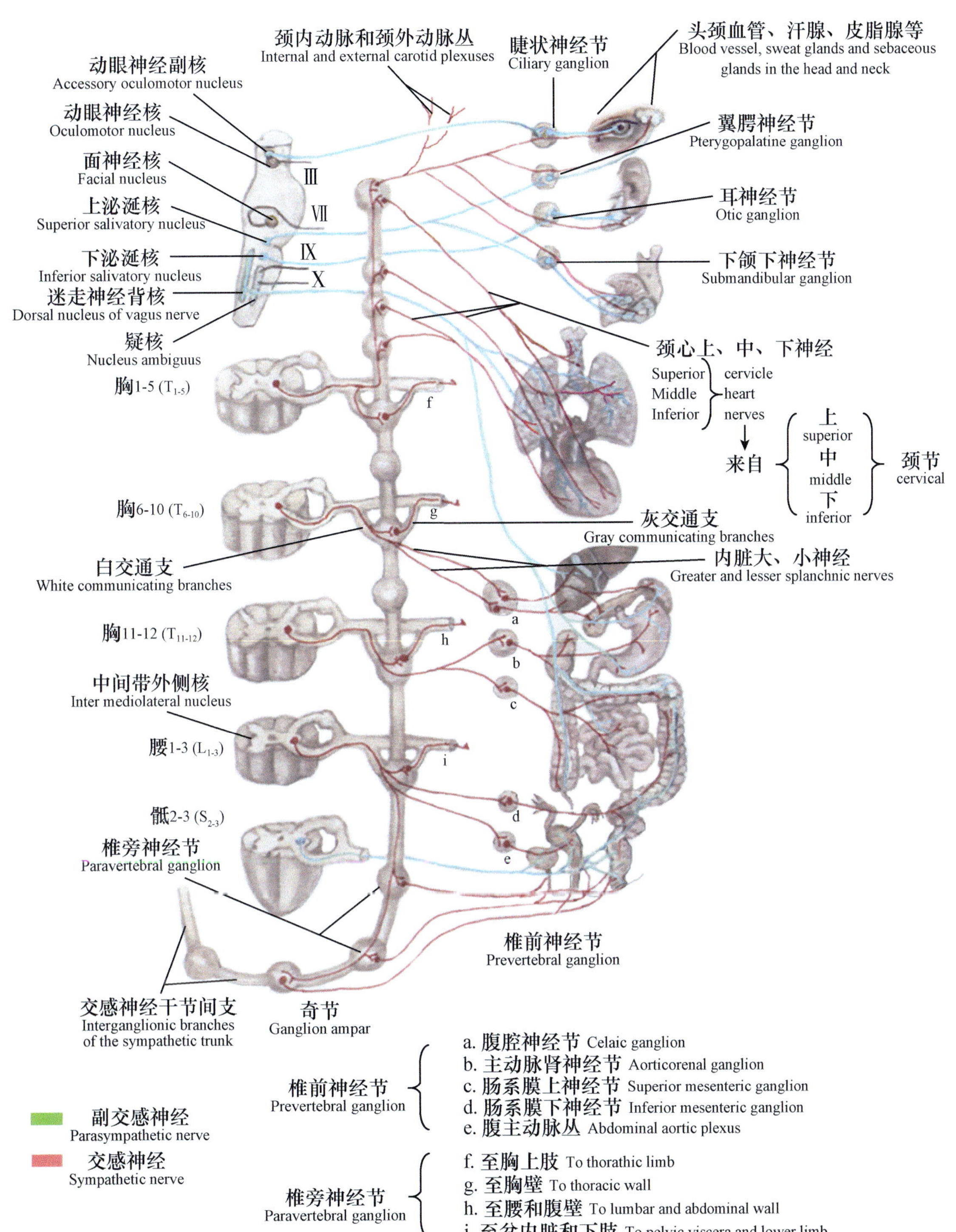

图 4-44　内脏神经传出示意图
A diagram of the efferent side of the autonomic nervous system

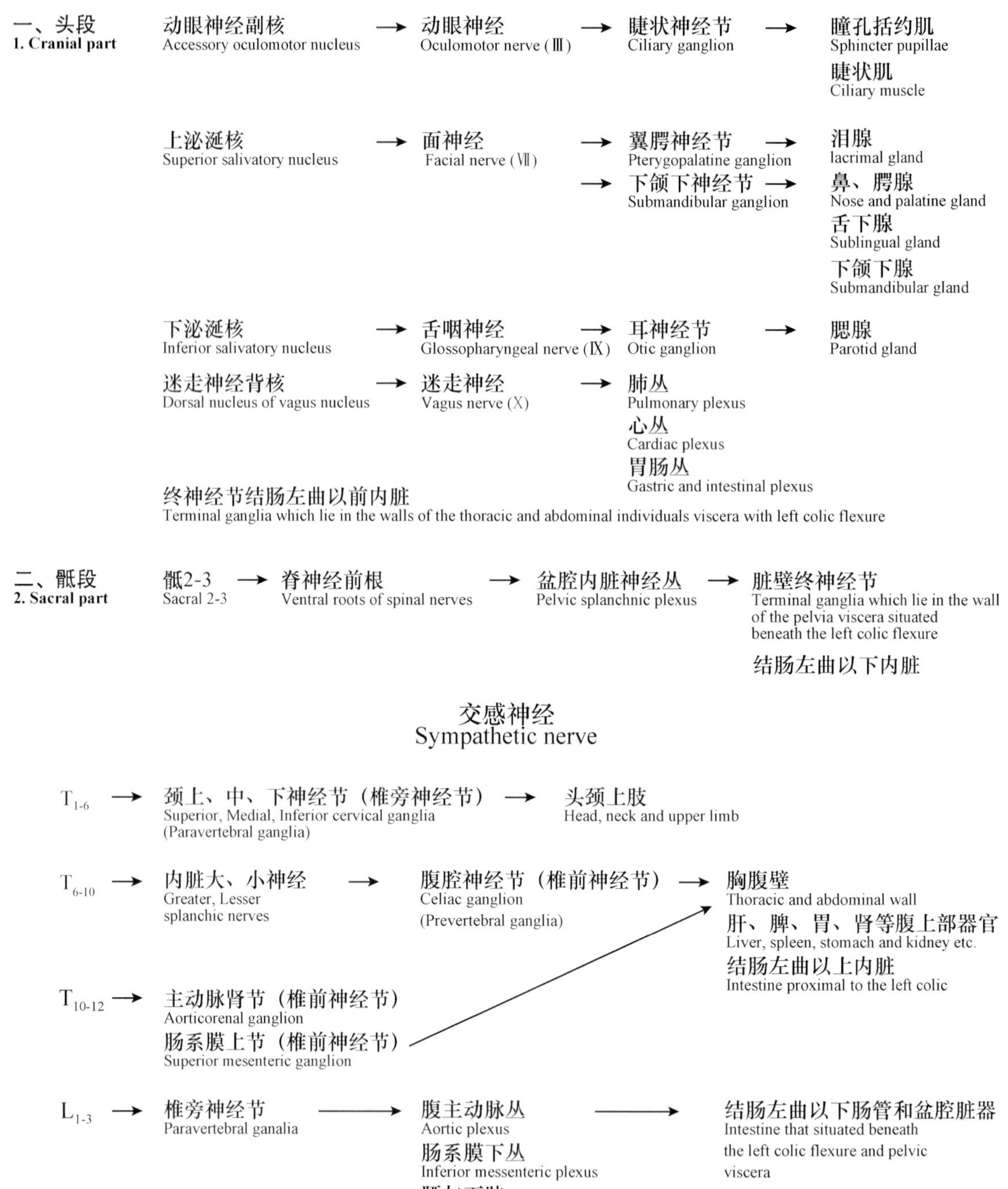

图 4-45 交感神经与副交感神经传导示意表
A table showing the pathways of sympathetic and parasympathetic nerves

感 觉 器

SENSORY ORGANS

第5章

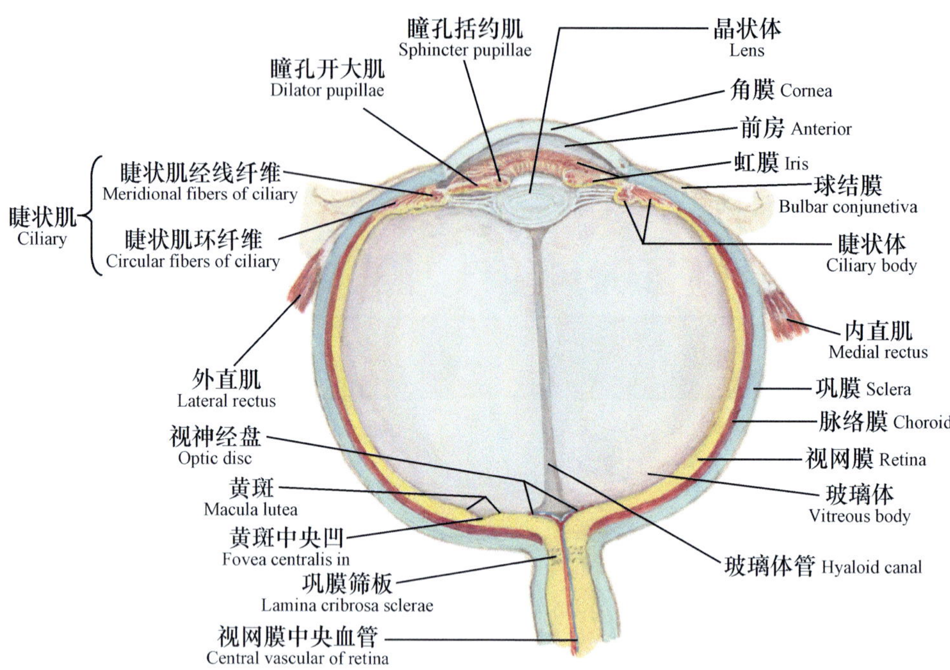

图 5-1 眼球水平切
Horizontal section of eyeball

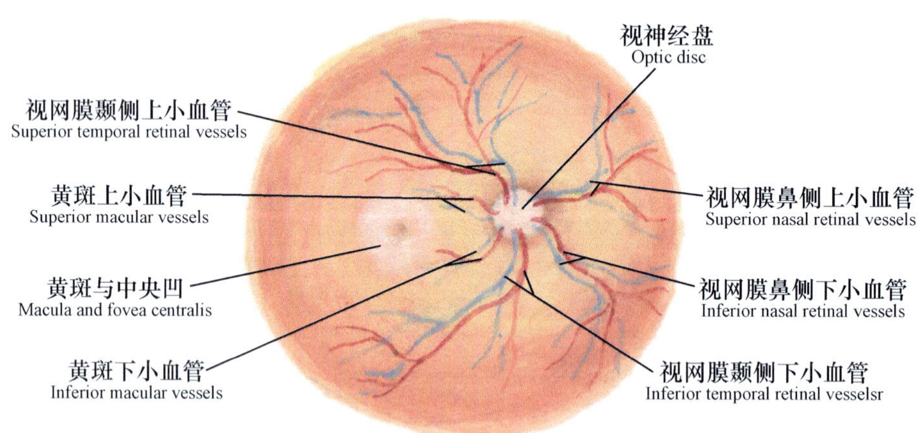

图 5-2 眼底镜所见（右侧）
Ophthalmoscopic view of fundus of the eyeball (Right side)

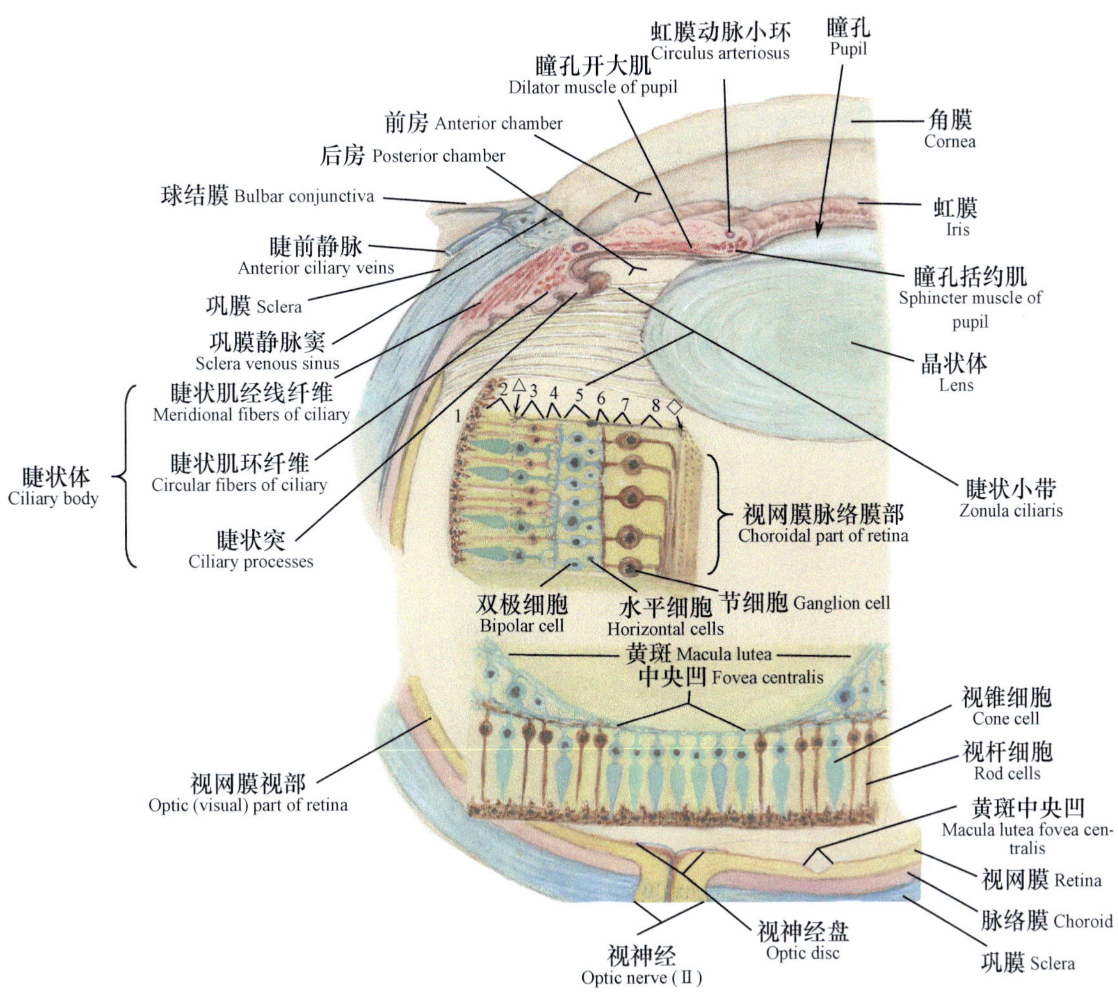

1. 色素上皮层 Pigment epithelium layer	2. 视细胞层 Visual cell layer
3. 外核层 Outer nuclear layer	4. 外网状层 Outer plexiform layer
5. 内核层 Inner nuclear layer	6. 内网状层 Inner plexiform layer
7. 节细胞层 Ganglion cell layer	8. 神经纤维层 Nerve fiber layer
△ 外界膜 Outer limiting membrane	◇ 内界膜 Internal limiting membrane

图 5-3 视网膜
Retina

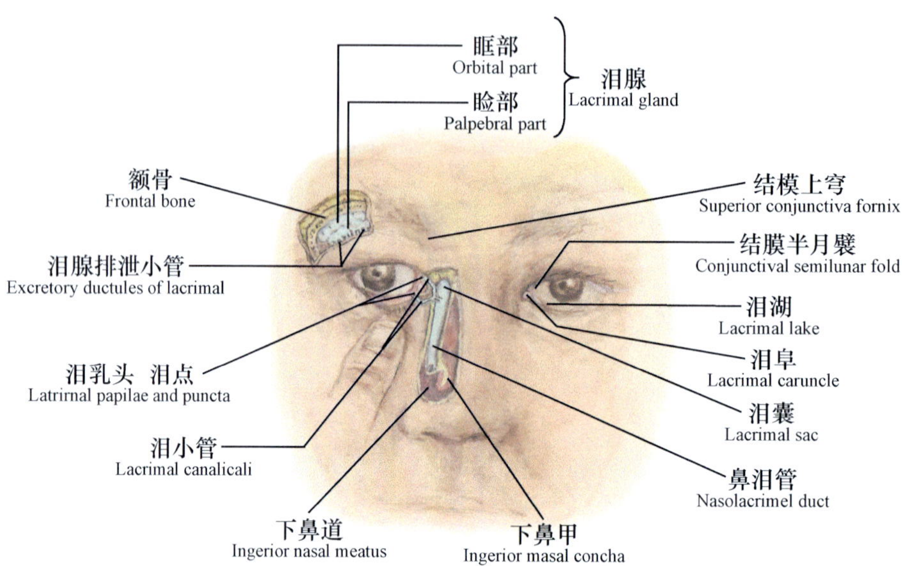

图 5-4 泪器
Lacrimal Apparatus

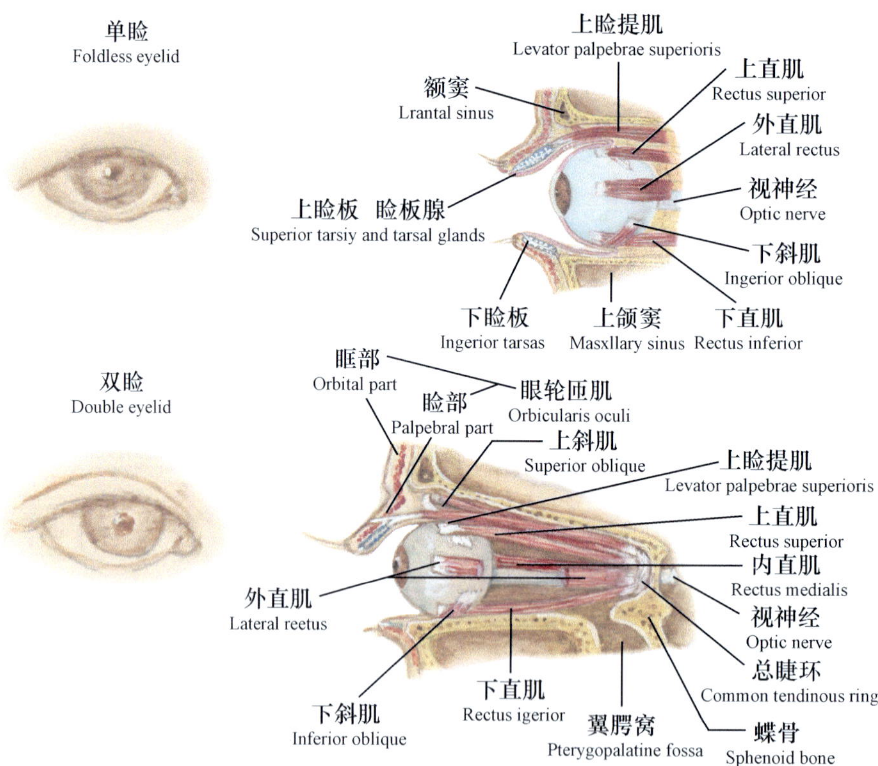

图 5-5 左侧睑和眼外肌
Left eyelid and extraocular muscles

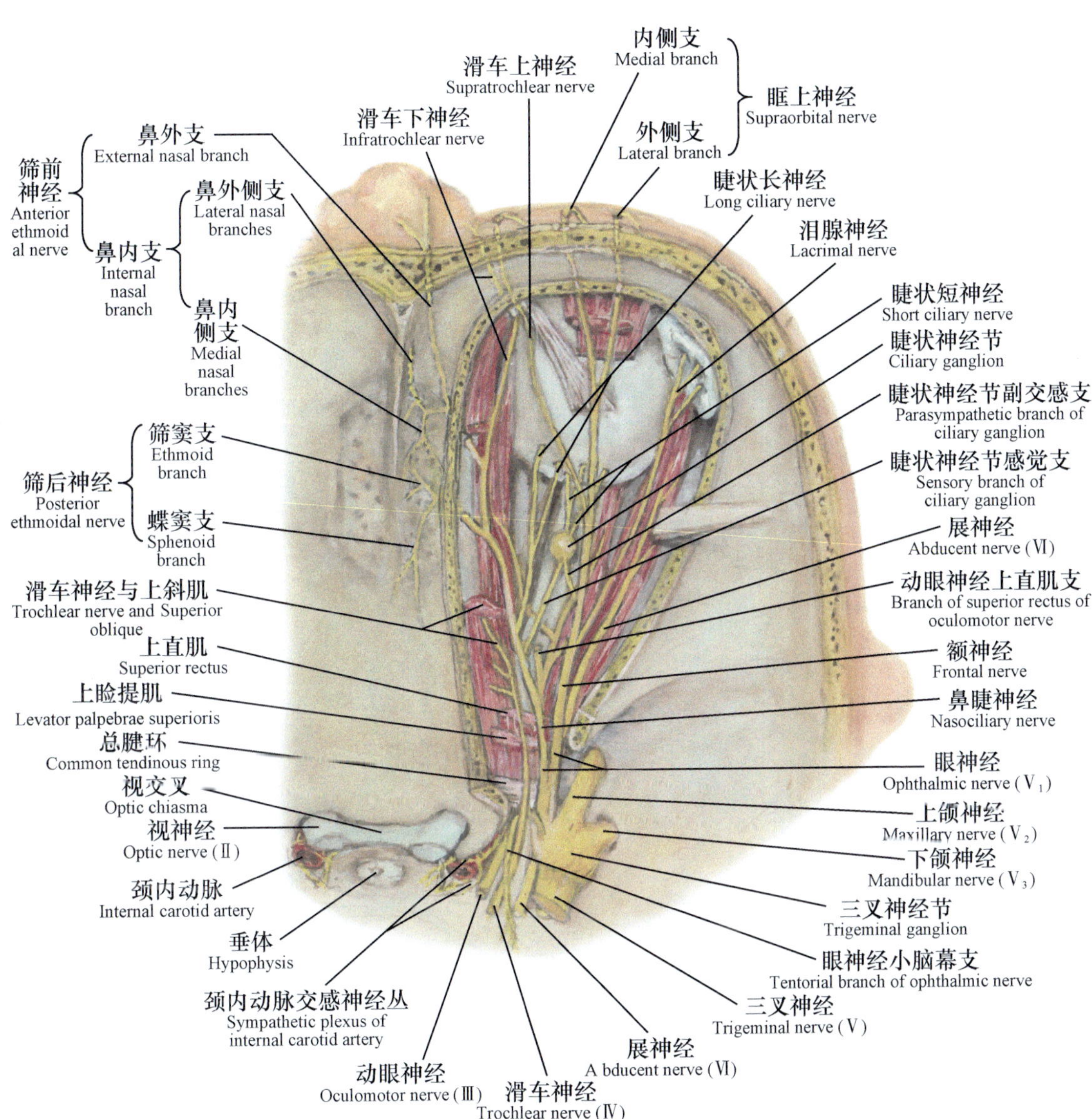

图 5-6 眶内神经（Ⅱ Ⅲ Ⅳ Ⅴ Ⅵ）
Intraorbital nerves（Ⅱ，Ⅲ，Ⅳ，Ⅴ，Ⅵ）

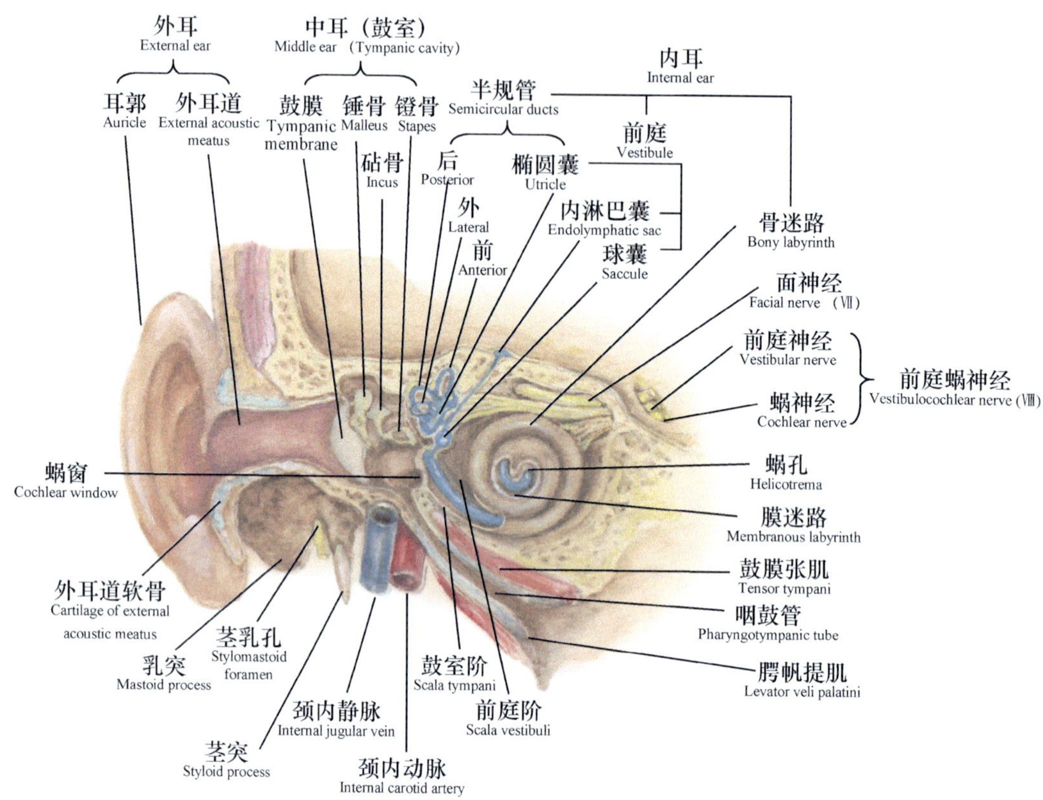

图 5-7 前庭蜗器额状观
Frontal section of vestibular cochlear organ

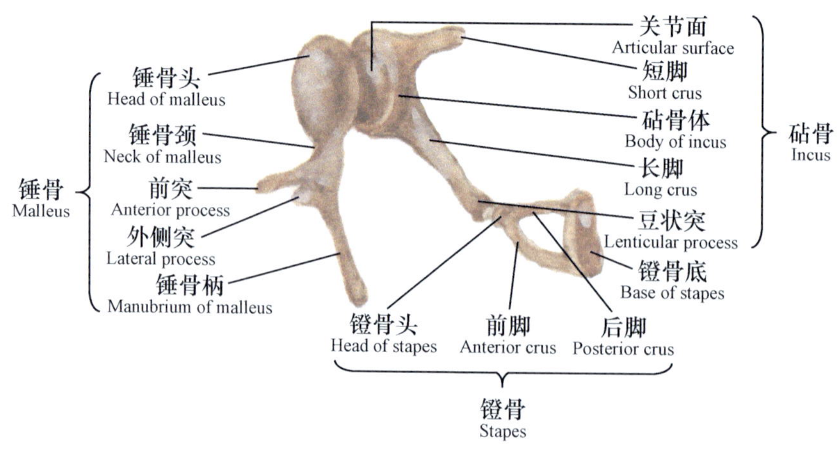

图 5-8 听小骨
Auditory ossicles

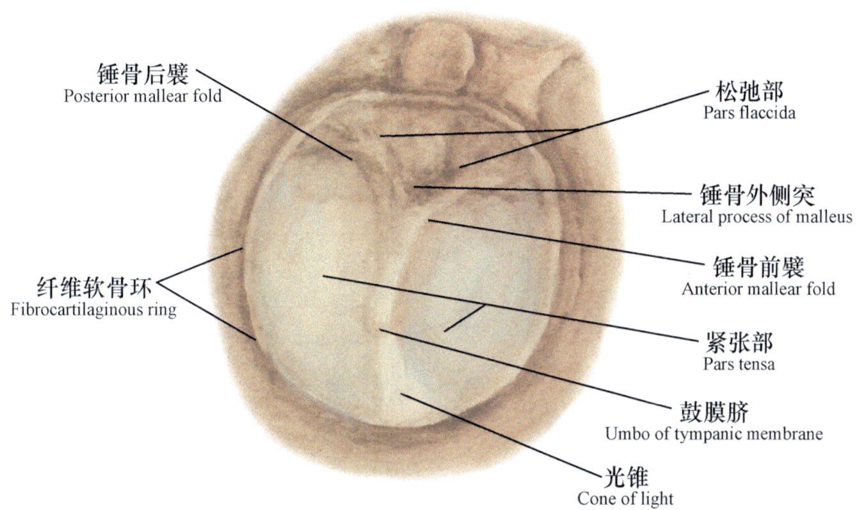

图 5-9 右侧鼓膜外侧观
Lateral view of the right tympanic membrane

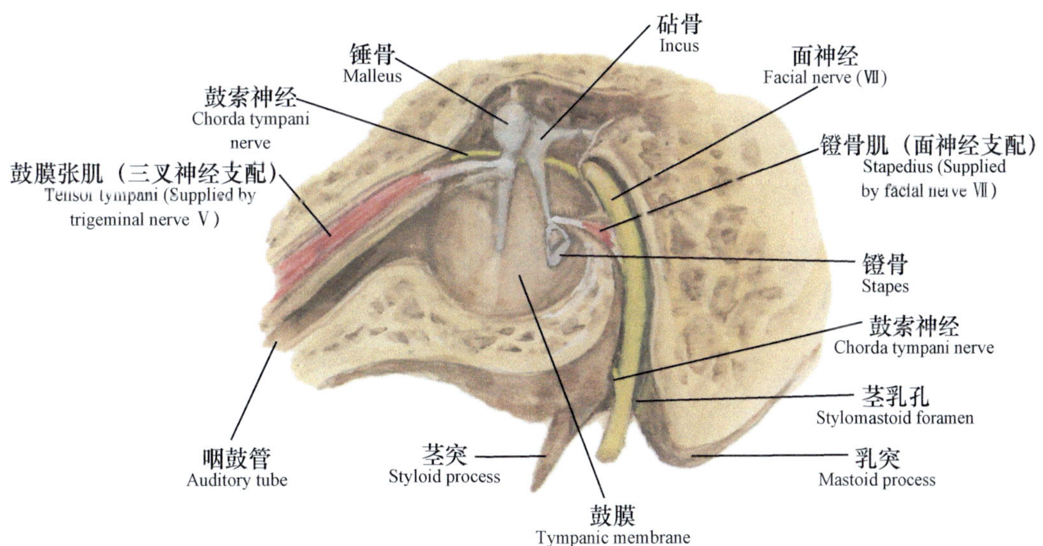

图 5-10 右侧鼓膜内侧观
Medial view of the right tympanic membrane

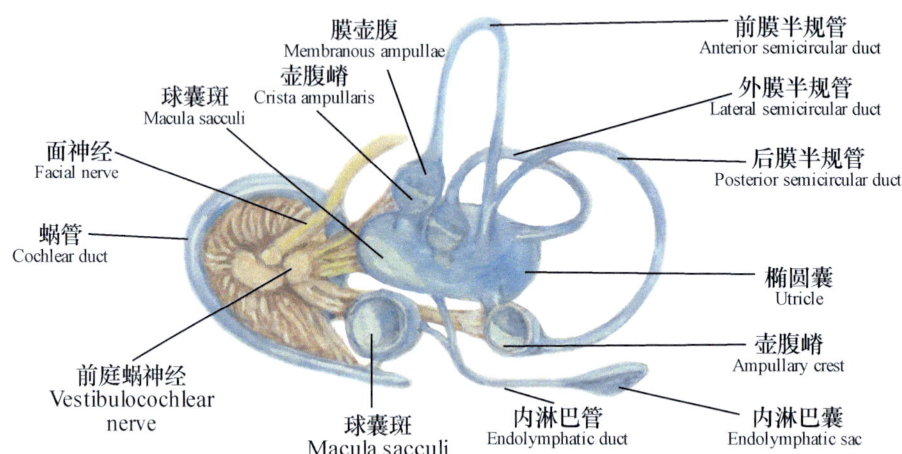

图 5-11　膜迷路示意图
Schematic diagram of the membranous labyrinth

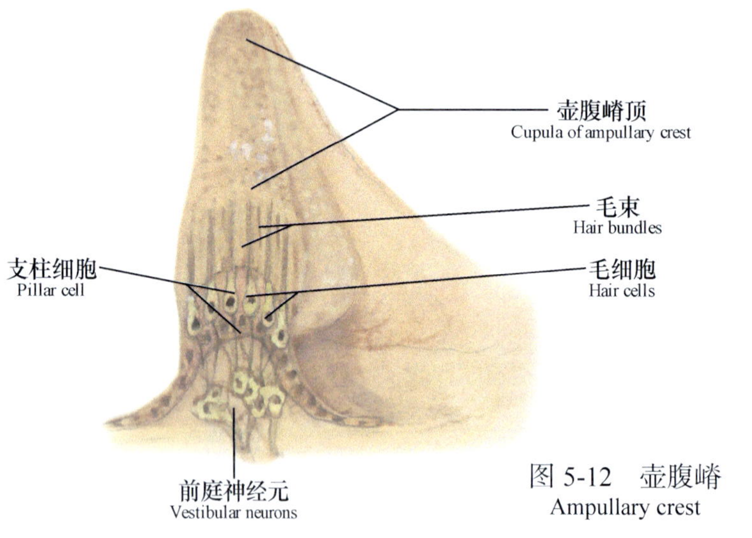

图 5-12　壶腹嵴
Ampullary crest

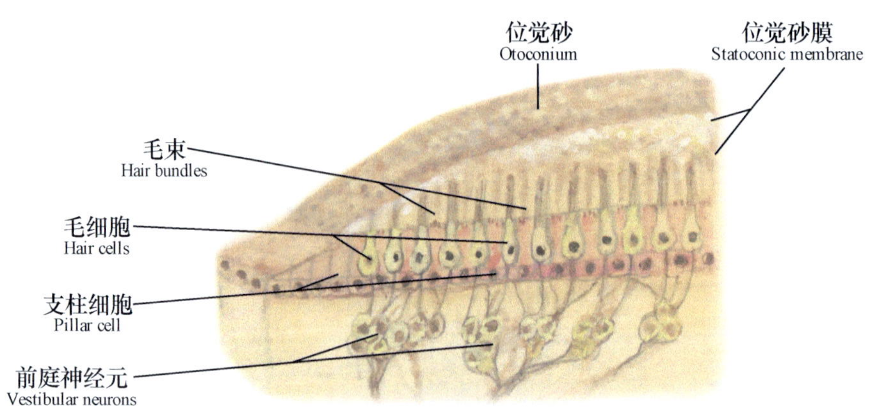

图 5-13　囊斑
Macula of saccula

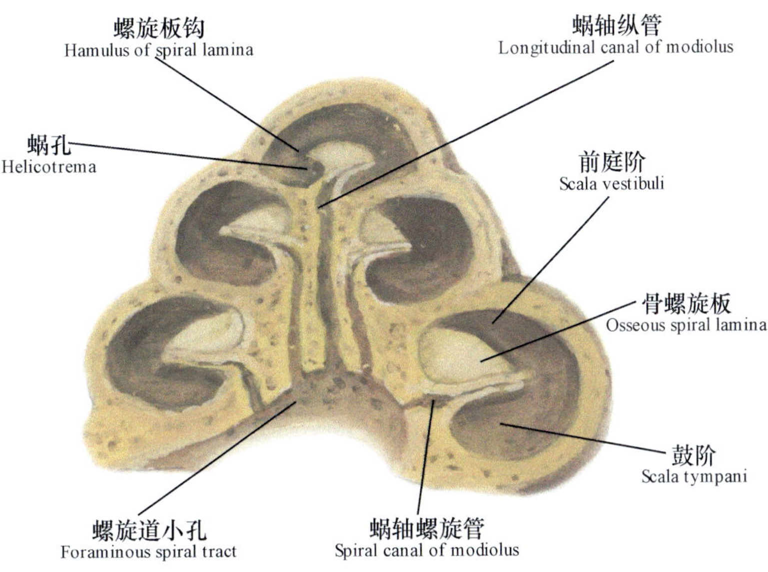

图 5-14 骨蜗管
Osseous cochlear duct

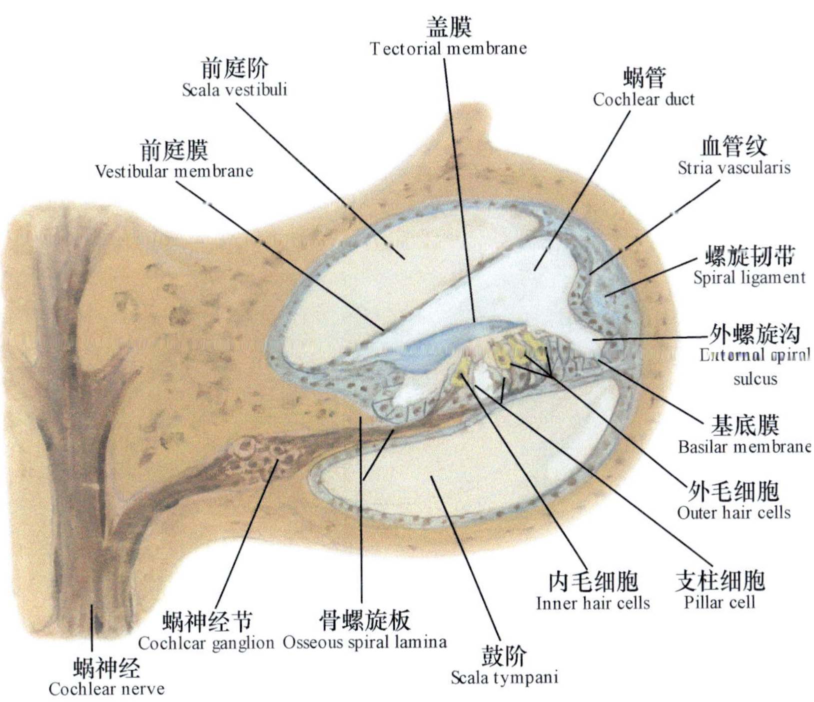

图 5-15 膜蜗管与螺旋器
Cochlear duct and spiral apparatus

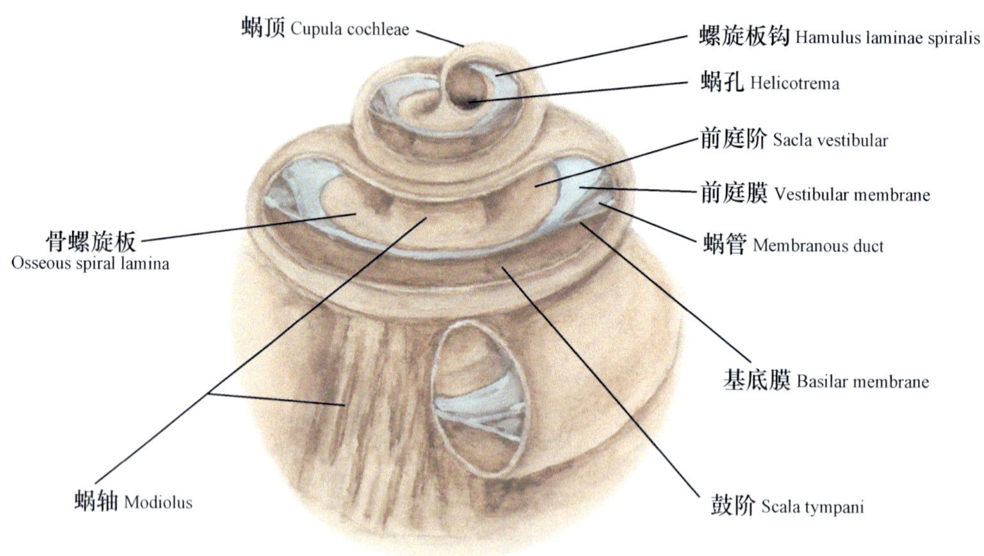

图 5-16 耳蜗
Cochlea

基底膜的两层上皮间有放射状的胶原性纤维组织，称听弦，约 24000 条。听弦长度逐渐加长，短听弦对高音起共鸣作用，长听弦对低音起共鸣作用。图中数字表示声音的频率

There are radial collagenous fibrous tissues between two epithelial layers of basilar membrane, called Auditory string, about 24,000. The length of the strings gradually lengthened, with the short strings resonating with the high notes and the long strings resonating with the low notes. The Numbers represent the frequency of sound.

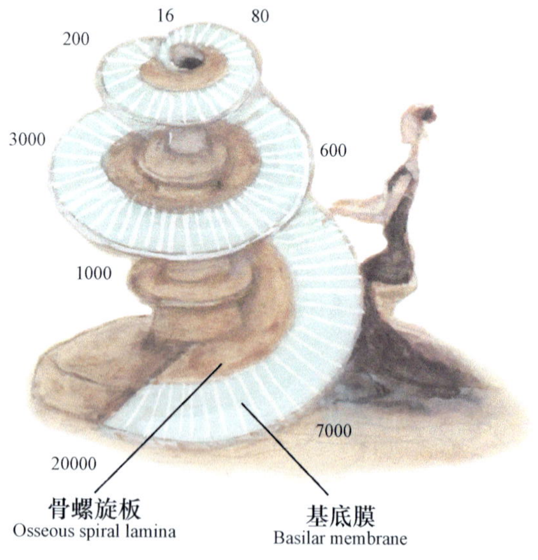

图 5-17 基底膜
Basilar membrane

毛干
Hair shafts
表皮
Epidermis
真皮
Dermis
皮下组织
Hypodermis
角质层
Stratum corneum
透明层
Stratum lucidum
颗粒层
Stratum granulosum
棘层
Stratum spinosum
基底层
Stratum basale
汗腺
Sweat gland
皮脂腺
Sebaceous gland
触觉小体
Tactile corpuscle
立毛肌
Arrectores pilorum
环层小体
Pacinian corpuscle
毛乳头
Hair papilla
毛母基
Hair papilla
结缔组织根鞘
Connective tissue root sheath
外根鞘
External root sheath
内根鞘
Internal root sheath
上皮根鞘
Epithelial root sheath

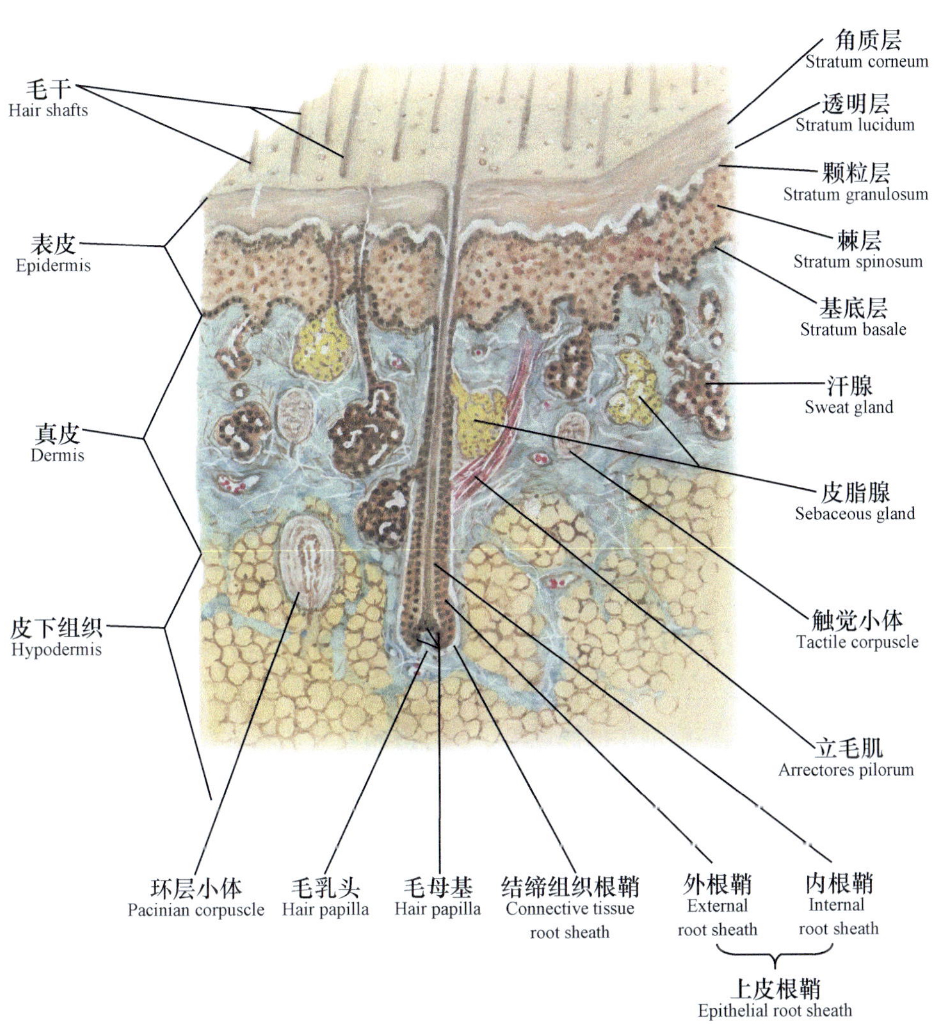

图 5-18 皮肤
Skin

编后致敬辞

——致敬郭连魁先生

《郭连魁人体解剖学图谱》的出版，完成了先生毕生心愿，是先生从教近半个世纪教学理念与人生追求的最佳见证，让我们深深地感受到先生的创作魅力。

先生笔名郭晓，意喻晓以事理，通晓达识；人生始终如晨晓日丽，蕴藏着炽热的生命力。

先生 1949 年入山西医学院。1952 年，响应国家号召，参加北京协和医学院“人体解剖学师资培训班”，从此，开始从事人体解剖学的教学科研事业。

先生倾毕生教学经验和长年美术技艺的积累，凭着百折不挠的韧劲和精益求精的追求，耗费 20 多年精力，日复一日伏案创作，为山西医科大学‘百年校庆’献上一份厚礼，为习医学子搭建了一座通往成功成才的桥梁。

除帧帧质朴写实画风的绘图作品外，先生力求将系统解剖学、局部解剖学及变异解剖学知识精密结合，同时，以解剖学家所独具的教学意识，在书中适当位置，加入纲领性总结概括文字，从而帮助初学者深入了解有关结构的功能，同时对已学者起到综合复习的作用。

先生可谓是“解剖学资深教授中的著名画家”，其所达令人敬仰之高度，无人企及。高度的背后，是先生自幼年始，对绘画的痴迷：临摹写生，笔不离手，持之以恒，经年磨砺，日积月累。

端详先生的每幅作品，以独具特色的工笔手法勾线，敷色典雅，明暗适度，融中西绘画手法于一体，传递经典人体解剖学的深邃与美妙，淋漓尽致地表达人体解剖学知识，是一部展现科学与艺术相结合的雄浑画卷。

无疑，《郭连魁人体解剖学图谱》的出版，呈现着先生难以估量的艰苦劳作、绘画的天赋，以及对人体解剖学教学理念的深刻理解。

谨以此文，向先生致敬！

山西医科大学
《郭连魁人体解剖学图谱》
编　委　会